❧ THE MEDIEVAL
ECONOMY OF SALVATION

THE MEDIEVAL ECONOMY OF SALVATION

CHARITY, COMMERCE, AND THE RISE OF THE HOSPITAL

ADAM J. DAVIS

CORNELL UNIVERSITY PRESS

Ithaca and London

First paperback printing 2021. Printed with corrections.
First published 2019 by Cornell University Press

Library of Congress Cataloging-in-Publication Data

Names: Davis, Adam Jeffrey, 1973– author.
Title: The medieval economy of salvation : charity, commerce, and the rise of the hospital / Adam J. Davis.
Description: Ithaca : Cornell University Press, 2019. | Includes bibliographical references and index.
Identifiers: LCCN 2019006494 (print) | LCCN 2019008000 (ebook) | ISBN 9781501742118 (pdf) | ISBN 9781501742125 (epub/mobi) | ISBN 9781501742101 | ISBN 9781501742101 (cloth)
Subjects: LCSH: Hospitals, Medieval—France—Champagne-Ardenne—History. | Charities—France—Champagne-Ardenne—History—To 1500. | Charity—Religious aspects—Christianity—History—To 1500. | Medical economics—France—Champagne-Ardenne—History—To 1500.
Classification: LCC RA989.F73 (ebook) | LCC RA989.F73 C48 2019 (print) | DDC 362.110944/31—dc23
LC record available at https://lccn.loc.gov/2019006494

ISBN 978-1-5017-5524-8 (paperback)

Dedicated, with love, to my parents,
Toni Hahn Davis
and David Brion Davis,
who exemplify generosity and kindness

❧ Contents

❦ Illustrations

❧ ACKNOWLEDGMENTS

A year-long fellowship from the National Endowment for the Humanities in 2014–15 provided critical time for the research and writing of this book. I am grateful to Paul Reitter of The Ohio State University for inviting me to be a visiting fellow at Ohio State's Humanities Institute during the very productive period of my NEH Fellowship. A Robert C. Good Fellowship from Denison University made it possible for me to spend the 2017–18 academic year as a visiting fellow at Clare Hall, Cambridge. The Cambridge University Library was an ideal place to complete this book, and Clare Hall provided a vibrant intellectual environment in which to think deeply and engage with other scholars. I'm grateful to David Ibbetson, the president of the College, and the fellows of Clare Hall, for such a fruitful and enjoyable residency in Cambridge, and to our Clare Hall neighbors—now the dearest of friends—Laura and Chris Batten, Efrat and Roi Granot, Lily Panoussi and Konstantinos Orginos, and Sílvia Gassiot Pintori and Lluís To Figueras.

I thank the archivists at the Bibliothèque Nationale de France, the Institut de Recherche et d'Histoire des Textes, the departmental archives of the Aube (Troyes), Seine-et-Marne (Dammarie-les-Lys), and Marne (Reims), the municipal archives of Provins and Reims, and closer to home, the librarians at Denison University and Ohio State. Portions of some chapters of this book include reworked material that was previously published, including "Preaching in Thirteenth-Century Hospitals," *Journal of Medieval History* 36, no. 1 (March 2010): 72–89 (https://www.tandfonline.com/doi/full/10.1016/j.jmedhist.2009.12.002); "The Economic Power of a Hospital in Thirteenth-Century Provins," in *Center and Periphery: Studies on Power in the Medieval World in Honor of William Chester Jordan*, ed. Katherine L. Jansen, G. Geltner, and Anne E. Lester (Leiden: Brill, 2013), 121–34; and "Hospitals, Charity and the Culture of Compassion in Medieval Europe," in *Approaches to Poverty in Medieval Europe: Complexities, Contradictions, Transformations, c. 1100–1500*, edited by Sharon Farmer (Turnhout: Brepols, 2016), 23–45.

I would not have been able to write this book without meaningful research support and leave time from Denison University. I'm grateful to my departmental colleagues at Denison for their generosity in reading and commenting on portions of this book. I also thank a group of Bexley/Columbus neighbors, who happen to also be fellow historians and friends, for their encouragement as I worked on this book: David Bernstein (who took the book's author photo), Michael Flamm, Robin Judd, Scott Levi, Jennifer Siegel, Mitchell Snay, and Karen Spierling. Other friends have been equally supportive along the way: Or and Sharon Mars, Jessica and Andrew Mills, Kenny Steinman, and Rayna and Isaac Weiner. Sam and Elizabeth Dyson, dear college friends, have served as valuable sounding boards about academic publishing and so much else. Rick and Susan Bradley, old family friends, who, in 1980, saved the day by lending my father a typewriter in Paris when the one he was using broke, again helped make a book possible by repeatedly opening up the *chambre de bonne* in their Paris apartment to me while I was in France doing research for this book.

Although researching and writing a book can be a solitary endeavor, it can also provide an opportunity for forging fruitful dialogue with other scholars. I was able to try out some of the arguments in this book at several invited talks, and I thank the conveners for the opportunity to share my work at Cambridge University; All Souls College, Oxford; the Israel Institute for Advanced Study in Jerusalem; the École des Hautes Études en Sciences Sociales in Paris; the University of Tennessee at Knoxville; Loyola University of Chicago; Wittenberg University; and the University of Dayton. I am particularly indebted to Ted Evergates, who has been a generous resource for my frequent questions about Champagne and the medieval aristocracy. I also thank a number of colleagues for their assistance while I worked on this book, whether providing me with an obscure reference or a draft of their own work in progress, serving as a sounding board, or offering suggestions on a chapter: the late John Baldwin, Arnaud Baudin, Elisheva Baumgarten, Federico Botana, Connie Bouchard, Elma Brenner, James Brodman, Michael Cusato, O.F.M., David d'Avray, Charles de Miramon, Sean Field, Lluis To Figuera, M. Cecilia Gaposchkin, Lindy Grant, Richard Firth Green, Dan Hobbins, Bill Jordan, Rick Keyser, Thomas Lacomme, Anne Lester, Amy Livingstone, Eyal Poleg, Julia Smith, Ben Soskis, Bertrand Taithe, Tamara Mann Tweel, John Van Engen, and Sethina Watson.

Sharon Farmer has been a generous interlocutor and reader of my work. Her own book on the survival strategies of the medieval poor was an early inspiration for this project, and a paper that I presented in Leeds in 2010, which was subsequently published in a collection that she edited, served as an important launching pad for some of the ideas in this book. I owe a debt of gratitude to John Arnold for his warm hospitality in Cambridge. Our discussions about medieval pious giving helped me sharpen my arguments in chapter 3. Judah Galinsky has been a devoted interlocutor and collaborator who has allowed me to think comparatively about Jewish and Christian charitable practices.

I'm deeply grateful to Miri Rubin, whose work I've long admired, for her careful reading of the manuscript for the press, for her important suggestions and words of encouragement, and for her and Gareth Stedman Jones's tremendously gracious hospitality to our entire family during our year in Cambridge. I also owe a debt of gratitude to Peter Brown, not only for what he taught me many years ago when I was in graduate school at Princeton, but for his recent work on Christian attitudes toward wealth and the afterlife in Late Antiquity, which has very much influenced my thinking about medieval ideas about charity. Finally, I wish to thank both the anonymous readers for their extremely valuable feedback, and Mahinder Kingra, who has been an unwaveringly supportive and responsive editor.

Noah and Ewa Davis, Naomi and Barry Schimmer, and Rebecca and Ben Kirshner have been enthusiastic cheerleaders during the years that I worked on this book project, and I thank them for their support. This book was what took our family to Cambridge for what was truly a magical year for us all. I'm especially grateful to Alexandra for being willing to embark on that year-long family adventure and for all of her love, wise counsel, and steadfast encouragement while I worked on this book. This project has spanned the lifetimes of our children, Jonah and Elena, who bring us endless joy and delight.

This book is dedicated, with love, to my parents, who have both been so supportive of this project and so much else. It is possible that my father's own scholarship on the history of abolitionism contributed in some small way to my own interest in the history of charity and the human impulse to provide assistance to the stranger. In recent years, as he has entered his nineties, my father has been on the receiving end of caregiving from a nursing home, care for which we are deeply appreciative, and which has often made me think about caretakers in distant times and places. The book's dedication is inspired by the example of my parents' own lifetime of generosity and kindness to others.

❧ Abbreviations

AD   Archives départementales
AMC   Archives municipales et communautaires
BM   Bibliothèque municipale
BnF   Bibliothèque Nationale de France
Dupraz   Dominique Dupraz, "Les cartulaires de l'Hôtel-Dieu de Provins: Édition critique" (Thèse, L'École Nationale des Chartes. Paris, 1973)
Mansi   J. D. Mansi, *Sacrorum Conciliorum nova et amplissima collectio* (31 vols., Florence, 1759–98)
PL   *Patrologiae cursus completus: Series Latina*, ed. J. P. Migne (221 vols., Paris, 1844–55)

❧ A Note on Monies and Measures

In much of medieval Europe, money was calculated in pounds (*l.*, French *livres*, Latin *libri*), shillings (*s.*, French *sous*, Latin *solidi*), and pence (*d.*, French *deniers*, Latin *denarii*). These denominations were related at the standard 12 *d.* = 1 *s.*, and 20 *s.* = 1 *l.* Most transactions in Champagne involved either the currency of the county, known as the *provinois* (*prov.*), or the French *tournois* (*t.*). The *provinois* held a higher silver content until ca. 1224, when it was debased to conform to the value of the *tournois*. Four *livres parisis* (*par.*), meanwhile, which was the standard currency of the French royal kingdom until 1203, was equivalent to five *livres tournois*. Unless otherwise indicated, references to money in this book are to the count's coins (*provinois* and, after 1284, *tournois*), which were minted in Troyes or Provins.

Although measures varied by locality, an *arpent* was a land measure roughly equivalent to an acre. A *muid* (*modius* in Latin) was a dry measure worth about 12 *setiers* (a *setier* being the equivalent of 12 bushels); a liquid *muid* was worth about 24 *setiers*. The *cens* was a nominal rent, usually paid in coin in recognition of a landlord's superior right to property.

THE MEDIEVAL
ECONOMY OF SALVATION

Introduction
A Charitable Revolution in an
Age of Commerce

It was a cold winter evening in 2010, and I had just arrived in Paris for a short research trip. The tiny hotel where I would be staying was on the fifth floor of the ophthalmological wing of the hôtel-Dieu (or hospital) just across from the cathedral of Notre Dame.[1] Given the subject of the book I was in France to research, it seemed appropriate that I should stay in a "hospital-hôtel," especially since some medieval hospitals not only housed the sick and poor but also functioned as hotels that charged their guests based on the length of their visits. As the TripAdvisor reviews warned, guests in this hotel often shared the elevator with patients in wheelchairs or on gurneys. When I arrived at the entrance to the hospital, however, what struck me was the large number of homeless Parisians who were using the hospital's heated foyer as a shelter for the night. I remember thinking that if this had been the thirteenth century, these homeless people, rather than relegated to the foyer, would have been admitted to the hôtel-Dieu and given a bed and a meal after they had confessed their sins.

---

1. The hôtel-Dieu that is still functioning today is in a nineteenth-century structure. The medieval hôtel-Dieu, built during the twelfth century, stood on the south side of the cathedral, between the cathedral and the Petit Pont, and housed up to two hundred poor and sick guests. See Ernest Coyecque, *L'hôtel-Dieu de Paris au moyen age: l'histoire et documents* (Paris: H. Champion, 1889), 159–61.

1

A few days later, I was sitting in an archive in Dammarie-lès-Lys (in the southeastern suburbs of Paris), just down the street from the hauntingly beautiful ruins of Le Lys, the royal Cistercian abbey for women, founded in 1251. The archive's holdings include two large cartularies for the main hospital of Provins, a martyrological obituary with the names of donors and members of the hospital personnel, and hundreds of original single-sheet charters that were subsequently copied into the cartularies. A testament from 1253 for Alice la Pelée, a bourgeois woman from Provins, records her bequests to the hospital of houses, land, a vineyard, her bedding, and the sum of 60 *livres* (l.). She also stipulated that bread should be distributed to the poor on the day of her death. In her testamentary bequests, Alice was more generous to the main hospital of Provins than to any churches, monasteries, houses of friars, or other hospitals or leprosaria. Did she have some connection to this hospital during her lifetime, I wondered?[2] Another testament found in the same archive, this one from 1260, came from Guillaume, a priest who served as the curate of Sceaux (in the Loiret) and the dean of Gâtinais. He also showed a strong propensity to give to various hospitals and leprosaries, particularly the main hospital of Provins.[3] His bequests included leaving a small sum for the marriage portion for ten poor girls in Sceaux and ten girls in Sourdun (near Provins), as well as funds to feed the poor in these towns and to buy them shoes. In his testament of 1219, Jacques de Hongrie, who served as sergeant to Countess Blanche, made bequests to a long list of religious and charitable institutions, including the brothers of Saint John of Jerusalem (the Hospitallers), the lepers of Crolebarbe (near Provins), a planned *domus Dei* in Provins for poor students, and various churches and monasteries.[4] But in addition to these gifts, Jacques showed a special attachment to the hospital of Provins, to which he not only made significant bequests of land but where he also planned to spend the last years of his life, serving the poor and sick as a *conversus*, having taken the religious habit while still married.[5] What explains the charitable impulses of Alice, Guillaume, and Jacques, which were so typical of their time?

During the twelfth and thirteenth centuries hundreds of hospitals and leper houses were founded all over Europe to care for the poor, sick, and vulnerable, and these new charitable institutions received broad support from

---

2. Dupraz, nos. 143, 323; AD: Seine-et-Marne, 11HdtA12 ("grand cartulaire" for the hospital of Provins), fol. 40v–41, 97.

3. The trust he placed in this hospital was further reflected in his choice of the hospital's master as one of the executors of his will. See Dupraz, no. 243; AD: Seine-et-Marne, 11HdtA12, fol. 73v.

4. Dupraz, no. 446; AD: Seine-et-Marne, 11HdtA12, fol. 129v–130.

5. *Obituaires de la province de Sens*, vol. 1, part 2, *Diocèses de Sens et de Paris*, ed. Auguste Molinier and Auguste Longnon (Paris: Imprimerie Nationale, 1902), 1:943.

townspeople, merchants, aristocrats, and ecclesiastics. To give a sense of the scale of new hospital foundations in France, Champagne's capital city of Troyes had five general hospitals during the thirteenth century as well as several hospitals run by other religious orders (the Antonines and Trinitarians); the diocese of Bourges had some 120 hospitals and 78 leprosaries; in the relatively small region of the lower Rhône valley, by the fourteenth century there were around 250 hospitals; by the later Middle Ages, there were as many as 360 hospitals in the provinces of Sens and Reims (not including leprosaries and houses for poor clerics).[6] First established mostly during the twelfth and early thirteenth centuries, these hospitals were founded by a wide range of actors: members of the royal family, aristocrats, merchants, townspeople, municipalities, bishops, cathedral chapters, monasteries, confraternities, and various kinds of religious orders, including the hospitaller orders. That these "houses of mercy" were often located in the heart of urban centers, at major points of circulation (on trade and pilgrimage routes; near bridges and rivers), and near areas of economic exploitation (markets and fairs, mills, and lands being cultivated) reflected the degree to which they were easily accessible, highly visible, and thoroughly enmeshed in the local society and economy.[7] As Miri Rubin has shown, hospitals were placed in the Jewish quarter of some towns "as an assertion of Christian faith," proudly showcasing for Jews Christian welfare in action.[8]

The word *hospital* is in some ways a problematic (but necessary) way of referring to what the medieval terms *domus Dei* or *meson Dieu* (house of God) and *hospitale* denoted.[9] As an institution, the medieval hospital was

---

6. Daniel Le Blévec, *La part du pauvre: L'assistance et charité dans les pays du Bas-Rhône du XIIe siècle au milieu du XVe siècle* (Rome: École Française de Rome, 2000), 599; François-Olivier Touati, "De l'infirmerie monastique à l'hôpital moderne: lieux, édifices et formes de l'assistance dans la France du Centre et de l'Ouest," in *Archéologie et architecture hospitalières de l'antiquité tardive à l'aube des temps modernes*, ed. Touati (Paris: La Boutique de l'Histoire, 2004), 399; Annie Saunier, *"Le pauvre malade" dans le cadre hospitalier médiéval: France du Nord, vers 1300–1500* (Paris: Éditions Arguments, 1993).

7. François-Olivier Touati, "La géographie hospitalière médiévale (Orient-Occident, IVe–XVe siècles): Des modèles aux réalités," in *Hôpitaux et maladreries au moyen âge: Espace et environnement. Actes du colloque international d'Amiens-Beauvais, 22, 23, et 24 novembre 2002*, ed. Pascal Montaubin (Publications du CAHMER, 2004), 13–14. For the specific example of the hospital of Amiens, which relocated in the early thirteenth century from the cathedral neighborhood to the new, bustling, highly commercial area of Saint-Leu, see Pascaul Montaubin, "Le déménagement de l'Hôtel-Dieu d'Amiens au XIIIe siècle: un hôpital dans les enjeux urbanistiques," in *Hôpitaux et maladreries au moyen âge*, 51–86.

8. Miri Rubin, *Charity and Community in Medieval Cambridge* (Cambridge: Cambridge University Press, 1987), 108.

9. On the danger of inferring too much about a hospital's function based on terminology, see François-Olivier Touati, "Problème d'histoire, d'architecture et d'archéologie hospitalière," in *Archéologie et architecture hospitalière*, ed. Touati, 7–23.

not conceived primarily in medical terms but rather functioned in a variety of ways, including as a religious house (often containing a chapel with an altar), a hostel, a shelter, a retirement home, or a temporary place for physical rehabilitation and convalescence. There was no clear definition of what constituted a hospital in medieval canon law, since not all hospitals were thought to belong to the church. Since hospitals could be subject to a wide range of different custodians and jurisdictions, the legal status of hospitals was clearly distinct from that of monasteries and religious orders.[10] Some medieval hospitals were quite specialized in terms of the categories of people they admitted; there were separate hospitals for the blind, for pilgrims, for the elderly, for those afflicted with ergotism, for lepers, for pregnant women, for orphans and abandoned children, for unwed mothers, for poor clerics, for poor students, and for reformed prostitutes. Hospitaller and military orders, lay confraternities, and penitential groups founded during this period were also actively engaged in charitable work, including working in hospitals, while some monastic orders increasingly conceived of caregiving as central to their spiritual identities.[11]

The "hospital movement" in Champagne—the subject of this book— was clearly connected to a broader pan-European religious culture of charity, reflected, for example, in hagiographical texts, preaching, devotional literature, vernacular didactic texts on the vices and virtues, an outpouring of representations of the works of mercy in the visual arts, and the growing sanctification of charity evident in saints of the period, many of whom were lay women who had founded or worked in a hospital.

---

10. In *On Hospitals: Welfare, Law, and Christianity in Western Europe, 400–1320* (Oxford: Oxford University Press, 2020), Sethina Watson fundamentally overturns the historiography on medieval hospitals and the law. She rejects, for example, Jean Imbert's contention that canon law's treatment of hospitals was based on a Roman-law model.

11. James W. Brodman, *Charity and Religion in Medieval Europe* (Washington, DC: Catholic University of America Press, 2009); Daniel Le Blévec, "Fondations et œuvres charitables au moyen âge," in *Fondations et œuvres charitables au moyen âge*, ed. Jean Dufour and Henri Platelle (Paris: Éditions du CTHS, 1999), 7–22; Le Blévec, *La part du pauvre*; Anne E. Lester, *Creating Cistercian Nuns: The Women's Religious Movement and Its Reform in Thirteenth-Century Champagne* (Ithaca: Cornell University Press, 2011); Lester, "Cares Beyond the Walls: Cistercian Nuns and the Care of Lepers in Twelfth- and Thirteenth-Century Northern France," in *Religious and Laity in Western Europe, 1000–1400: Interaction, Negotiation, and Power*, ed. Janet Burton and Emilia Jamroziak (Turnhout, Belgium: Brepols, 2006), 197–224; François-Olivier Touati, *Maladie et société au moyen âge: La lèpre, lépreux et les léproseries dans la province ecclésiastique de Sens jusqu'au milieu du XIVe siècle* (Paris: De Boeck Université, 1998); Jean Richard, "Les Templiers et les Hospitaliers en Bourgogne et en Champagne méridionale (XIIe–XIIIe siècles)," in *Die geistlichen Ritterorden Europas*, ed. Manfred Hellmann and Josef Fleckenstein (Sigmaringen, Germany: Thorbecke, 1980), 231–42; Malcolm Barber, "The Charitable and Medical Activities of the Hospitallers and Templars," in *A History of Pastoral Care*, ed. G. R. Evans (London: Cassell, 2000), 148–68.

In the words of André Vauchez, the twelfth and thirteenth centuries witnessed "a veritable revolution in charity" and the emergence of "an authentic spirituality of benevolence," a turning point in the way that women and men thought about and acted toward their poor and needy neighbors.[12] In addition to drawing new and much-needed attention to the charitable revolution of the high Middle Ages, a period whose legacy of persecution and religious violence (the Crusades, the violent repression of heretics, the massacres and expulsions of European Jews) tends to be far better known, this book is the first to explore the relationship between the European charitable revolution and the commercial revolution that was unfolding simultaneously. Until now, no one has examined the evolution of medieval ideas about charity, the outpouring of charitable giving, and the creation of new charitable institutions through the lens of the concomitant commercial explosion. This book explains how these two revolutions gave rise across Europe to the medieval hospital, a new type of social welfare institution.

My study of the emergence of hospitals in Champagne casts new light on the nature of religious charity during Europe's first great age of commerce. Using hospitals in the region of Champagne as a case study, *The Medieval Economy of Salvation* explores the connection between the robust profit economy of the time and the flowering of new charitable institutions. In tracing the emergence of hospitals during a period of intense urbanization that saw the transition from a gift economy to a commercial one, this book demonstrates that far from eroding the power of the gift, the new commercial economy infused charitable giving and service with new social and religious meaning and a heightened expectation of reward.

The county of Champagne, southeast of Paris, provides the ideal stage for illuminating the connections between charity and commerce. With its international trade fairs and robust markets for credit and currency exchange, Champagne was the epicenter of European commerce and international exchange at the time, bringing together merchants from all over northern Europe and the Mediterranean basin. The twelfth and thirteenth centuries witnessed enormous demographic and economic expansion across Latin Christendom, including the clearing of lands for commercial cultivation, the founding of new markets and towns, the enlargement of existing towns, the expansion of trade, the growth of the money supply, and the development of systems

---

12. André Vauchez, *La spiritualité du moyen âge occidental (VIIIe–XIIIe siècle)*, 2nd ed. (Paris: Seuil, 1994), 118.

of credit.[13] In this context, Champagne's fairs played a critical role both in the commercialization of the medieval economy and in the stimulation of economic development.[14] Champagne's international trade fairs are well recognized as "a standard-bearer of the medieval Commercial Revolution," and "the undisputed fulcrum of international exchange in Europe for much of the thirteenth century."[15] The four principal Champenois fairs, which took place six times a year, each for a period of about six weeks, rotating among the towns of Bar, Lagny, Provins, and Troyes, served both as "the money-market of Europe," and as "an emporium for the trade in wares," most especially the exchange of cloth and wool supplied by Flemish and northern French traders for items provided by Italian and Provençal merchants from Mediterranean markets.[16] Thus, studying the emergence of new charitable institutions in Champagne during the twelfth and thirteenth centuries makes it possible to probe the interplay between the charitable revolution and the concomitant commercial revolution. This book does not often venture into the fourteenth century, which was marked by dramatic demographic and economic changes, concentrating instead on the twelfth and thirteenth centuries, the golden age of hospital foundations. Much of this book focuses on the southern part of Champagne (Troyes, Provins, and Bar-sur-Aube), since this region was the site of the major trade fairs and thus provides an ideal window for exploring the nexus between commerce and charity. This southern part of Champagne, south of the Marne River, was also the base of comital power, with the counts playing a significant role both in overseeing the fairs and in founding, patronizing, and protecting hospitals.[17] But this book also draws on examples

---

13. Richard H. Britnell and Bruce M. S. Campbell, "Introduction," in *A Commercialising Economy: England 1086 to c. 1300*, ed. Britnell and Campbell (Manchester: Manchester University Press, 1995), 3, 5.

14. John H. Munro, "The 'New Institutional Economics' and the Changing Fortunes of Fairs in Medieval and Early Modern Europe: The Textile Trades, Warfare, and Transaction Costs," *Vierteljahrschrift fur Sozial- und Wirtschaftsgeschichte* 88 (2001): 1–47.

15. Jeremy Edwards and Sheilagh Ogilvie, "What Lessons for Economic Development Can We Draw from the Champagne Fairs?" *Explorations in Economic History* 49 (2012): 131. On the evolution of the Champenois fairs, see Robert-Henri Bautier, "Les foires de Champagne: Recherches sur une évolution historique," in *La Foire*, vol. 5 of *Recueils de la Société Jean Bodin* (Brussels: Editions de la Librairie Encyclopédique, 1953), 97–147. See also Elizabeth Chapin, *Les villes de foires de Champagne, des origines au début du XIVe siècle* (Paris: H. Champion, 1937); M. Félix Bourquelot, *Études sur les foires de Champagne: sur la nature, l'étendue et les règles du commerce qui s'y faisait aux XIIe, XIIe et XIVe siècles*, 2nd ser., vol. 5 of *Mémoires présentés par divers savants à l'Académie des Inscriptions et Belles-Lettres de l'Institut Impérial de France* (Paris: Le Portulan, 1865).

16. Edwards and Ogilvie, "What Lessons for Economic Development," 132.

17. As Michel Bur has shown, it was only in the later twelfth century that the counts of Champagne began acquiring greater power in the diocese of Reims. See Michel Bur, "Le comte de

from elsewhere in Champagne, such as Reims (in the north of the county), an archiepiscopal city, which makes for an interesting point of comparison with the comital cities of Troyes and Provins. In considering evidence from other parts of northern France and Europe, I have sought to embed developments in Champagne within a larger charitable and commercial context, pointing to some of the ways that the county was distinctive while also demonstrating that the emergence of hospitals in Champagne was part of a broader pan-European phenomenon.

On several levels, Champagne's commercial context is crucial for under-standing the emergence of its hospitals. First, the fairs generated some of the capital needed to support these institutions. Hospitals received revenue from the fairs directly, and the hospitals benefited even more indirectly from the commercial prosperity that made pious bequests possible. Second, Cham-pagne witnessed a great deal of traffic of peoples and goods due to the criss-crossing of merchants and their wares. Foreign merchants, migrants in search of work, and others in need of accommodation often turned to Champagne's hospitals for assistance. More generally, though, the greater economic pros-perity experienced by some during this period did little to reduce widespread poverty, and in fact may have contributed, along with urban transformation, to an increase in the number of people who were visibly living on the mar-gins. As one medieval economic historian put it, "Among the costs of com-mercialization was a more precarious life for perhaps a fifth or more of the population."[18] This is borne out by chronicles of the time and even more so by tax records from different regions, which suggest that a significant percent-age of rural and urban households (peasants, urban migrants, single women, and so on) were considered to be living below what was considered a taxable level.[19] Finally, although the Christian religious imagination had drawn on the language of commerce as a conceptual framework from the time of the

---

Champagne dans le diocèse de Reims au XIIe siècle," in *La Champagne médiévale: Recueil d'articles*, ed. Michel Bur (Langres, France: Dominique Guéniot, 2005), 239–56. See also Pierre Desportes, *Reims et les Rémois aux XIIIe et XIVe siècles* (Paris: Picard, 1979), 52–53.

18. Richard H. Britnell, "Commercialisation and economic development in England, 1000–1300," in *A Commercialising Economy: England 1086 to c. 1300* (Manchester: Manchester University Press, 1995), 23.

19. Sharon Farmer, *Surviving Poverty in Medieval Paris: Gender, Ideology, and the Daily Lives of the Poor* (Ithaca: Cornell University Press, 2002); Philipp Schofield, "Approaching Poverty in the Medieval Countryside," in *Poverty and Prosperity in the Middle Ages and the Renaissance*, ed. Cynthia Kosso and Anne Scott (Turnhout, Belgium: Brepols, 2012), 100–101; Christopher Dyer, "Poverty and Its Relief in Late Medieval England," *Past and Present* 216 (2012): 41–78; Dyer, "The Experience of Being Poor in Late Medieval England," in *Experiences of Poverty in Late Medieval and Early Modern Europe*, ed. Anne M. Scott (Aldershot, U.K.: Ashgate, 2012), 20–39.

Gospels and the early Church Fathers, the profit economy of the high and later Middle Ages, as Giacomo Todeschini, Jacques Chiffoleau, and others have shown, also left its imprint on the spiritual realm, infusing the notions of spiritual rewards, exchange, and reciprocity with heightened meaning, particularly within the context of charitable institutions and practices.[20] During a period of commercial effervescence, but also increasingly visible poverty, ideas about commerce and markets were redeployed in the spiritual realm of charitable giving and service.

As this book shows, far from being oppositional forces, commerce and charity were remarkably symbiotic. At the same time that Champagne's economy was becoming monetized and that the number of commercial transactions was increasing, the amount of voluntary, pious giving was also on the rise, particularly in the form of gifts to charitable causes such as hospitals.[21] That this period was marked by a renewed focus on the redemptive aspects of almsgiving and on the way that gifts and charitable service were thought to generate rewards can be seen both in the language of donation charters to Champagne's hospitals and in the writings of biblical exegetes about pious giving.[22] Archival evidence indicates that pious *pro anima* gifts were understood at the time as reciprocal and dynamic exchanges, whereby the donor reaped valuable and calculable assets in the form of spiritual benefits.[23]

---

20. Giacomo Todeschini, *Il prezzo della salvezza: Lessici medievali del pensiero economico* (Rome: La Nuova Italia Scientifica, 1994); Todeschini, "I vocabolari dell'analisi economica fra alto e basso medioevo: Dai lessici della disciplina monastica ai lessici antiusurari," in *Rivista storica Italiana* 110, no. 3 (1998): 781–833; Todeschini, *Les marchands et le temple: La société Chrétienne et le cercle vertueux de la richesse du moyen age à l'époque moderne,* trans. Ida Giordano and Mathieu Arnoux (Paris: Albin Michel, 2017), particularly chs. 3–4; Jacques Chiffoleau, "Pour une économie de l'institution ecclésiale à la fin du moyen âge," *Mélanges de l'École française de Rome* 96, no. 1 (1984): 247–79.

21. As I demonstrate in chapter 3, the continued vitality of *pro anima* gifts to Champagne's hospitals during the thirteenth century stood in contrast to a decline in the number of pious gifts to Champagne's monasteries, as Richard Keyser has shown. As a result, monasteries came to rely more on acquisitions from purchases, exchanges, and quittances. Léopold Genicot noted a similar pattern with respect to gifts to the abbeys of the county of Namur. Gifts to these abbeys declined precipitously from 1280 onwards, and donors in the thirteenth century placed far more conditions on their gifts. See Genicot, "L'évolution des dons aux abbayes dans le comté de Namur du Xe au XIVe siècle," *XXXe Congrès de la Fédération archéologique et historique de Belgique, Bruxelles, 28 Juillet—2 Août 1935: Annales* (Brussels, 1936), 133–48.

22. Emmanuel Bain, *Église, richesse et pauvreté dans l'occident médiéval: L'exégèse des Évangiles aux XIIe–XIIIe siècles* (Turnhout, Belgium: Brepols, 2014).

23. As Jacques Chiffoleau demonstrated in his study of Avignon, the notion that it was possible to calculate the price of salvation only became fully developed during the later Middle Ages. See Chiffoleau, *La comptabilité de l'au-delà: Les hommes, la mort et la religion dans la région d'Avignon à la fin du moyen âge (vers 1320–vers 1480)* (Rome: École Française de Rome, 1980). For the north of France, see Catherine Vincent, "Y-a-t-il une mathématique du salut dans les diocèses du nord de la France à la veille de la réforme?" *Revue d'histoire de l'Église de France* 77, no. 198 (1991): 137–49.

By analyzing the complex and overlapping motives that led women and men to support hospitals, this book probes what giving meant to medieval people and thereby provides a window into a pivotal moment in European history when care for the sick and poor became popularized and institutionalized. Champagne's hospitals served as visible symbols of piety and the works of mercy, and as a result, they were popular objects of benefaction—so popular that they increasingly eclipsed monastic houses in the number and size of the donations they received from a broad segment of society. These institutions also presented lay women and men with a new penitential opportunity to personally perform the works of mercy. Working in a hospital was embraced as a pious way to earn salvific rewards without necessarily taking monastic vows, while still acquiring the security that came with living and working in a fraternal community dedicated to mutual assistance.

Some of the new significance of gifts and charitable service, I argue, was related to religious developments, such as growing Eucharistic piety, a preoccupation with Purgatory, and the rise of a confessional society, all of which fueled a greater demand for the celebration of Masses, which was sometimes a condition for pious gifts. Charity was also widely regarded as an antidote to the vice of avarice, which was associated with commerce. In this way, Champagne's thriving commercial economy helped fuel the perceived moral need for charity. Indeed, in an effort to promote the value of almsgiving, some preachers cast the practice as a potentially lucrative alternative to commerce, both in the temporal and spiritual sense, with almsgivers promised the hundredfold reward referenced in Matthew 19:29.[24] Almsgiving was itself increasingly conceived and described in commercial terms, with God even cast as a debtor and the almsgiver as a virtuous moneylender. While some potential donors might have been reluctant to give away a portion of their wealth to the poor, preachers sought to reassure them that they were making the wisest kind of investment by earning credit with God and funding "a heavenly treasure." As this book demonstrates, the notion of charitable gifts as loans to God with the strong potential for a redemptive reward played a crucial factor in fostering charitable behavior in the monetized and commercial economy of thirteenth-century Europe. Moreover, support for charitable institutions may have been fueled by spiritual anxiety about growing prosperity, with charity serving to justify profit-making when some of

---

24. Spencer E. Young, "More Blessed to Give and Receive: Charitable Giving in Thirteenth and Early Fourteenth-Century *Exempla*," in *Experiences of Charity, 1250–1650*, ed. Anne M. Scott (Farnham, U.K.: Ashgate, 2015), 77.

those profits were channeled toward alms.[25] In that sense, the pursuit of profit, it was believed, could advance the pursuit of salvation. In this vein, some Franciscan and Dominican preachers defended the money used for almsgiving and donations to hospitals as "virtuous wealth."[26] The foundation of so many hospitals in the twelfth and thirteenth centuries is thus a manifestation of the tension between traditional Christian morality and the new profit-oriented economy, a penitential expression in a society increasingly preoccupied with acquisition.

This book also seeks to shed new light on the diverse and often surprising roles that hospitals played and the impact that they had on the larger society. For instance, as chapter 4 shows, Champagne's hospitals were engaged in significant profit-making of their own and served as creditors, landlords with large numbers of tenants and serfs, holders of fiefs with lordly rights (including justice), cultivators of crops for sale, and owners of commercial stalls at trade fairs. Account books from some of Champagne's hospitals disclose how they managed their finances, how they sought to juggle their expenses and revenues, caring for those in need of assistance while aggressively participating in the agricultural and rent markets. To fully understand hospitals' relationships with their patrons, it is necessary to learn more about the diverse services that they provided to the larger community (such as providing money loans, leasing mills and ovens, and distributing life annuities in return for donations), the social networks that hospitals were part of, and the ways they functioned as power brokers. Pious gifts made to Champagne's hospitals during the thirteenth century at times had conditions placed on them that obligated the hospital to perform a service, such as paying a lifetime annuity to one of the donor's relatives. As a result, it was the wishes and needs of donors that shaped a hospital's manifold functions, requiring the institution to perform services well outside of its original charitable and religious mission.[27] As Paul Bertrand has shown, hospitals even served as economic partners to members of mendicant orders (who might otherwise have

---

25. Lester K. Little, *Religious Poverty and the Profit Economy in Medieval Europe* (Ithaca: Cornell University Press, 1978).

26. Nicole Bériou, "L'esprit de lucre entre vice et vertu: Variations sur l'amour de l'argent dans la prédication du XIIIe siècle," in *Actes des congrès de la Société des historiens médiévistes de l'enseignement supérieur public* 28, no. 1 (1997): 267–87.

27. This same phenomenon can be seen in the late medieval and Renaissance hospitals of Italian lay confraternities. See Nicholas Terpstra, *Lay Confraternities and Civic Religion in Renaissance Bologna* (Cambridge: Cambridge University Press, 1995); Matthew Thomas Sneider, "The Bonds of Charity: Charitable and Liturgical Obligations in Bolognese Testaments," in *Poverty and Prosperity in the Middle Ages and Renaissance*, ed. Cynthia Kosso and Anne Scott (Turnhout, Belgium: Brepols, 2012), 129–42.

not been connected to a hospital at all), with hospitals serving as intermediaries between donors and individual friars, distributing pensions to friars
so that they did not violate their vows of poverty.[28] By creating a social taxonomy of those who engaged in various kinds of transactions with hospitals
(gifts, exchanges, sales and purchases, loans), this book demonstrates how
these charitable institutions were enmeshed in complex webs of reciprocity.

In exploring the rise of Champagne's hospitals, I have also tried to uncover
as much as possible about the individuals that hospitals served, including the
vulnerable, the needy, and the sick as well as the newly arrived migrants with
no familial or neighborly support. Drawing on scattered pieces of evidence,
this book seeks to deepen our understanding of these people and their experiences living on the margins of medieval society. Why did an individual in
need of help turn to a particular institution or for that matter, certain groups,
neighbors, or family members? What constituted hospital care, and what
forms of assistance did hospitals provide to those living outside the hospital
walls? And how were the recipients of hospital care thought to play a critical
role in the economy of salvation for a hospital's benefactors and its personnel? In short, this book asks what it was that held together a hospital's dense
network of relations, including the institution's benefactors, its personnel,
and those for whom it cared.

While the benefaction of medieval monasteries has been studied extensively, far less attention has been paid to the significant charitable support
given to hospitals, notwithstanding some studies of hospitals in particular
regions.[29] We still need to learn more about the social networks involved in

---

28. Paul Bertrand, *Commerce avec dame pauvreté: Structures et fonctions des couvents mendiants à Liège (XIIIe–XIVe siècles)* (Geneva: Droz, 2004), 215–16, 472.

29. Jean Imbert, ed., *Histoire des hôpitaux en France* (Toulouse: Privat, 1982); Alain Saint-Denis, *L'hôtel-dieu de Laon, 1150–1300* (Nancy, France: Presses Universitaires de Nancy, 1983); Le Blévec, *La part du pauvre*; Jacqueline Caille, *Hôpitaux et charité publique à Narbonne au Moyen Age* (Toulouse: Privat, 1977); Saunier, *"Le pauvre malade"*; Pierre de Spiegeler, *Les hôpitaux et l'assistance à Liège (Xe–XVe siècles): Aspects institutionnels et sociaux* (Paris: Société d'Edition "Les Belles Lettres," 1987); Jean Imbert, *Les hôpitaux en droit canonique (du décret de Gratien à la sécularisation de l'administration de l'Hôtel-Dieu de Paris en 1505)* (Paris: J. Vrin, 1947); Irène Dietrich-Strobbe, "Sauver les riches: La charité à Lille à la fin du Moyen Âge," (thesis, l'Université Paris-Sorbonne, 2016); Sally Mayall Brasher, *Hospitals and Charity: Religious Culture and Civic Life in Medieval Northern Italy* (Manchester: Manchester University Press, 2017); G. G. Merlo, *Esperienze religiose e opere assistenziali nei secoli XII et XIII* (Turin, 1987); John Henderson, *The Renaissance Hospital: Healing the Body and Healing the Soul* (New Haven: Yale University Press, 2006); James W. Brodman, *Charity and Welfare: Hospitals and the Poor in Medieval Catalonia* (Philadelphia: University of Pennsylvania Press, 1998); Brodman, *Charity and Religion*; Gisela Drossbach, *Christliche Caritas als Rechtsinstitut: Hospital und Orden von Santo Spirito in Sassia (1198–1378)* (Paderborn, Germany: Schöningh, 2005); Benjamin Laqua, *Bruderschaften und Hospitäler während des hohen Mittelalters: Kölner Befunde in westeuropäisch-vergleichender Perspektive*

the giving and receiving of charitable support. How did a particular family come to patronize certain charitable institutions or organizations, including institutions that were at times located some distance away? In addition to closely examining patterns of hospital patronage, this book interrogates the identities of those who worked in Champagne's hospitals, who, in some cases, had themselves been benefactors before joining the hospital's religious community. What propelled them to join a hospital's personnel? Were there any gender or class patterns as to those who patronized and worked inside hospitals? A plethora of untapped primary source material for Champagne provides tantalizing clues as to what hospitals meant to people of various social classes and what motivated charitable giving and service. Institutions never simply emerge in a given society but are created by individuals and groups, often in response to problems. Institutions thus reflect the social and cultural values, beliefs, and aspirations of a particular place and time. This study of medieval charity and charitable institutions illuminates broader questions about the nature of social relationships and lived experiences.

Explaining the Emergence of a Charitable Revolution

The popularization of charitable giving and service as religious ideals emerged as part of the larger apostolic movement of the twelfth and thirteenth centuries, which included an outpouring of lay religious devotion. Charitable giving and service were very much tied to a growing concern with personal salvation and the penance that it was believed was needed to achieve it. Those making pious bequests often explicitly linked their giving

---

(Stuttgart: Anton Hiersemann, 2011); Brigitte Resl-Pohl, *Rechnen mit der Ewigkeit: Das Wiener Bürgerspital im Mittelalter* (Munich: Oldenbourg Verlag, 1996); Neithard Bulst and Karl-Heinz Spieß, eds., *Sozialgeschichte mittelalterlicher hospitäler* (Ostfildern, Germany: Jan Thorbecke Verlag, 2007); Lucy C. Barnhouse, "The Elusive Medieval Hospital: Mainz and the Middle Rhine Region," (PhD dissertation, Fordham University, 2017); Lies Vervaet, "Goederenbeheer in een veranderende samenleving: Het Sint-Janshospital van Brugge ca. 1275–ca. 1575," (PhD dissertation, University of Ghent, 2015); Rubin, *Charity and Community*; Margaret Webster and Nicolas Orme, *The English Hospital, 1070–1570* (New Haven: Yale University Press, 1995); Carole Rawcliffe, *Medicine for the Soul: The Life, Death, and Resurrection of an English Medieval Hospital, St. Giles's, Norwich, c. 1249–1550* (Stroud, U.K.: Sutton, 1999); Rawcliffe, *The Hospitals of Medieval Norwich* (Norwich, U.K.: Centre of East Anglian Studies, University of East Anglia, 1999); Sheila Sweetinburgh, *The Role of the Hospital in Medieval England: Gift-Giving and the Spiritual Economy* (Dublin: Four Courts Press, 2004); Gisela Drossbach, ed., *Hospitäler in Mittelalter und früher Neuzeit: Frankreich, Deutschland und Italien: Eine vergleichende Geschichte* (Munich: R. Oldenbourg Wissenschaftsverlag, 2007); Martin Scheutz, Andrea Sommerlechner, Herwig Weigl, and Alfred Stefan Weis, eds., *Europäisches Spitalwesen: Institutionelle Fürsorge in Mittelalter und Früher Neuzeit* (Vienna: R. Oldenbourg, 2008); Peregrine Horden, "A Discipline of Relevance: The Historiography of the Later Medieval Hospital," *Social History of Medicine* 1 (1988): 359–74.

to the welfare of their souls, thereby reflecting a belief in the intercessory powers of the sick and poor recipients of their gifts. Moreover, the traditional theological notion of an almost quantifiable link between salvation and almsgiving became all the more vital with the development of the doctrine of Purgatory during the twelfth century.[30] As Jacques Le Goff put it, "at the heart of the economy of salvation and its social functioning were 'mercy, *caritas* and the gift.'"[31]

The growing sanctification of charity is evident in the large number of saints from this period who were venerated for their acts of compassion, which often included founding and working in a hospital.[32] André Vauchez has shown that "a new category of saint" emerged as part of the apostolic movement, with sanctity increasingly tied to the practice of charity as opposed to contemplation.[33] Many of these charitable saints were lay men and women (as opposed to monastic or clerical saints), and quite a few, like St. Elizabeth of Hungary, came from aristocratic or even royal backgrounds.[34] Even apart from those who were formally canonized, however, charity became a central feature of lay spirituality, an opportunity to do penance without renouncing the world by joining a monastic order or going on crusade. Even crusading, however, was seen by contemporaries as a charitable endeavor, an expression of one's love of God and one's fellow Christians in the East who were in need of assistance. As Jonathan Riley-Smith put it in his classic essay, "Crusading as an Act of Love," "the crusades were as much the products of the renewed spirituality of the central Middle Ages, with its concern for living the *vita apostolica* and expressing Christian ideals in the active works of charity, as were the new hospitals, the pastoral work of the Augustinians and Premonstratensians and the service of the friars."[35]

The penitential aspect of both charity and crusading can certainly be seen in the descriptions of Saint Louis, the thirteenth-century king of France, who twice went on crusade and patronized religious houses, the mendicant

---

30. Jacques Le Goff, *The Birth of Purgatory*, trans. Arthur Goldhammer (Chicago: University of Chicago Press, 1984).

31. Jacques Le Goff, *Money and the Middle Ages: An Essay in Historical Anthropology*, trans. Jean Birrell (Cambridge: Polity Press, 2012), 132.

32. André Vauchez, *Sainthood in the Later Middle Ages*, trans. Jean Birrell (Cambridge: Cambridge University Press, 1997); Jonathan Riley-Smith, "Crusading as an Act of Love," *History* 65, no. 214 (1980): 177–92.

33. Vauchez, *Sainthood*, 199. On the relationship between charity and female sanctity, see Daniel Le Blévec, "Le rôle des femmes dans l'assistance et la charité," in *La femme dans la vie religieuse du Languedoc (XIIIe–XIVe s.)*, Cahiers de Fanjeaux, vol. 23 (Toulouse: Privat, 1988), 171–90.

34. Vauchez, *Sainthood*.

35. Riley-Smith, "Crusading as an Act of Love," 192.

orders, and numerous leprosaria and hospitals, even founding a hospital for the blind in Paris.[36] Louis IX's hagiographers stressed that his extraordinary generosity and concern for the downtrodden were evidence of his sanctity, but his charity was in fact rooted in a Capetian tradition of giving generously not only to religious houses but also hospitals, leprosaries, and other charitable causes: Louis's grandfather, Philip Augustus, left 21,000 *l. par.* for "poor, orphans, widows and lepers" in his testament of 1222; his father, Louis VIII, bequeathed 10,000 *l. par.* in 1225 for some two thousand leprosaries; and in 1269 Louis IX left 2,000 *l. par.* for eight hundred leprosaries and 2,000 *l. par.* for two hundred hôtels-Dieu.[37] The Book of Hours of Jeanne of Evreux (Louis's great-granddaughter) gave visual expression to Saint Louis's charity, with the humble king depicted caring for the sick in hospital beds, washing the feet of the poor, and so forth.[38] Interestingly, Louis's hagiographers cast his charity as central to his style of royal governance and his sense of responsibility to God for the administration of justice in his kingdom. One of Louis's hagiographers described him as "the father of the poor," and late medieval "mirrors for princes" often used this same phrase to underscore that charity was not just a religious virtue but also a royal responsibility.[39] In trying to account for the popular outpouring of charitable giving during this

---

36. See M. Cecilia Gaposchkin, *The Making of Saint Louis: Kingship, Sanctity, and Crusade in the Later Middle Ages* (Ithaca: Cornell University Press, 2008).

37. François-Olivier Touati, *Archives de la lèpre: Atlas des léproseries entre Loire et Marne au moyen age* (Paris: Edition du C.T.H.S., 1996), 70. As Bautier has shown, the formalized annual distributions by the French almonry to monasteries, hospitals, leprosaries, and the poor of individual towns and cities, as established by Louis IX in 1260, continued into the fifteenth century. See R.-H. Bautier, "Les aumônes du roi aux maladreries, maisons-Dieu et pauvres établissements du royaume: Contribution à l'étude du réseau hospitalier et de la fossilisation de l'administration royale de Philippe Auguste à Charles VII," in *Assistance et Assistés jusqu'à 1610. Actes du 97ᵉ congrès des Sociétés savantes, Nantes 1972* (Paris: Bibliothèque Nationale, 1979), 37–106. On Louis IX's patronage and protection of the hospitals of Normandy, see François Neveux, "Naissance et développement des hôtels-Dieu en Normandie (XIIe–XIVe siècle)," in *Hôpitaux et maladreries au moyen âge: Espace et environnement. Actes du colloque international d'Amiens-Beauvais, 22, 23 et 24 novembre 2002*, ed. Pascal Montaubin 17 (2004): 247–48.

38. Gerald B. Guest, "A Discourse on the Poor: The Hours of Jeanne d'Evreux," *Viator* 26 (1995): 153–80; Joan A. Holladay, "The Education of Jeanne d'Evreux: Personal Piety and Dynastic Salvation in her Book of Hours at the Cloisters," *Art History* 17, no. 4 (December 1994): 585–611. Some doubt, however, has been cast on whether a king such as Saint Louis really was as charitable as his hagiographers would suggest. The number of royal gifts to charitable institutions in Normandy, for example, actually declined quite sharply in the mid-thirteenth century. See Damien Jeanne, "Le roi charitable: Les politiques royales envers les établissements d'assistance de la Normandie centrale et occidentale, XIIIe–XVe siècle," in *Une histoire pour un royaume, XIIe–XVe siècle: Actes du colloque Corpus Regni, organisé en hommage à Colette Beaune*, ed. Anne-Hélène Allirot and Colette Beaune (Paris: Perrin, 2010), 119–55.

39. Priscille Aladjidi, "L'idéal politique du roi 'père des pauvres,'" in *Une histoire pour un royaume*, 88–101.

period, one wonders whether the example of the royal patronage of charitable institutions may have played a role in inspiring greater lay (and even clerical) generosity. In a region like Champagne, the continued patronage of counts and countesses, who founded several of the largest and wealthiest hospitals (and who, more generally, were deeply involved in ecclesiastical affairs, regularly confirming the election of abbots and abbesses), was absolutely vital for the success of these charitable institutions.

As Michel Mollat, André Vauchez, and others have shown, medieval social and religious attitudes toward the sick and poor were ambivalent, often combining feelings of scorn and fear with reverence toward those considered the "poor of Christ," who were widely regarded as powerful spiritual intercessors and were credited with making charity and its attendant spiritual benefits possible.[40] As these scholars readily acknowledge, the poor continued to be stigmatized and harassed, and there was suspicion that some beggars were able-bodied and therefore "undeserving" of assistance. The hagiographic topos of a saint's humble, personal ministry to the sick poor continued to have force in the high Middle Ages precisely because the *miserabiles* were still met with disdain, and it was thus considered unnatural for someone to care for them. Yet in terms of collective attitudes, poverty was also increasingly regarded as a sign of divine election, with the poor seen as Christ's vicars on earth.[41] It was common in medieval *exempla*, for example, for a poor man (or leper) to appear as Christ in disguise. The status of the *pauperes Christi*, traditionally those who took religious vows of voluntary poverty, was gradually extended to include the *miserabiles*, a category that, according to the churchman Jacques de Vitry (d. 1240), included the involuntary poor, the hungry, the leprous, those with various kinds of disabilities, and those who cry.[42] In this way, the *miserabiles* came to supplant monks and nuns as sought-after intermediaries between this world and the next, as the natural agents of collective redemption. The new spiritual power ascribed to the poor, sick, and disabled, and to the works of mercy performed on their behalf reflects what

---

40. Jean Longère, "Pauvreté et richesse chez quelques prédicateurs durant la seconde moitié du xiie siècle," in *Études sur l'histoire de la pauvreté*, ed. Michel Mollat (Paris: Publications de la Sorbonne, 1974), 1:255–73; Michel Mollat, *The Poor in the Middle Ages: An Essay in Social History*, trans. Arthur Goldhammer (New Haven: Yale University Press, 1986); Vauchez, *Spiritualité du moyen âge occidental*, 118–23.

41. In his study of the problem of wealth in late antiquity, Peter Brown likewise cites examples of the poor being both the objects of scorn and admiration. The fantastically wealthy Pinianus and Melania the Younger so wished to identify with the poor that they enlisted on the poor roll of the church of Jerusalem in 417. See Brown, *Through the Eye of a Needle: Wealth, the Fall of Rome, and the Making of Christianity in the West, 350–550 AD* (Princeton: Princeton University Press, 2012), 300.

42. Mollat, *Poor in the Middle Ages*, 102.

the French historian François-Olivier Touati has called nothing short of a "mutation de conscience" on the part of the medieval laity.[43] This "transformation of conscience" is evident not only in the frequency of twelfth- and thirteenth-century charitable giving and the mushrooming of hospital foundations but also in the decision of some women and men to dedicate their lives to caring for the *miserabiles* in these institutions.

In trying to understand medieval Christians' expressions of support for new charitable institutions like hospitals, we ought to consider how specific cultural and devotional experiences might have conditioned people to feel compassion and behave charitably toward those in need of assistance. The historian Lynn Hunt has proposed a causal relationship between the rise of humanitarian concerns during the eighteenth century and cultural experiences such as the reading of epistolary novels.[44] Just as these novels provoked "imagined empathy" in their readers for the plight of the novels' characters, the medieval faithful projected their own "imagined relationship" with a suffering Jesus and a compassionate Mary, evoked in preachers' sermons and in visual representations in churches, onto the *miserabiles* of their own community. In short, developments in medieval spirituality, including a greater emphasis on the humanity of Jesus and Mary, may have made it easier for medieval Christians to empathize with a suffering stranger, to see themselves, a family member, or Jesus in the sufferer (or, for that matter, in the one seeking to alleviate the suffering).

There remains a need to explore the relationship between charitable practices and developments in devotion that expanded medieval Christians' capacity for imagination and empathy. Beginning in the late eleventh century and continuing through the twelfth and thirteenth centuries—the very period that saw the mushrooming of hospital foundations and the creation of new charitable organizations—compassion became a pervasive theme in devotional literature, so much so that J. A. W. Bennett argued that the popularity of the literary genre of affective meditation on Christ's Passion represented a "revolution in feeling."[45] Likewise, Sarah McNamer has credited affective meditations on the Passion with "the invention of compassion." According to McNamer, "The cultivation of compassion in the devotional realm . . . clearly had the potential to effect ethical thinking and behavior on

---

43. Touati, *Maladie et société*, 214.

44. Lynn Avery Hunt, *Inventing Human Rights: A History*, 1st ed. (New York: Norton, 2007).

45. J. A. W. Bennett, *Poetry of the Passion: Studies in Twelve Centuries of English Verse* (Oxford: Clarendon Press, 1982), 32.

a wider scale."[46] The objective of meditations such as the pseudo-Bonaventurean *Meditationes vitae Christi* was "to teach their readers, through iterative affective performance, how to feel."[47] This imitative devotion and affective identification with Jesus and Mary could also be stimulated with help from the painted rood screens and crucifixes that were ubiquitous in medieval churches (and hospitals) or the scenes of the crucifixion and the Man of Sorrows in psalters, missals, and Books of Hours. Scenes from the evangelical past, whether visual or textual, sought to elicit a sense of compassion and above all empathy from the meditant.

While it is impossible to establish a direct causal link, it is possible that affective devotional experiences made it easier for some people to empathize with their needy neighbors. Moreover, material support for charitable causes such as hospitals may be related to developments in meditative and devotional practices. Did meditations on the Passion and a growing preoccupation with the figure of the suffering Jesus create an enlarged capacity for feelings of compassion for fellow Christians in need?[48] In this vein, is there any connection between women's (especially widows') high rate of charitable giving and service in hospitals, as we will see in chapters 3 and 5, and the fact that, as McNamer and others have shown, affective devotion was so gendered, with compassion for the suffering Christ associated with "feeling like a woman"?[49]

Institutionalizing a Charitable Ideal: The Medieval Reinvention of the Hospital

The ideology of charity that served as the basis for the support medieval hospitals received was rooted in scriptural and patristic thought that emphasized the responsibility of all Christians to perform charitable works. Medieval sources often cited the words of Jesus in Matthew 25:35–36, enumerating what came to be understood as the six corporal works of mercy: "For I was hungry, and you gave me to eat: I was thirsty, and you

---

46. Sarah McNamer, *Affective Meditation and the Invention of Medieval Compassion* (Philadelphia: University of Pennsylvania Press, 2010), 150.

47. McNamer, *Affective Meditation*, 2.

48. McNamer, *Affective Meditation*, 150. Admittedly, it was one thing for a Passion narrative to elicit devotion to Christ and another for that compassion to be translated into concrete works of mercy directed at strangers in one's own midst. As Miri Rubin and others have shown, meditations on the Passion could just as easily lead to horrific violence against Jews as inspire acts of compassion for a fellow Christian.

49. McNamer, *Affective Meditation*, 119–49.

gave me to drink: I was a stranger, and you took me in: naked, and you covered me: sick, and you visited me: I was in prison, and you came to me." Jesus's words in Matthew 25:40 ("As long as you did it to one of these my least brethren, you did it to me") represented a central tenet of Christian charity, namely that to help the poor and needy is to help Jesus himself. Christians believed that if Christ was to show them mercy, they had to show beneficence to their neighbors in need, since they considered the poor and powerless to be Christ's representatives on earth. While the medieval theological concept of *caritas* referred to the love of God, it was believed that one way to show one's love of God was by providing assistance to one's needy neighbors.[50] Charity was understood as an act of mercy and love that could take the form of hospitality, personal acts of service, or a specific material gift or bequest (coin, food, clothing, property). Gifts to churches and monasteries were also considered a form of charity, a way of fulfilling one's duties both to Christ and the poor, since churches and monasteries were thought to redistribute the gifts they received as alms to the poor. Yet as we shall see in chapter 3, during the twelfth and thirteenth centuries lay donors and testators increasingly directed their bequests to hospitals, which were thought, even more so than churches and monasteries, to embody the performance of the seven corporal works of mercy. Church Fathers such as Ambrose and Augustine had earlier popularized the notion that almsgiving and benefaction of the poor had the capacity to erase sin and deliver the almsgiver from death, and this idea of redemptive almsgiving remained a central force underlying charity during the medieval period and beyond.[51]

Although the notion of serving others and seeing Christ in those who are suffering was a central part of New Testament teaching, Peter Brown has argued that it was only during the late fourth century that "the poor," a category essentially created by late Roman bishops, became objects of material and religious concern, as reflected in the emergence of the first hospitals, or *xenodocheia*.[52] From the fourth to the seventh centuries, these Christian charitable institutions, which cared for the sick, leprous, disabled, and strangers, developed in the Byzantine Levant and Asia Minor, supported by both the

---

50. Eliza Buhrer, "From *Caritas* to Charity: How Loving God Became Giving Alms," in *Poverty and Prosperity in the Middle Ages and the Renaissance*, ed. Cynthia Kosso and Anne Scott (Turnhout: Brepols, 2012), 113–28.

51. Abigail Firey, "'For I Was Hungry and You Fed Me': Social Justice and Economic Thought in the Latin Patristic and Medieval Christian Traditions," in *Ancient and Medieval Economic Ideas and Concepts of Social Justice*, ed. S. Todd Lowry and Barry Gordon (Leiden: Brill, 1998): 333–70.

52. Brown, *Through the Eye of a Needle*, 53–90.

Byzantine Church and emperors.[53] Above all, late antique bishops founded and patronized hospitals as a way of asserting their role as protectors of the poor.[54] Giving gradually shifted from the traditional, pagan civic generosity, in which the wealthy gave large gifts to their city, to a new Christian model in which the "middling" classes gave what modest gifts they could to the poor and their local church. As the pages that follow will show, a second wave of this "democratization of charity" was to take place in twelfth and thirteenth-century Europe, but on a completely different scale.

Already in late antiquity, however, charitable practices were redefining the relationship between the spiritual and the material. Institutionalized charity in the form of *xenodocheia* provided the church with a way of legitimizing its own growing wealth. Peregrine Horden has argued that late antique hospitals allowed the church to draw a distinction between accumulated wealth and wealth that was distributed to those most in need, a kind of "down-payment on salvation."[55] Hospitals in the Byzantine world developed earlier and in different ways than those in the less urbanized early medieval Latin West.[56] By the twelfth century, the Pantocrator Xenon-Hospital in Constantinople, a royal hospital foundation that was unusual even for Byzantium in its size and in the degree of its medicalization, was serving as a teaching facility with a medical staff (including an elaborate hierarchy of physicians)

53. Timothy S. Miller, *The Birth of the Hospital in the Byzantine Empire* (Baltimore: The Johns Hopkins University Press, 1985); Mark Alan Anderson, "Hospitals, Hospices, and Shelters for the Poor in Late Antiquity," (PhD dissertation, Yale University, 2012).

54. Brown, *Through the Eye of a Needle*, 81.

55. Peregrine Horden, "Cities within Cities: Early Hospital Foundations and Urban Space," in *Stiftungen zwischen Politik und Wirtschaft: Ein Dialog zwischen Geschichte und Gegenwart*, ed. Sitta von Reden (Munich, 2015), 160. Even the so-called "Spiritual Franciscan," Peter John Olivi, known for what was seen as his radical understanding of the meaning of ecclesiastical poverty, would make a similar point at the end of the thirteenth century, arguing that commerce could be beneficial to society so long as the wealth it generated was distributed rather than accumulated. See Sylvain Piron, "Le devoir de gratitude: Émergence et vogue de al notion d'*antidora* au XIIIe siècle," in *Credito e usura fra teologia, diritto e amministrazione: Linguaggi a confront (sec. XII–XVI)*, ed., Diego Quaglioni, Giacomo Todeschini, and Gian Maria Varanini (Rome: École Française de Rome, 2005), 97–99.

56. Although there has been some debate about the extent to which Byzantine hospitals were medicalized, there were clearly some Byzantine hospitals that provided professional care for the sick, regardless of their social class. Timothy Miller has been criticized for the extent to which he described Byzantine hospitals as medicalized and for arguing that the institutional origins of the "modern hospital" can be traced back to Byzantine hospitals. For an example of this critique, see Vivian Nutton, review of *The Birth of the Hospital in the Byzantine Empire*, *Medical History* 30 (1986): 218–21; Peregrine Horden, "How Medicalised Were Byzantine Hospitals?" in *Hospitals and Healing from Antiquity to the Later Middle Ages*, ed. Peregrine Horden (Aldershot, U.K.: Ashgate, 2008), 213–35. For a comparison of the treatment of leprosy in Byzantium and the Latin West, see Timothy S. Miller and John W. Nesbitt, *Walking Corpses: Leprosy in Byzantium and the Medieval West* (Ithaca: Cornell University Press, 2014).

numbering close to one hundred and housing up to sixty-one patients.[57] In terms of medicalization, there was nothing during this period remotely like this in the Latin West, where hospitals rarely had physicians. By the ninth and tenth centuries, many cities in the Islamic world, from Egypt and the Levant, to Baghdad, also had hospitals, or *bimaristans* (a Persian word), charitable and pietistic institutions that cared for the sick and poor. As was true in the Byzantine world, some *bimaristans* were remarkably medicalized and served as centers of medical education, although the principal function of many *bimaristans* was to house the poor.[58]

Although the *xenodocheia* and *bimaristans* of the early medieval Byzantine and Islamic world were clearly more medicalized and systematized than the institutional forms of poor relief that existed in the Latin West at the time, one should not discount the role of both episcopal and monastic poorhouses that fed, clothed, and sheltered the poor and strangers. Several hospitals had been established in Rome by as early as 400, including one founded by Jerome's disciple, Fabiola.[59] Various bishops (Caesarius of Arles, Praeiectus of Clermont) and kings (Childebert I) in Merovingian Gaul are known to have founded hospitals.[60] During the ninth century, the Carolingians sought to reform social welfare by tying the management of hospitals to cathedral chapters and the canonical life, and this association would persist during the high Middle Ages.[61] Meanwhile, the connection between monasticism and charity was inscribed in the Rule of Saint Benedict, which cast hospitality as an obligation of the religious life. Benedictine guesthouses and infirmaries were standard features of monasteries in the Latin West during the early Middle Ages and up through the high and later Middle Ages.[62] During the

---

57. Horden, "How Medicalised Were Byzantine Hospitals?"

58. Ahmed Ragab, *The Medieval Islamic Hospital: Medicine, Religion, and Charity* (Cambridge: Cambridge University Press, 2015).

59. Guenter B. Risse, *Mending Bodies, Saving Souls: A History of Hospitals* (New York: Oxford University Press, 1999), 94–95.

60. Michel Mollat, "Les premiers hôpitaux (VIe–XIe siècles)," in *Histoire des hôpitaux en France*, ed. Jean Imbert (Toulouse: Privat, 1982), 16–32. Ragab, *Medieval Islamic Hospital*, 67.

61. Risse, *Mending Bodies*, 95.

62. Julie Kerr, *Monastic Hospitality: The Benedictines in England, c. 1070–c. 1250* (Woodbridge, U.K.: Boydell Press, 2007); Daniel Le Blévec, "Les moines et l'assistance: L'exemple des pays du Bas-Rhône (XIIe–XIIIe siècles)," in *Moines et monastères dans les sociétés de rite Grec et Latin*, ed. Jean-Loup Lemaitre, Michel Dmitriev, and Pierre Gonneau (Geneva: Droz, 1996), 335–45; Philippe Racinet, "Les infirmeries monastiques: perspectives de recherche," in *Hôpitaux et maladreries au moyen âge: Espace et environment. Actes du colloque international d'Amiens-Beauvais, 22, 23 et 24 novembre 2002*, ed. Pascal Montaubin (Amiens, France: CAHMER, 2004), 21–34; Daniel Le Blévec, "Maladie et soins du corps dans les monastères cisterciens," in *Horizons marins, itinéraires spirituels*, vol. 1, *Mentalités et sociétés. Mélanges offerts à Michel Mollat* (Paris, 1987): 171–82.

early Middle Ages, monasteries were also the exclusive centers of medical learning. The famous early ninth-century monastic plan for the monastery of St. Gall, although never executed, nonetheless reflects the significant charitable role that was envisioned for the monastery, including serving as a "hospitale pauperum" as well as a regular distributor of food and clothing to the poor.[63] During the high Middle Ages, bishops and monasteries continued to play an active role as dispensers of charity, whether by building new hospitals to house the traveling poor and sick, making regular distributions of bread and clothing to the poor (particularly in ritualized, liturgical forms, such as the *mandatum* on Holy Thursday, when thirteen poor people were received, had their feet washed, and were given alms), or managing hospitals that they appropriated.[64] However, with the proliferation of new charitable institutions during this period, monks increasingly played only a secondary role in the provision of charity.[65]

The same cannot be said, however, for nuns and other religious women, many of whom were zealous in their pursuit of charitable and caretaking roles. As Anne Lester has shown, during the late twelfth and thirteenth centuries Cistercian nuns in Champagne were frequently associated with caregiving, which was seen as a defining feature of their spiritual activities. There are numerous cases of Cistercian nuns taking over a struggling hospital or founding a new monastic house next to a preexisting hospital.[66] Charitable work was also a central element of the beguines' activities in northern France and the Low Countries, enabling them to marry their spiritual ideals with pressing social needs.[67] Indeed, some beguinages were founded as hospitals for sick, elderly, or needy women, and outside the beguinages, it was common for beguines to work as nurses for individual women in their homes or in hospitals. More generally, the religious reform movements of the twelfth century and the aspiration to lead an apostolic life gave new energy to the longstanding tradition of religious women serving as caregivers.

---

63. Risse, *Mending Bodies*, 97–100.

64. Kerr, *Monastic Hospitality*; "Le Blévec, Les moines et l'assistance"; Eliana Magnani, "Le pauvre, le Christ et le moine: la correspondance de rôles et les cérémonies du *mandatum* à travers les coutumiers du XIe siècle," in *Les clercs, les fidèles et les saints en Bourgogne médiévale*, ed. Vincent Tabbagh (Dijon: Éditions universitaires de Dijon, 2005): 11–26.

65. Le Blévec, "Les moines et l'assistance," 345.

66. Lester, "Cares Beyond the Walls"; Lester, *Creating Cistercian Nuns*.

67. Tanya Stabler Miller, *The Beguines of Medieval Paris: Gender, Patronage, and Spiritual Authority* (Philadelphia: University of Pennsylvania Press, 2014); Walter Simons, *Cities of Ladies: Beguine Communities in the Medieval Low Countries, 1200–1565* (Philadelphia: University of Pennsylvania Press, 2001); Le Blévec, "Le rôle des femmes."

Also central to the emergence of the hospital movement of the twelfth and thirteenth centuries was the growing influence of the canons regular, who sought to revive the apostolic ideal by embracing a life of monastic-like poverty and communal living without withdrawing from the world. These canons regarded pastoral service, particularly to the poor living outside the cloister, as central to the apostolic life and therefore to their mission and identity.[68] The reform of many chapters, including cathedral chapters, which often involved the "regularization" of the canons such that they became subject to the Augustinian Rule, gave new impetus to charitable activity. In this context, the apostolic aspirations of the clergy simultaneously involved a new inward-looking religious discipline as well as outward-looking service to others, evident in canons' role overseeing hospitals.[69]

The reformer and promoter of the canonical movement, Yves de Chartres (d. 1116), who himself served as head of an abbey of canons regular before becoming the bishop of Chartres and an influential canon lawyer, was particularly preoccupied with the value of almsgiving and performing the works of mercy, as evidenced by his prolific letters (a staggering 298 of which are extant) and sermons, which exhorted monks, canons, and members of the laity to do more to share their wealth with the poor and feed and house the stranger.[70] Yves regarded the canons regular as the ideal managers and moral stewards of charitable institutions. He was instrumental in reorganizing hospitals and leprosaria in various parts of Europe under the aegis of canons regular, and he invoked the charitable and pastoral activities of these canons in claiming their superiority over monks.[71] Some communities of canons regular specialized in caretaking, and the early charitable activities of canons regular also served as models for the new charitable orders that emerged during the thirteenth century, such as the Canons Regular of the Holy Cross (who ran inns for pilgrims and travelers), the Penitents of Saint Mary Magdalen (who sought to reform repentant prostitutes), the Trinitarians and Mercedarians (who ransomed captives), and the Val-des-Écoliers, founded

---

68. On the expansion of the canons regular, see Michel Parisse, ed., *Les chanoines réguliers: Émergence et expansion (XIe–XIIIe siècles). Actes du sixième colloque international du CERCOR, Le Puy en Velay, 29 juin–1er juillet 2006* (Saint-Étienne: Publications de l'Université de Saint-Étienne, 2009).

69. François-Olivier Touati, "Aime et fais ce que tu veux: Les chanoines réguliers et la révolution de charité au moyen âge," in *Les chanoines réguliers: Émergence et expansion (XIe–XIIIe siècles)*, ed. Michel Parisse (Saint-Étienne: Publications de l'Université de Saint-Étienne, 2009), 175, 188–93, 205. See also Mathieu Arnoux, *Des clercs au service de la réforme: Études et documents sur les chanoines réguliers de la province de Rouen* (Turnhout, Belgium: Brepols, 2000), 119–27.

70. François-Olivier Touati, *Yves de Chartres (1040–1115): Aux origines de la révolution hospitalière médiévale* (Paris: Les Indes Savantes, 2017), 12–15, 40–44.

71. Touati, *Yves de Chartres*; Touati, "Aime et fais ce que tu veux," 183–91.

in Champagne in the early thirteenth century by masters and students from Paris to address worldly problems, including caring for the sick poor.[72] In Champagne, the Val-des-Écoliers oversaw hospitals and leprosaria at Meaux (1262), Traînel (northeast of Sens), Reims, and Louppy-le-Château (by 1220), near Bar-le-Duc.[73] The activities of this order are perhaps the most concrete example from this period of scholastics not just giving serious thought to the pressing moral and social problems of the day, such as poverty, but also actively working to alleviate those problems.

Let us consider just one example of a hospital whose foundation was clearly an outgrowth of the ecclesiastical reform movement of the twelfth century. In late December of 1120, the famed Parisian scholastic and reforming bishop of Châlons-en-Champagne, Guillaume de Champeaux, whose most famous pupil (and bitter rival) had been Peter Abelard, must have sensed that the end of his days was near. On Christmas Day, just a few weeks before he made a deathbed conversion to Cistercianism, he composed what was essentially a testament, in which he founded a "hospitalis domus" for the poor, adjoining the cathedral chapter of Châlons.[74] As Guillaume made clear, the foundation of this hospital was directly tied to his desire to curb corrupt customs, including the sale of prebends, the sale or pledging of liturgical vessels from the cathedral's treasury, the holding of induction banquets for new canons, and the payment of a fee ("feodum") for new deans and cantors. Among the gifts that Guillaume bequeathed to his new hospital foundation, his testament stipulated that henceforth, whenever a cathedral canon died or departed, the hospital would receive the fruits of the canon's prebend for "the use of the poor." It is noteworthy that Guillaume, who decades earlier had converted to the religious life to become a canon regular, did not channel these annates to the Augustinian chapter, but instead chose to use these funds to endow a hospital for the poor. Given Guillaume de Champeaux's association with the canons regular (and his defense of Saint Bernard of Clairvaux and the Cistercians), it is in some ways not surprising that at the very end of his life he founded a hospital essentially as an act of pious reform, an antidote to the avarice and corruption that he felt was all too ubiquitous.

---

72. Touati, "Aime et fais," 209. See also James W. Brodman, *Ransoming Captives in Crusader Spain: The Order of Merced on the Christian-Islamic Frontier* (Philadelphia: University of Pennsylvania Press, 1986); Brodman, *Charity and Religion*, 150–72, 174–75.

73. Touati, "Aime et fais," 210 and note 182.

74. Charles de Miramon, "Quatre notes biographiques sur Guillaume de Champeaux," in *Arts du langage et théologie aux confins des XIe et XIIe siècle*, ed. I. Rosier-Catach (Turnhout, Belgium: Brepols, 2011): 45–82.

Whereas in some regions, confraternities, guilds, or parishes played a leading role in the provision of charity, in Champagne the principal institutional form of charity during the twelfth and thirteenth centuries were hospitals run by canons regular and lay sisters and brothers, who like the canons, frequently lived according to the Augustinian Rule. These hospitals provide a fascinating window into the intersection of the religious and lay life, a way for lay women and men to participate in the evangelical and fraternal life alongside the clergy. Indeed, both the growing desire of the laity to devote themselves to charitable service and the increased "regularization" of lay women and men who worked in hospitals—the hospital sisters and brothers—often reflected the inspiration of the canons regular. Jean de Montmirail, for example, who was a Champenois lord and counsellor to King Philip Augustus, decided, after befriending a canon regular, to abandon the life of the court and build a hospital near his castle, where he and his wife would care for the sick and leprous.[75] Here, too, Yves de Chartres played a leading role not just in promoting the canonical life but also in carving out what François-Olivier Touati has called a "third way," a religious life open to lay women and men who wished to devote themselves to caring for the poor without the constraints of becoming a canon, monk, or nun.[76] The Augustinian Rule, which was the most widely observed rule among the canons regular, provided the ideal structure, flexibility, and charitable spirit for institutions that cared for the needy and the vulnerable.[77] Yet, as Touati has rightly warned, we should not assume that hospitals that were, at least on the surface, "Augustinian" shared any institutional ties with each other or were part of an organized network. It was common for hospitals to draw on monastic vocabulary and inspiration without being administratively connected.[78]

The creation of hospital orders associated with the crusading movement may also have contributed to the popularization of hospitals as religious and charitable institutions worthy of benefaction in the Latin West.[79] The Knights of Saint John, or Hospitallers, founded in Jerusalem before the Latin

---

75. Touati, "Aime et fais," 207.

76. Touati, *Yves de Chartres*, 15, 58, 79.

77. Touati, *Yves de Chartres*, 19, 55–56.

78. François-Olivier Touati, "Les groupes des laïcs dans les hôpitaux et les léproseries au moyen âge," in *Les mouvances laïques des ordres religieux*, ed. Nicole Bouter (Saint Étienne: Publications de l'Université de Saint-Étienne, 1996), 131–32; "Aime et fais," 205–6 and note 171.

79. Questions have been raised about the possible mutual influences between Islamic, Byzantine, and crusader hospitals. While it is likely that some crusader hospitals were influenced by existing *bimaristans* in the Levant, the *bimaristan* al-Salahi in Jerusalem was partially built on the grounds of the Christian hospital of Saint John of Jerusalem. See Ragab, *Medieval Islamic Hospital*, 59.

conquest of the city, were originally established to house and care for pilgrims, and even after the order became militarized, it continued to manage a large network of hospitals not only in the Levant but all over Latin Christendom as well, including in Champagne.[80] Reflective of the influence of the crusading movement on hospitals in the West, it was common for hospitals in Europe to be dedicated to the Holy Sepulchre or to Saint John the Baptist, the name of the Order's famous hospital in Jerusalem.[81] There is some debate about the extent to which the Templars engaged in charitable activities in the Latin West, but it is clear that some Templar commanderies were established in preexisting hospitals, that hospitals were at times placed under the protection of Templars, which occurred in Champagne, and that such hospitals served as a source of income for the Order.[82] In France and elsewhere in Europe, the military orders helped shape the urban landscape of the twelfth and thirteenth centuries, engaging both in the pastoral ministry and a range of charitable activities (which included involving members of the laity, through their orders' lay confraternities, in the provision of charity) as well as participating actively in the new urban economy.[83] Far less well known are the networks of hospitals managed by canons from particular churches in the Levant, such as the Church of the Nativity in Bethlehem

---

80. On the Hospital of Saint John of Jerusalem's influence on the hospital movement in the Latin West, see Timothy S. Miller, "The Knights of Saint John and the Hospitals of the Latin West," *Speculum* 53, no. 4 (October 1978): 709–33. For the charitable activities of the Hospitallers in the Lower Rhone, see Le Blévec, *La part du pauvre*, 85–124. On the role of women in hospitals in Europe managed by the Hospitallers, see Damien Carraz, "Présences et devotions féminines autour des commanderies du Bas-Rhône (XIIe–XIIIe siècle)," in *Les orders religieux militaires dans le Midi (XIIe–XIVe siècle)*, *Cahiers de Fanjeaux*, vol. 41 (Toulouse: Privat, 2006), 71–99; Anthony Luttrell, "Les femmes hospitalières en France méridionale," *Les orders religieux militaires dans le Midi (XIIe–XIVe siècle)*, *Cahiers de Fanjeaux*, vol. 41 (Toulouse: Privat, 2006), 101–13; Anthony Luttrell and Helen J. Nicholson, eds., *Hospitaller Women in the Middle Ages* (Aldershot, U.K.: Ashgate, 2006).

81. Touati, "La géographie hospitalière," 18.

82. Alan Forey has argued that the Templars did not manage hospitals in Europe. See Alan Forey, "The Charitable Activities of the Templars," *Viator* 34 (2003): 109–41. There is clear evidence, however, of hospitals, such as those at Possesse (dep. Marne), Chappes (dep. Aube), and Tilchâtel (dep. Côte-d'Or), being donated to the Order of the Temple, and presumably managed by its members. See Jochen Schenk, *Templar Families: Landowning Families and the Order of the Temple in France, c.1170–1307* (Cambridge: Cambridge University Press, 2012), 36 and note 27, 131–32, 139–40, 251n2; Damien Carraz, *L'ordre du Temple dans la basse vallée du Rhône (1124–1312): Ordres militaires, croisades et sociétés méridionales* (Lyon: Presses Universitaires de Lyon, 2005), 508–9; Michael Moseph Peixoto, "Growing the Portfolio: Templar Investments in the Forests of Champagne," in *L'économie Templière en Occident: Patrimoines, Commerce, Finances: Actes du colloque international (Troyes—Abbaye de Clairvaux, 24–26 octobre 2012*, ed. Arnaud Baudin, Ghislain Brunel and Nicolas Dohrmann (Langres, 2013): 207–24.

83. Damien Carraz, "Templars and Hospitallers in the Cities of the West and the Latin East (Twelfth to Thirteenth Centuries)," *Crusades* 12 (2013): 103–20.

and the Church of the Annunciation in Nazareth, both of which possessed dependent hospitals in Champagne.[84] Although hospital orders and churches based in the Levant possessed dependent hospitals in the Latin West, it is not clear that the line of influence for the hospital movement in the West came principally from the Levant. Indeed, Jean Richard has argued that hospitals in the West also exerted their own influence on Levantine hospitals.[85]

The twelfth and thirteenth centuries were clearly the golden age for new hospital foundations in the Latin West, and many of these hospitals were not attached either to a monastery or to a bishop's palace. Champagne very much reflects this trend, with hospitals being founded during this period by counts and countesses, aristocrats, cathedral chapters, and various kinds of monastic houses.[86] In charting the remarkable scale of leprosaria and hospital foundations during this period, François-Olivier Touati has documented the massive wave of leper hospitals that swept across Europe as early as the eleventh century, somewhat earlier than the foundations of general hospitals for the sick poor during the twelfth and thirteenth centuries. Leprosy was considered a permanent condition, with lepers being required to take religious vows upon being received in a leprosarium. The majority of Europe's leprosaria were very small, many containing only one or two lepers, with the number of personnel often outnumbering the lepers.[87] In contrast, those admitted to general hospitals were regarded as temporary guests, and many hospital statutes barred entry to those with chronic conditions, such as leprosy, a disability, or chronic illness, fearing that these individuals might never leave and would pose a permanent financial strain on the institution.[88] The sick and poor in hospitals generally outnumbered the personnel, although

---

84. Jean Richard, "Hospitals and Hospital Congregations in the Latin Kingdom During the First Period of the Frankish Conquest," in *Outremer: Studies in the History of the Crusading Kingdom of Jerusalem*, ed. B. Z. Kedar, H. E. Mayer, and R. C. Smail (Jerusalem: 1982), 89–100. The regular canons of Nazareth had dependent hospitals in Chambry, Evergnicourt (until it was later transferred to the hospital of Laon), Pierrepont-en-Laonnois (until it was turned over to the bishop of Laon), and Chappes. The bishop of Hebron also established the hospital of Saint-Abraham in Troyes in the twelfth century. See also Brodman, *Charity and Religion*, 172–74.

85. Richard, "Hospitals and Hospital Congregations." See also Touati, "La terre sainte: Un laboratoire hospitalier au moyen age?" *Sozialgeschichte mittelalterlicher Hospitäler*, ed. Neithard Bulst and Karl-Heinz Spieß (Ostfildern, Germany: Jan Thorbecke Verlag, 2007), 169–212.

86. Unlike in other parts of France and Europe, Champagne does not seem to have had hospitals that were founded or run by town officials.

87. Touati, *Maladie et société*, 298, 360. On leper hospitals, see also Carole Rawcliffe, *Leprosy in Medieval England* (Woodbridge, U.K.: Boydell, 2006); Elma Brenner, *Leprosy and Charity in Medieval Rouen* (Woodbridge, U.K.: Boydell, 2015).

88. Touati, *Maladie et société*, 380.

there were certainly a good number of tiny rural almshouses that might contain only one or two guests.

Interpretative Approaches to Understanding Charitable Practices

Scholarship on medieval charity has been influenced by a broader anthropological literature on the meaning of gifts.[89] Scholars have examined how the practice of giving gifts promoted social bonding, enforced social cohesion among the aristocracy, and reinforced personal ties.[90] How much social and physical distance separated givers and takers? How did the process of giving and receiving affect the social dynamic and power relations between different groups, either to reaffirm hierarchy and deepen social divisions or to undermine them? Some scholars, meanwhile, have argued that preindustrial charity functioned as a kind of strategy and social negotiation between elites and the poor, part of a broader pattern of reciprocity and exchange, since there was almost always an expectation on the part of the giver to receive something in exchange for a gift, thereby placing pressure on the recipient of the gift to repay the donor.[91] It is clear that charitable practices and the emergence of charitable organizations were not merely responses to demographic changes or greater demands from those in need of assistance. Rather, the practice of charity often reflected developments in patronage networks and divisions among social elites, including conflicts over family wealth or competition over prestige.[92]

This book addresses many of these important questions, paying close attention to the language of gifts, counter-gifts, and service, and traces

89. For a critique and "problematization" of some of the anthropological models for explaining gift-giving during the early Middle Ages, see the edited collection, Wendy Davies and Paul Fouracre, eds., *The Languages of Gift in the Early Middle Ages* (Cambridge: Cambridge University Press), 2010. See also Eliana Magnani, ed., *Don et sciences sociales: Théories et pratiques croisées* (Dijon: Éditions de l'Université de Dijon, 2007).

90. Barbara H. Rosenwein, *To Be the Neighbor of Saint Peter: The Social Meaning of Cluny's Property, 909–1049* (Ithaca: Cornell University Press, 1989); Arnoud-Jan Bijsterveld, "The Medieval Gift as Agent of Social Bonding and Political Power: A Comparative Approach," in *Medieval Transformations: Texts, Power, and Gifts in Context*, ed. Esther Cohen and Mayke B. De Jong (Leiden: Brill, 2001), 123–56.

91. Marco H. D. van Leeuwen, "Logic of Charity: Poor Relief in Preindustrial Europe," *The Journal of Interdisciplinary History* 24, no. 4 (April 1994): 589–613.

92. Sandra Cavallo, *Charity and Power in Early Modern Italy: Benefactors and Their Motives in Turin, 1541–17* (Cambridge: Cambridge University Press, 1995); Cavallo, "The Motivations of Benefactors: An Overview of Approaches to the Study of Charity," in *Medicine and Charity Before the Welfare State*, ed. Colin Jones and Jonathan Barry (London: Routledge, 1991), 46–62.

records of earlier gifts and transactions between the same parties. A systematic analysis of the bequests made to Champagne's hospitals, the identities of donors, and other types of transactions involving these hospitals reveals that gifts to hospitals were rarely one-way transfers but rather often multi-directional and at times multi-generational, often involving the building and nurturing of long-term relationships. While drawing on a rich, anthropologically informed literature, the arguments in this book remain grounded in the particular social and cultural context of medieval Champagne. The universalist Maussian model of gift exchange clearly cannot be applied to all societies, since charitable practices and the motivations underlying them are highly variable and are tied to particular social, cultural, and institutional forces. Nor can we simply apply the latest findings from the field of neuroscience, which suggest that most humans are biologically hardwired to be altruistic, a sharp departure from the long-received *homo economicus* model of human nature which assumed "rational," narrowly self-interested behavior as the norm.[93] Even if we now know that to provide care to a needy stranger or to voluntarily give up one's property does not run counter to human nature, there is compelling evidence that these are learned behaviors fulfilling the particular social roles of a given community. The nature and scale of charitable practices has varied across space and time, and the challenge is to explain how so and why.

Another historiographical trend in the study of medieval charity has been a shift away from focusing on the institutional provision of charity to instead consider the role the poor themselves played in the provision of welfare services and the systems of support they relied upon from family members, friends, and neighbors.[94] In her study of the survival strategies employed by the poor in thirteenth-century Paris, Sharon Farmer used an inquest into the posthumous miracles of Saint Louis to reconstruct the daily lives of the poor witnesses to and the beneficiaries of alleged miracles. When a

---

93. For a review of the vast literature on this subject, see Jennifer L. Goetz, Dacher Keltner, and Emiliana Simon-Thomas, "Compassion: An Evolutionary Analysis and Empirical Review," *Psychological Bulletin* 136 (2010), 351–74. E. O. Wilson and others have advanced a controversial theory called "group selection" to explain how altruism and self-sacrifice benefit a group at the expense of an individual. See Jonah Lehrer, "Kin and Kind: A Fight About the Genetics of Altruism," *The New Yorker* (March 5, 2012), 36–42. For a critique of this theory, see Steven Pinker, "The False Allure of Group Selection," *Edge: Conversations on the Edge of Human Knowledge*, June 18, 2012.

94. During the 1970s, Michel Mollat pioneered the study of the medieval poor. See especially, Mollat, ed., *Études sur l'histoire de la pauvreté: Moyen age—XVIe siècle)*, 2 vols. (Paris: Publications de la Sorbonne, 1974). See also Bronislaw Geremek, *The Margins of Society in Late Medieval Paris* (Cambridge: Cambridge University Press, 1987). For a more recent approach, see Farmer, *Surviving Poverty*.

forty-two-year-old widowed Parisian laundress became paralyzed in 1272, for instance, she received assistance from a circle of female friends, who not only helped dress and feed her but also took her to Saint Louis's tomb in Saint-Denis in the hopes that she would be cured, as she allegedly was.[95] While the focus of the present book is on the people who received institutional care as well as on those who worked in and supported these institutions, the issue of neighborly and familial support nonetheless arises frequently, since hospitals were very much part of other networks of care. Moreover, some of the very recipients of familial or neighborly care who appeared in Farmer's study also received institutional care. Hospitals were not remote and foreign entities that the sick and poor turned to only in dire need or when one lacked familial assistance. One might have a relative or friend who worked in, had spent time in, or even supported the local hospital, and the person who turned to a hospital for temporary assistance might well have interacted at an earlier point with the hospital in some capacity, receiving a distribution of food or clothing, purchasing something at one of the hospital's stalls at a trade fair, or even hearing Mass in the hospital's chapel. In short, this book, which is just as much about individuals, families, and neighborhoods as it is about institutions, demonstrates that there was not as stark a divide as is sometimes suggested between familial or neighborly forms of support and what we think of as institutional forms of charity.

Reconstructing the motivations behind charitable activity, while notoriously difficult to do, is crucial for understanding social relations and the medieval *mentalité*. In trying to understand medieval charity, scholars have considered the mingling of self-interest and self-sacrifice, of paternalism and humility. While some have argued that charity was principally spurred by economic and material forces and a burgeoning urban culture, others have suggested that developments in spirituality and devotional culture are central to understanding what charity meant to its practitioners. Was medieval charity embedded in a larger culture of reciprocity and exchange? Or was it primarily a reflection of religious devotion and an attempt to secure salvation by imitating the life of Christ? Did it represent neighborliness and concern for the less fortunate, or was it instead an assertion of power, a way to elevate one's social status and affirm existing hierarchies of power?

Underlying these questions about what lay behind medieval charitable practices is a fundamental disagreement over just how charitable medieval society was. Some have expressed skepticism that medieval charity was ever

---

95. Farmer, *Surviving Poverty*, 136–38.

performed without an expectation of reward. Miri Rubin is surely right in observing that "Charity cannot be satisfactorily understood as a purely altruistic act since gift-giving is so rich in rewards to the giver."[96] Teofilo Ruiz, however, has gone even further. First, in his study of medieval northern Castile, he argued that charitable bequests generally represented a tiny proportion of overall bequests and appeared "as an afterthought" to the testators, who were generally far more focused on "secular concerns," such as their family, friends, and business obligations.[97] Second, Ruiz has challenged the notion that limited, "ceremonialized" giving even constituted a form of charity, since it was so routinized: "It was bread and vestments given without love. It was not charity."[98] Far from bringing benefactors and recipients of charity together, "ritualized giving," according to Ruiz, "reaffirmed the existing social distance between rich and poor, reminding those receiving charity of their place in a well-defined hierarchy of eating and dressing."[99] By highlighting the instrumental aspects of medieval charity, scholars have at times echoed the suspicion with which Enlightenment *philosophes* viewed religious charity as a form of outright *égoïsme,* stemming solely from the giver's concern with his or her own social status and prospects for salvation (as opposed to the recipient's material or spiritual state).[100] What this explanatory model ignores, however, is that a donor's concern with his or her own salvation or social status could easily coexist with genuine concern for the recipient's material or spiritual state.[101] Rarely can human behavior be reduced to a simple explanation or single cause, such as power, gender, status, or piety. Charity is and was an inherently complex and multi-layered phenomenon.

Unlike much of the work done on medieval charity, this book does not regard giving as merely ceremonial or as a self-serving, calculated display of the giver's power and prestige. Rather, I contend that multiple factors and motivations could simultaneously be at play in charitable giving and service,

---

96. Rubin, *Charity and Community*, 1.

97. Teofilo F. Ruiz, *From Heaven to Earth: The Reordering of Castilian Society, 1150–1350* (Princeton: Princeton University Press, 2014), 121; Ruiz, "The Business of Salvation: Castilian Wills in the Late Middle Ages," in *On the Social Origins of Medieval Institutions: Essays in Honor of Joseph F. O'Callaghan,* ed. Donald J. Kagay and Theresa M. Vann (Leiden: Brill, 1998), 86.

98. Ruiz, "Business of Salvation," 89.

99. Ruiz, "Business of Salvation," 67.

100. Whereas the *philosophes* associated religious charity with *égoïsme,* they argued that *bienfaisance* represented a more pure, selfless form of altruism, in large part because it was stripped of religious values. See Colin Jones, *Charity and Bienfaisance: The Treatment of the Poor in the Montpellier Region 1740–1815* (New York: Cambridge University Press, 1982), 2–3.

101. For a fuller discussion of these issues, see Adam J. Davis and Bertrand Taithe, "From the Purse and the Heart: Exploring Charity, Humanitarianism, and Human Rights in France," *French Historical Studies* 34, no. 3 (Summer 2011), 413–32.

including religious devotion. While it is difficult to know what moved a particular donor to make a bequest or decide to join a hospital community, I pay close attention to the language of charters, the parties involved, and the circumstances of these decisions. Wherever possible, I try to reconstruct the relationship between a donor and a hospital and the particular context for a gift or a decision to join a hospital community. While closely examining the particular circumstances and relationships that may have informed an individual's choices and interactions, I also consider the spiritual and devotional dimensions of charitable service and giving.

The medieval culture of reciprocity and exchange was just as evident in devotional practices as in the marketplace. Yet it would be unfair to impose our own modern discomfort with "the economics of salvation" onto the people of the past or to cynically cast aspersions on the motivations behind their pious gifts. As is true of all historical inquiry, our task is to understand what charitable giving and service meant *to them*. Peter Brown has observed that while early Christians in the West viewed wealth as a conduit between this earthly world and the heavenly world to come, many people living in the twenty-first century are reflexively made uncomfortable by Jesus' suggestion to the rich young man in Matthew 19:21 that almsgiving might bring about the transfer of treasure to heaven.[102] For well over a millennium, however, this notion was considered "a metaphor to live by."[103] As Brown has put it in describing the late antique religious imagination, almsgiving was understood as being like the "paradoxical joining of heaven and earth, of base money and eternity, and of God with humanity."[104] While drawing on a long intellectual tradition that stretched back to the Hebrew Scriptures, the commercialization of charity in the religious imagination of thirteenth-century Christians also reflected the commercial and monetized economy of their own day.[105] For medieval Christians, almsgiving was in some respects seen as another economic transaction that involved exchange, like buying, selling, exchanging, or lending property or money. What differentiated almsgiving from these other economic transactions, however, was the possibility of its being spiritually redemptive.

The county of Champagne, southeast of Paris, provides an excellent case study for addressing these issues. There is unusually abundant documentary

---

102. Peter Brown, *The Ransom of the Soul: Afterlife and Wealth in Early Western Christianity* (Cambridge: Harvard University Press, 2015), 27–30.

103. Brown, *Ransom of the Soul*, 30.

104. Brown, *Ransom of the Soul*, 32.

105. Bain, *Église, richesse et pauvreté*, 368–69.

evidence for the many Champenois hospitals founded during this period. Until now, no one has utilized these many documents—hundreds of single-sheet charters (records of property dealings), lengthy cartularies, hospital statutes, donor and personnel records, visitation records, financial inventories and account books, and comital records—that exist for the dozens of hospitals in Troyes, Provins, Bar-sur-Aube, Nemours, Meaux, Châlons, and Reims. These rich, untapped sources help illuminate the identity of hospital donors, the economic power of hospitals, the nature of hospital religious life, the life details of the personnel, the annual expenditures on a hospital's food and supplies, and even the use and organization of a hospital's space. A careful analysis of these sources reveals how embedded hospitals were in the wider social, cultural, religious, and economic fabric of Champagne.

At the center of this story about the charitable practices and institutions in medieval Champagne are the counts and countesses and other members of the aristocracy who served as significant institutional benefactors. However, the largesse of the urban bourgeoisie and various kinds of clerics, ranging from parish priests to cathedral canons, was also critical and reflects the democratization of charity during this period. Since Champagne was such a hub of monastic life, particularly reformed monasticism, using the county as a case study permits us to consider the relationship between contemporary monastic currents and the hospital movement. How did the foundation (and reform) of chapters of canons regular in Champagne contribute to the institutionalization of charity? Finally, how did the county's economic prosperity—a product of its role as an international center of commerce and banking, featuring annual trade fairs, a constant flow of people and goods, and a mint that produced the dominant coin of international commerce—sustain this culture of charity?

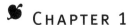

CHAPTER 1

Medieval Understandings of Charity

From Penance to Commerce

Although the sanctity of Count Thibaut II of Champagne (d. 1152) was never formally recognized, his reputation for performing works of charity, including visiting the sick and poor in hospitals (some of which he had founded), was popularized by several thirteenth-century *exempla* collections. One of the most repeated stories involved the count's close friendship with a certain leper in Sézanne, whom the count frequently visited. According to Étienne de Bourbon, when the count was asked why he personally gave shoes and clothes to Champagne's poor, he responded that he believed doing so would increase his compassion for the poor, make him more humble, and encourage others to imitate his example. The count also hoped that the poor "would be moved to remember him and pray for him."[1] Jacques de Vitry, also a native of Champagne, meanwhile, underscored Count Thibaut's fixation on the promise of redemption while performing works of charity, a trait found less often among those the church canonized for their pious charity. Moreover, according to Jacques, the count reportedly told his knights to stop acting so surprised by his personal almsgiving, as if it were somehow out of the ordinary for him, for "I will be quite

---

1. Stephani de Borbone, *Tractatus de diversis materiis praedicabilibus*, ed. Jacques Berlioz, *Corpus Christianorum. Continuatio Mediaevali*, vol. 124A (Turnhout, Belgium: Brepols, 2015), 332.

angry if I do not receive my reward."[2] Here, the "economy of salvation" was in plain view.

This chapter does not focus on Champagne but rather on religious and moral ideas about charity, sanctity, and salvation, largely emanating from the University of Paris during the thirteenth century. These ideas, however, are crucial for understanding the culture of charity that emerged in Champagne and elsewhere during this period. The county of Champagne was politically, economically, and culturally interconnected with Paris long before being incorporated into the French royal domain in 1285. The arguments and ideas that will be discussed in this chapter, which were contained in model sermon and *exempla* collections and didactic texts, largely produced in Paris, covering proper and improper ways to perform the works of mercy, were disseminated, often by mendicant preachers, in nearby Champagne. The texts analyzed in this chapter thus help illuminate the rationale for charitable giving and service being articulated by preachers and churchmen at the time.

Scholars have explored the intellectual and cultural impact of the monetization of the economy, whether in a growing interest in measurement and scientific thought or the increasing quantification of sin, penance, and the virtues in a confessional society obsessed with Purgatory.[3] This chapter argues that the traditional notion of redemptive almsgiving also took on new meaning in the highly commercial context of thirteenth-century Europe, with almsgiving increasingly conceived and described in commercial terms. In framing charitable giving as an integral part of the economy of salvation, preachers and theologians placed great emphasis on the potential rewards for charity, primarily in terms of spiritual redemption in the world to come, but some preachers and moralists also pointed to the material rewards that they argued would result from charitable giving. Perhaps in an effort to appeal to commercially minded listeners, mendicant preachers and theologians used a vocabulary that was replete with market terminology to describe redemptive almsgiving as a kind of usurious loan to God that would be repaid a hundredfold.[4] Medieval

---

2. Jacques de Vitry, *The Exempla or Illustrative Stories from the Sermones Vulgares of Jacques de Vitry*, ed. Thomas Frederick Crane (London, 1890; reprint, New York, 1971), 127n2.

3. Joel Kaye, "The Impact of Money on the Development of Fourteenth-Century Scientific Thought," *Journal of Medieval History* 14 (1988): 251–70; Kaye, *Economy and Nature in the Fourteenth Century: Money, Market Exchange, and the Emergence of Scientific Thought* (Cambridge: Cambridge University Press, 2009); Chiffoleau, *La comptabilité de l'au-delà*; Simon Kemp, "Quantification of Virtue in Late Medieval Europe," *History of Psychology* 21, no. 1 (2018): 33–46.

4. This language included several terms—*pretium*, *pensio*, *merces*, and *gagium*—that were increasingly being used in the language of remuneration for work in various kinds of "documents of practice" at the time. See Patrice Beck, Philippe Bernardi, and Laurent Feller, eds., *Rémunérer le travail au moyen âge: Pour une histoire sociale du salariat* (Paris: Picard, 2014).

sermon *exempla* further developed the notion that the needy recipients of charity were themselves stand-ins for Christ (or Christ in disguise), thereby reinforcing the notion, found in Matthew 25:40, in which Jesus announces, "Truly I tell you, whatever you did for one of the least of these brothers and sisters of mine, you did for me." In this way, assisting those who were most vulnerable was thought to offer a way both to repay Christ and to be further repaid by him in the future.

One also finds, however, particularly among the members of Peter the Chanter's circle and some thirteenth-century mendicant preachers, an argument that for charity to be spiritually meritorious it needed to be performed with pure and pious intentions. While emphasizing the spiritual value of the works of mercy and, in particular, encouraging members of the laity to perform these works, these preachers in a sense sought to "raise the bar" in their insistence that the works be performed under particular conditions. These churchmen stressed that not all forms of almsgiving and charity were equally meritorious, and they expressed anxiety both about the motivations underlying almsdeeds and the possibility that the works of mercy would be performed incorrectly. These concerns included the sense that charity had become overly transactional, was being performed begrudgingly, involved tainted alms, benefited undeserving recipients, or was performed to win acclaim or in the expectation of some other recompense. Even while seeking to contrast pious almsgiving with other, seemingly more worldly economic transactions, however, many of these preachers and theologians paradoxically used market terminology and concepts to describe the act of almsgiving and how it could reshape the human-divine relationship. By exploring the evolution of Christian ideas about charitable giving and service, this chapter seeks to explain the ideological and cultural underpinnings of the broad support given to hospitals during the twelfth and thirteenth centuries and underscores the profound interconnectedness between economic ideas and the notion and practice of redemptive almsgiving.

After tracing the biblical and patristic foundations of the Christian ideology of charity, this chapter considers the influence of the late twelfth-century Parisian schoolman Peter the Chanter and his circle as well as the role of the mendicants in working out what they viewed as the logic of charity. In reflecting on what might be termed "the laicization of charity" during the high Middle Ages, which is crucial for understanding the rise of the hospital as an institution, this chapter considers how the charitable ideal was taught and learned both through didactic texts on the proper (and improper) ways of performing the works of mercy and through the examples of charitable saints, many of whom were lay women and men. What ideas about charity were taught to the medieval laity, how were these ideas transmitted, and what impact did religious and cultural representations of charity have on charitable practices?

Medieval representations of charity tended to focus on the almsgiver, not the recipient of charity. Much of the discussion about charity built on a long tradition of associating charity and the works of mercy with penance for sin. Thirteenth-century developments in confessional practices and a growing preoccupation with Purgatory as a real and terrifying place heightened the significance of the works of mercy. Moreover, confessional manuals and treatises on the virtues and vices identified charity as the virtue that most closely corresponded to the vice of avarice; in the increasingly commercial, profit-oriented economy of thirteenth-century Europe, charity therefore had additional social and religious appeal. The growing veneration for charitable work, for example, is reflected in "the sanctification of charity" during the late twelfth and thirteenth centuries, as sanctity increasingly became tied to the practice of charity. As we shall see, popular representations of the saints canonized during this period depicted their extraordinary willingness to make personal sacrifices, debasing themselves and suffering in an effort to alleviate the suffering of others. Hagiographical accounts exalted these charitable saints' selfless service as holy and Christ-like and served as a role model for others to follow.

A Theology of Almsgiving and Charitable Service

Late twelfth- and thirteenth-century theologians and canonists drew on scriptural and patristic texts in developing a theology of charity that reflected the new cultural ethos of giving and recognized the involuntary poor as a class of people with important status.[5] It was only in the early twelfth century that the six good deeds in Matthew 25:35–36 were established as the canonical corporal works of mercy, along with burying the dead (from Tobit 12:12), which was added in the late twelfth century.[6] The pastoral orientation of the "biblical-moral" school in Paris during the late twelfth and early thirteenth centuries under the influential theologian Peter the Chanter and his circle

---

5. Imbert, *Les hôpitaux en droit canonique*; Brian Tierney, *Medieval Poor Law: A Sketch of Canonical Theory and Its Application in England* (Berkeley: University of California Press, 1959); Brian Tierney, "The Decretists and the 'Deserving Poor,'" *Comparative Studies in Society and History* 1, no. 4 (June 1959): 360–73.

6. Federico Botana, *The Works of Mercy in Italian Medieval Art, c.1050–c.1400* (Turnhout: Brepols, 2012), 1–2.

showed a strong interest in economic as well as moral questions, and charity encompassed both. These interests persisted throughout the thirteenth century, particularly under the influence of the mendicants, as theologians at the University of Paris sought to connect academic questions to practical, contemporary issues facing those with the *cura animarum*. A good illustration of the application of pastoral concerns to the subject of almsgiving can be found in a university sermon Ranulphe de la Houblonnière preached on the feast day of Saint Nicolas.[7] In many respects a typical scholastic sermon, with its citation of *auctoritates* and its subdivided format, Ranulphe's sermon was also squarely focused on what one might call the mechanics of proper almsgiving, ensuring that alms be given with the right intention; that there be no delay; that the alms be given cheerfully; that they be rightfully owned; that the giving be done voluntarily and discreetly; and that the almsgiver show humility. These same points on the proper mechanics of giving were laid out by Étienne de Bourbon, the Paris-trained Dominican preacher and inquisitor, in his collection of preaching material, and they were also taken up by other members of Peter the Chanter's circle.[8] For example, Innocent III, who as a young man had studied in Paris with the Chanter, argued in his *Libellus de eleemosyna*, that alms should be given with joy ("hilaritate"). The pope warned his listeners that they would lose all the merit of giving alms if they did so with a sad face ("tristem vultum"); to acquire merit, one had to give with a visibly joyful countenance.[9] The influence of these scholastic ideas about the proper mechanics of almsgiving is even evident in the *Breviari d'amor*, an encyclopedic poem composed in Occitan verse ca. 1288 by Matfre Ermengaud, a jurist and troubadour from Béziers who had ties to the Franciscan Order. With textual and visual demonstrations that sought to make scholastic ideas more accessible to the laity, the *Breviari* contained a

---

7. Nicole Bériou included this sermon in *La prédication de Ranulphe de la Houblonnière: Sermons aux clercs et aux simples gens à Paris au XIIIe siècle*, vol. 2 (Paris: Études Augustiniennes, 1987), 265–78.

8. See Stephani de Borbone, *Tractatus de diversis materiis praedicabilibus*, ed. Jacques Berlioz, *Corpus Christianorum. Continuatio Mediaevali*, vol. 124A (Turnhout, Belgium: Brepols, 2015), 323–33. These were also central themes in the *Speculum morale*, for a long time wrongly attributed to Vincent of Beauvais. The *Speculum* contains numerous *exempla* illustrating proper and improper forms of almsgiving, visiting the sick, and so forth. See Vincent of Beauvais, *Bibliotheca mundi seu speculi maioris Vincentii Burgundi* (Douai, 1624), 3:246–71, 1463–90.

9. Innocent III, *Libellus de eleemosyna*, in PL 217, col. 754d. A twelfth-century Latin text, the "Moralium dogma philosophorum," enumerated many of the same expectations about what constituted proper almsgiving and, among others, warned donors not to delay their gifts; not to give more than they could afford; not to create jealousy among other would-be donors; and not to give for the wrong reasons. See Richard Newhauser, "Justice and Liberality: Opposition to Avarice in the Twelfth Century," in *Virtue and Ethics in the Twelfth Century*, ed. Richard Newhauser and Istvan P. Bejczy (Leiden: Brill, 2005), 301.

lengthy discussion of "how and to whom alms should be given." Like Ranulphe de la Houblonnière, Étienne de Bourbon, and Innocent III, the Occitan verses of the *Breviari* stressed the need for alms to be given with piety, with humility (ideally, in secret), without being asked, and so forth.[10]

It was Peter the Chanter and his circle that first initiated a systematic moral theology of charity. Peter was educated in the cathedral schools of Reims and then Paris, went on to become a master and canon at Notre Dame in Paris, and returned to Reims as a dean shortly before his death in 1197. He argued that mercy is exalted above every other virtue and that the way to imitate Christ is through the performance of works of mercy.[11] Addressing the regular clergy in his *Verbum abbreviatum*, the Chanter warned of the danger that the offices and prayers—the *horae vocales*—recited in the cloister, would be done at the expense of the seven *horae reales*, the active hours outside of prayer time, which corresponded, he argued, to the seven works of mercy. In addressing a point that had long been debated by Christians—the relative merits of the active and contemplative life—the Chanter here emphasized the value of the active life and the supreme importance of the works of mercy.[12] In his discussion of almsgiving, he argued that "the piety of giving makes the alms, not the quantity of the gift."[13] For the Chanter and many of his students, simply giving alms was not sufficient, since they believed that not all forms of almsgiving and charity were equally meritorious. The context for a gift, including the extent to which it represented a sacrifice on the part of the giver, determined the type of spiritual benefit the giver earned. If a rich man and a poor man both gave the same amount of alms, they likely would not receive the same remission of enjoined penance.[14] These theologians, who sought to apply the Bible to pressing contemporary social and economic concerns, expressed anxiety about the motivations underlying almsgiving and the conditions under which alms were given. As Spencer

---

10. For a translation of these passages into modern French, see René Nelli, "L'aumone dans la littérature occitane: Le 'Breviari d'amor' de Matfre Ermengau," in *Assistance et charité, Cahiers de Fanjeaux* 13 (1978): 51–56. See also Matfre Ermengaud, *Le breviari d'amor*, ed. Peter T. Ricketts (Leiden: Brill, 1976); Botana, *Works of Mercy*, 58.

11. Peter the Chanter, *Verbum adbreviatum: Textus conflatus*, ed. Monique Boutry, *Corpus Christianorum*, vol. 196 (Turnhout, Belgium: Brepols, 2004), 638–39.

12. Botana, *Works of Mercy*, 30, 37–39; Peter the Chanter, *Verbum adbreviatum*, 525–26.

13. Peter the Chanter, *Verbum adbreviatum*, 660.

14. Robert W. Shaffern, *The Penitents' Treasury: Indulgences in Latin Christendom, 1175–1375* (Scranton: University of Scranton Press, 2007), 95–97. This was a point made in the *Breviari d'amor* as well. According to the poet, Matfre Ermengaud, "God finds it more meritorious for a poor man to give without hesitation one *maille* [a coin of little value]—and God will be more grateful for it—than for a rich man to give one hundred *sous*." Nelli, "L'aumône dans la littérature occitane," 55.

E. Young has put it, "For the most part, theologians shared this view that alms were not simply a means for purchasing salvation on the cheap or a substitute for good works, but rather a means for transforming the very character of the sinner. Intentions mattered and the redemptive power of alms derived from the act, rather than the fact, of giving them."[15] Jacques de Vitry, for example, who was part of the Chanter's circle and composed several model sermons directed at hospital audiences, echoed his teacher on the importance of intention and motivation in almsgiving. According to Jacques, the giving of alms should not be done to win praise, to obtain indulgences, or to secure one a place in heaven. In a sermon to hospital workers, a group that likely included alms collectors, Jacques argued that what mattered most was not the amount of alms collected but the inner state and motivations of the almsgiver.[16]

This emerging focus on the inner state and intentionality of the almsgiver was connected to a broader shift during the twelfth century in attitudes toward penance, and as Nicholas Vincent has observed, a "far greater emphasis upon contrition rather than penance as the defining feature of repentance."[17] In some respects, this may have represented an early backlash against the development of indulgences, which were thought to remit "enjoined penance" and which were often described in mercantile language.[18] The thirteenth century, for example, saw the development of the notion of a "treasury of merit," which the mendicants in particular did much to popularize.[19] The sufferings and merits of Christ and the saints were thought to have been transferred to the church in the form of this inexhaustible "treasury of merit," from which popes and bishops doled out indulgences. The system of indulgences, however, had early critics in the schools, with Peter Abelard, Peter of Poitiers, Peter the Chanter, and others casting such pardons both as an illogical practice and as a crass, for-profit strategy that ignored the need for genuine, interior contrition as opposed

---

15. Spencer E. Young, *Scholarly Community at the Early University of Paris: Theologians, Education, and Society, 1215–1248* (Cambridge: Cambridge University Press, 2014), 156.

16. Jessalynn Bird, "Texts on Hospitals: Translation of Jacques de Vitry, *Historia Occidentalis* 29, and Edition of Jacques de Vitry's Sermons to Hospitallers," in *Religion and Medicine in the Middle Ages*, edited by Joseph Ziegler and Peter Biller (York: York University Press, 2001), 129.

17. Nicholas Vincent, "Some Pardoners' Tales: The Earliest English Indulgences," *Transactions of the Royal Historical Society*, series 6, vol. 12 (2002): 30.

18. Vincent, "Some Pardoners' Tales," 32–33. On indulgences, see Shaffern, *The Penitents' Treasury*; R. N. Swanson, *Indulgences in Late Medieval England: Passports to Paradise?* (Cambridge: Cambridge University Press, 2007); R. N. Swanson, ed., *Promissory Notes in the Treasury of Merits: Indulgences in Late Medieval Europe* (Leiden: Brill, 2006).

19. Shaffern, *Penitents' Treasury*, 81–84, 102–6.

to merely visible good works.[20] For these critics, indulgences threatened to corrupt the spiritual function of penance with "the intrusion of a financial consideration linking indulgences to the payment of alms."[21] At the same time that bishops and popes were granting indulgences, schoolmen were arguing for a less "mechanical conception of penance."[22] Despite the growing popularity of indulgences and the related idea of a treasury of merit—or perhaps precisely because of these developments—the old penitential system of numerically determined tariffs was replaced by "a new style of penance, placing greater emphasis upon the sinner's inner contrition and the sincerity with which any penitential act was performed."[23] These developments in the Christian penitential system, as well as the tension between two different conceptions of penance, would have significant implications for pious giving and its future role in the economy of salvation.

Although thirteenth-century theologians expressed a desire that almsgiving be more generous and widespread, they were increasingly committed to the principle that alms by definition be voluntary, since they believed that voluntarism was at the core of what made a gift pious and potentially spiritually redemptive.[24] A number of theologians from Peter the Chanter's circle in Paris also questioned whether pious almsgiving could be coerced and still be considered meritorious. Peter himself frowned on forced almsgiving, which he believed was not pleasing to God, since it is "charity that makes alms, moreover, not the necessity of giving."[25] In commenting on Count Thibaut of Champagne's decision to force the rich to support the poor during a famine under threat of exacting a tax, Peter acknowledged the arguments in favor of this kind of coercion during a crisis but maintained that a secular ruler still needed the consent of his subjects.[26] His student, Robert of Courson, who himself became a teacher and a cardinal legate, argued that charity is by definition a voluntary act and cannot be forced but conceded that ecclesiastics could be coerced to give alms from goods belonging to the church.[27]

---

20. Shaffern, *Penitents' Treasury*, 95–97; Vincent, "Some Pardoners' Tales," 32–34.

21. Vincent, "Some Pardoners' Tales," 33.

22. Vincent, "Some Pardoners' Tales," 31.

23. Vincent, "Some Pardoners' Tales," 30.

24. This argument was echoed by Ranulphe de la Houblonnière, who argued that by definition, almsgiving could not be forced. See Bériou, *La prédication de Ranulphe*, 2:267.

25. Peter the Chanter, *Verbum adbreviatum*, 660.

26. Peter the Chanter, *Summa de sacramentis et animae consiliis*, ed. Jean-Albert Dugauquier (Louvain, France: Nauwelaerts, 1954), para. 204: III (2a), 147; para. 205: III (2a), 149, 150; and para. 251: III (2a), 255; Brodman, *Charity and Religion*, 16–17.

27. Brodman, *Charity and Religion*, 16–17; John W. Baldwin, *Masters, Princes, and Merchants: The Social Views of Peter the Chanter and His Circle* (Princeton: Princeton University Press, 1970), 1:237.

Pope Innocent III, who came from the same intellectual circle, insisted that for a charitable gift to be worthy of spiritual rewards, it had to be given freely and out of a spirit of empathy and sincere love, and so he asserted that even the clergy could not be coerced to make contributions.[28]

A number of preachers and reformers expressed concern that alms not be given in order to win acclaim.[29] In his *Dialogus miraculorum*, Caesarius of Heisterbach, a Cistercian, recounted a story that illustrated this point.[30] In the story, an apparition resembling a wealthy official of the duchy of Bavaria appears before his wife after his death to complain about having received eternal punishment in the afterlife; for her part, his wife is unable to understand how someone who had given so many alms and had been so hospitable to pilgrims during his lifetime could end up being denied salvation. "Are your good deeds of no avail?" the wife asks her husband. Her husband replies that he had given alms out of vainglory instead of charity and is therefore destined to suffer eternal punishment.[31] Both Jacques de Vitry and Étienne de Bourbon argued that alms should ideally be given in secret to avoid any possibility that a donation would be given in order to enhance one's earthly reputation.[32]

Another dimension to pious giving was its timing. Jacques de Vitry warned his audience not to delay in making charitable gifts, lest the poor have to wait: "For he who delays today will perhaps not give or minister tomorrow, with death unexpectedly having arrived or grave illness."[33] A late thirteenth-century *exemplum* composed (or repeated) by a sack friar in Provence placed alms in four categories based on when the alms were given. Alms that were given in one's youth were categorized as gold, alms given in youth and maturity were considered silver, lead alms were those given while an almsgiver was ill, and the least valuable alms in God's eyes, testamentary alms, given after death, were regarded as mud. The older one was when the alms were given, they had less value, since (so the reasoning went) it was primarily fear of the Last Judgment that served as the impetus for giving, rather than

---

28. Brodman, *Charity and Religion*, 21; Baldwin, *Masters, Princes, and Merchants*, 1:237.

29. See Innocent III, *Libellus de eleemosyna*, in PL 217, col. 754a.

30. Caesarius of Heisterbach, *Dialogus miraculorum*, ed. Josephus Strange, vol. 2 (Cologne: J. M. Heberle, 1851; repr. Ridgewood, NJ: Gregg Press, 1966), distinct. 12, p. 329

31. Young, *Scholarly Community*, 156.

32. Stephani de Borbone, *Tractatus de diversis materiis praedicabilibus*, 329; Jessalynn Bird, "Medicine for Body and Soul: Jacques de Vitry's Sermons to Hospitallers and Their Charges," in *Religion and Medicine in the Middle Ages*, ed. Joseph Ziegler and Peter Biller (York: York Medieval Press, 2001), 101.

33. Bird, "Texts on Hospitals," 129.

love of one's neighbor. Alms given after death also required less sacrifice than those given during one's youth.[34] The question of personal sacrifice also arose in debates among theologians about whether alms need only come from one's surplus, or whether, to earn merit, alms should come from one's own necessities, a debate that in the mid-thirteenth century was closely tied to the secular-mendicant controversy over the value of voluntary poverty.[35]

It has sometimes been suggested that whereas in the early modern period charity tended to be targeted to specific groups or individuals (and was therefore supposedly more "rational" and "organized"), Christian charity in the high Middle Ages was indiscriminate as to the recipient.[36] It is true that thirteenth-century Christian testaments often directed bequests to a long list of institutions, causes, and generic categories of people, such as "the poor" who, for instance, might be entitled to collect a pittance at a donor's funeral. Yet already during this period, one also finds a heightened concern about charitable donations ending up in the wrong hands.[37] Peter the Chanter and his student, Thomas of Chobham, both railed against false beggars who claimed to be poor, sick, or disabled in order to elicit the sympathies of potential donors; false beggars then showed great avarice in hoarding the alms they collected rather than using the alms for their necessities.[38] This is why some Christian communities sought to regulate almsgiving by distributing poor tokens to "legitimate," known beggars.[39] Moreover, open-handed, unquestioning distributions were relatively rare during the thirteenth century. Christian preachers, canon lawyers, and theologians laid out what they believed constituted the category of the deserving poor and warned of the need to be discriminating in one's charitable giving, since the worthiness of the recipient was directly related to the spiritual reward that the donor could expect and to the utility ("commodum") of the gift.[40] Although Gratian included discordant canons in his *Decretrum* on the subject of whether

---

34. Le Blévec, *La part du pauvre*, 177–78.

35. Young, *Scholarly Community*, 144–48.

36. For a historiographical review of the history of charity and its periodization by historians, see Adam J. Davis, "The Social and Religious Meaning of Charity in Medieval Europe," *History Compass* 12, no. 12 (December 2014): 935–50.

37. On the history of Christian attitudes toward indiscriminate almsgiving, see Young, *Scholarly Community*, 134–35.

38. Farmer, *Surviving Poverty*, 60–70. See also Thomas of Chobham, *Summa de arte praedicandi*, ed. Franco Morenzoni, *Corpus Christianorum, Continuatio Mediaevali*, vol. 82 (Turnhout: Brepols, 1988), 88.

39. William J. Courtenay, "Token Coinage and the Administration of Poor Relief in the Later Middle Ages," *Journal of Interdisciplinary History* 3 (1972/73): 275–95.

40. Todeschini, *Les marchands et le temple*, 170–71, 176–77.

charity should be given indiscriminately or discriminately, most canonists agreed that not all poor people were equally deserving of charity.[41] Drawing on patristic writings, some canonists developed a hierarchy of which classes of people should receive priority in the provision of charity. The moralist and preacher Jacques de Vitry argued that if one had to prioritize as to the preferred recipients of charity, the dishonest and the blasphemous (actors, vagabonds, ribalds) ought to be turned away. He stressed, however, that if one did give alms to sinners, it was obviously not to support their sins but to provide assistance to fellow humans in need.[42] The influential Bolognese canonist Huguccio maintained that while members of vile professions should be eligible for charity, the able-bodied poor who chose not to work should be refused (even when there were sufficient charitable funds), since to provide for them would only reward them for their idleness.[43] Despite disagreements among canonists, most agreed that when there were limited funds, the righteous and deserving poor should be provided for before the wicked, and that family members should be provided for before strangers.[44] The canonist Rufinus cited a saying from Ecclesiasticus 12:4 that was often repeated by later canonists: "May the alms sweat in your hands until you find a righteous person to whom to give them."[45]

Pope Innocent III's treatise on charity, *Libellus de eleemosyna*, reflects the tension between the ideal of indiscriminate charity and the widespread conviction that some recipients were more deserving than others.[46] Innocent suggested that ideally almsgiving should never be restricted, that alms should be given equally to the good and the wicked, an argument that some Church Fathers had earlier made. But Innocent also made clear that charity should only be given indiscriminately if there were unlimited resources, which he recognized would rarely be the case. Given this, he believed that almsgiving needed to be done according to a system based on the worthiness of the recipient.[47] After addressing one's own material needs, Innocent argued, a

---

41. Tierney, "The Decretists and the 'Deserving Poor,'" 370.

42. Bird, "Medicine for Body and Soul," 104.

43. Tierney, "The Decretists and the 'Deserving Poor,'" 369–70.

44. Young, *Scholarly Community*, 148–50.

45. Tierney, "The Decretists and the 'Deserving Poor,'" 363 and note 15. Pope Innocent III quoted this line to support the notion that priests were best suited to distribute alms, since they were the best judges of who was a deserving recipient.

46. Brenda Bolton, "Hearts Not Purses? Pope Innocent III's Attitude to Social Welfare," in *Innocent III: Studies on Papal Authority and Pastoral Care* (Aldershot, U.K.: Variorum, 1995), 123–45.

47. This notion of an "order of charity" (*ordo caritatis*) or prioritization of charitable recipients was introduced as early as the fourth century by Origen of Alexandria, although it was often misattributed to Ambrose. See Young, *Scholarly Community*, 135.

donor should next look after his or her parents, then friends and relatives, and then, all things being equal, the righteous stranger.[48] A gift given to the wrong person, he suggested, had no merit whatsoever and might even be considered a sin.

A central focus of many medieval theologians was the role of a potential recipient's need in the duty to give alms. Many theologians argued that a certain level of need mandated almsgiving (notwithstanding the value ascribed to voluntary giving), and sufficient need even rendered usurious alms permissible.[49] Much earlier, several of the Church Fathers had suggested that providing necessities to the poor was not so much the almsgiver parting with his own property but in a sense returning property that rightfully belonged to the poor or even to God. This idea was popularized during the twelfth and thirteenth centuries by Gratian, Robert of Courson, Guillaume d'Auxerre, and others, who argued that "in necessity everything is common."[50] Various theologians then engaged in discussions about different levels of need and hypothetical cases of competing needs, including the needs of the almsgiver and the needy recipient. Eudes de Châteauroux devoted one of his university "disputed questions" to the issue of "to whom should alms be given," and since he was addressing an audience of mostly future clerics, one of his central goals was to convey the pastoral responsibility of providing for those under one's charge, many of whom had pressing material needs in addition to spiritual ones.[51] Theologians, preachers, and various kinds of writers also invoked the image of the *corpus mysticum* to suggest that just as the various organs and members of the human body are interdependent, so too does a Christian society require that all of its members assist one another in a spirit of charity.[52] For example, in his thirteenth-century *Summa de poenitentia*, the Franciscan Servisanto of Faenza urged the members of the spiritual body to look after their neighbors, just as the various parts of a physical body work in tandem.[53]

---

48. Innocent III, *Libellus de eleemosyna*, in PL 217, col. 745–764. William of Auxerre and Eudes de Châteauroux also developed an "ordo caritatis," which outlined who should have priority in receiving alms. See Young, *Scholarly Community*, 148–50.

49. Odd Langholm, *Economics in the Medieval Schools: Wealth, Exchange, Value, Money and Usury According to the Paris Theological Tradition, 1200–1500* (Leiden: Brill, 1992), 76–77, 91–92.

50. Langholm, *Economics in the Medieval Schools*, 75–76.

51. Young, *Scholarly Community*, 149–50.

52. Botana, *Works of Mercy*, 182–84.

53. Botana, *Works of Mercy*, 183. As Botana has shown, this application of the *corpus mysticum* to the works of mercy was also used both by the Occitan poet and jurist Matfre Ermengaud in his *Breviari d'amor*, and in a Tuscan translation of *La somme le roi*.

As he did in so many domains, Thomas Aquinas established a science of *caritas*. Although Thomas agreed that it was natural to give alms to family members and those to whom one was most closely tied, he also argued that the potential recipient's righteousness, level of material need, and usefulness to the community were also relevant and even more important factors in the person's deservedness. Thomas wrote in his *Summa theologiae* that it behooved the almsgiver to be discriminating in giving alms, since the eternal rewards for almsdeeds depend on the recipient's worthiness and the recipient's prayers for the giver.[54] More generally, though, as Giacomo Todeschini has put it, Thomas viewed "Christian society as literally animated by *caritas*," which he regarded as a kind of social glue that promoted the common good and held people together: "*caritas* and the market are both inscribed in the great game of debts and credits, which, according to Thomas, links humans to God just as much as linking humans to each other in a system of obligations and dependencies that only acquires through *amicitia*, a civic variant of *caritas*, a productive and positive meaning in the history of salvation."[55]

In Peter Lombard's *Sentences*, which was to become the standard theological textbook used in universities, Peter pointed out that Saint Augustine had considered almsgiving as a form of justice, providing for the needs of the poor. Following Peter Lombard (and Augustine), a number of thirteenth-century theologians, notably Guillaume d'Auxerre, in his widely read *Summa aurea*, framed charity as a matter of justice.[56] But as Peter Lombard also pointed out, Augustine had elsewhere characterized almsgiving as a work of mercy, and so medieval theologians were left to reconcile these competing notions of almsgiving. On this score, Alexander of Hales differentiated between an almsgiver's giving his excess or surplus wealth, which he regarded as a form of justice, and an almsgiver's giving what he himself needed, which he believed thus involved self-sacrifice and therefore represented an act of mercy.[57] Although it was widely accepted that the payment of alms could remit sins, it was far less clear whether alms owed as a matter of justice merited the same spiritual rewards as alms given mercifully, and thus voluntarily.[58] Some theologians, such as Philip the Chancellor, believed that it was not enough to simply give alms from one's surplus wealth. In a

---

54. Thomas Aquinas, *Summa theologica*, trans. the Fathers of the English Dominican Province (New York: Benziger Bros., 1947), 2.31.3, 2.32.9.

55. Todeschini, *Les marchands et le temple*, 268, 277.

56. Langholm, *Economics in the Medieval Schools*, 75–78.

57. Langholm, *Economics in the Medieval Schools*, 127.

58. Young, *Scholarly Community*, 140.

sermon that he preached to the canons of St. Victor, he asserted that alms-giving should entail making personal sacrifice, that is, giving from one's own necessities, not just from one's surplus.[59] In viewing most ordinary almsgiv-ing as a form of justice, given in response to the pressing needs of the poor and given from the almsgiver's surplus wealth, theologians cast charity as an integral part of all economic transactions, such as buying, selling, and exchanging property, which were also thought to be conducted, at least ide-ally, according to mutual needs. As Odd Langholm has put it, in describing Henry of Ghent's theology of charity, "the duty to share with one's fellow man is not limited to the virtue of charity and the function of charity in the form of almsgiving; it extends to the function of economic exchange and to the virtue of justice in exchange."[60]

Treating charitable giving as an economic exchange, like buying and sell-ing, however, posed problems for some canonists and theologians. As alms-giving became increasingly associated with penance and actually came to be seen as the most powerful form of penance, superior to fasting and prayer, its role in the spiritual economy became even more crucial.[61] In the eyes of some, almsgiving risked being regarded in instrumental terms, as a kind of currency given with an expectation of a certain result. Already in the early twelfth century, Anselm of Laon warned that charity should never be treated as just another vulgar form of economic exchange, since for Anselm, what differentiated charity from all economic transactions was that the chari-table act was inherently disinterested.[62] Precisely because they were aware of the social implications of the gift, including the expectation that pious gifts would result in some kind of service or counter-gift, the Chanter and the members of his circle focused on the spiritual value of those gifts given solely "on account of God."[63] Guillaume d'Auvergne asked whether a sup-posedly charitable gift given with the expectation that the recipient would give something in return could even be considered a form of Christian char-ity when the action had little or nothing to do with God.[64] In both his *Historia occidentalis* and his sermons, Jacques de Vitry attacked the belief that alms-giving would automatically lead to salvation, even though it was precisely the promise of salvation that preachers often invoked as an argument in

---

59. Young, *Scholarly Community*, 144.
60. Langholm, *Economics in the Medieval Schools*, 254.
61. Young, *Scholarly Community*, 157–62.
62. Saint-Denis, *L'hôtel-Dieu de Laon*, 55–56.
63. Bain, *Église, richesse et pauvreté*, 312.
64. Piron, "Le devoir de gratitude," 89–91.

favor of almsgiving and charity more generally. In this regard, as Emmanuel Bain has argued, some theologians worried that the church was in danger of being replaced as the center of the economy of salvation, with some lay Christians believing that they could be saved simply by performing works of mercy.[65] In the eyes of these theologians, the works of mercy had come to be seen as almost too powerful and efficacious. Pious motivations, they argued, had to underlie almsgiving for it to be spiritually redemptive.

Seven centuries before the anthropologist Marcel Mauss wrote his landmark essay on the gift and the attendant expectation that a giver receive some form of counter-gift, some theologians and canonists acknowledged the existence of a natural law of reciprocity or a sense of obligation to do good to one's benefactor, something they referred to as "antidora" (or "antidota"). Sylvain Piron has shown that medieval anxiety about the obligation to show one's gratitude for a gift was closely tied to the growing hostility toward usury and the figure of the usurer, itself reflective of "a crisis of conscience for the Christian West faced with the first monetization of its economy."[66] For some theologians and canonists, the prohibition of usury seemed to call into question the morality of the law of reciprocity. As Thomas of Chobham and others argued, the law of reciprocity seemed to represent the very kind of Maussian counter-gift that Luke 6:35 ("do good, and lend, hoping for nothing thereby") seemed to oppose.[67] Was a pious and purely gratuitous gift even possible, however, within the framework of the economy of salvation that lay at the heart of medieval Christianity? Even Luke 6:35, after enjoining the love of one's enemies and the lending to them without any hope of receiving anything in return, went on to promise, "your reward shall be great, and you shall be the sons of the Highest." The subsequent verses continued: "Judge not, and you shall not be judged; condemn not, and you shall not be condemned; give, and it shall be given to you."

At the same time that there was a growing emphasis on what was regarded as free and pure almsgiving given solely on account of God, preachers and moralists were describing almsgiving in economic terms and highlighting the divine recompense that almsgivers could expect to receive. Indeed, as we shall see later in this chapter, some of the same moralists and preachers who fixated on the role of pious intention in giving simultaneously stressed the rewards that would be given to almsgivers if they gave alms correctly. Many

---

65. Bain, *Église, richesse et pauvreté*, 326.
66. Piron, "Le devoir de gratitude," 99.
67. Piron, "Le devoir de gratitude," 84, 87.

of these churchmen, however, drew an important distinction between the law of reciprocity when it involved God rather than merely another human being. In his *Libellus de eleemosyna*, Innocent III stressed the contrast between worldly and spiritual rewards, suggesting that the pauper profits the rich more than the rich profits the poor, because whereas the rich gives the pauper temporal alms, the poor repays the rich with eternal, spiritual rewards.[68] Innocent went on to underscore that alms should be given on account of eternal rewards, not to win worldly favor or the repayment from others. He cited Luke 14:12–14, in which Jesus enjoins his listeners in the house of a Pharisee not to invite rich friends for dinner with the hope of receiving a counter-invitation and recompense from them; rather, Jesus tells his listeners, invite the poor and disabled, and you shall be blessed and your recompense will be at the resurrection of the just. Building on this passage, Innocent III declared, "It is on account of this end, this recompense, this reward, that alms should be made."[69] Likewise, the Dominican biblical exegete, Hugues de Saint-Cher, made clear that Luke 6:38 ("give and it will be given to you") did not mean, as some sermon *exempla* seemed to suggest, that the same thing that was given in alms would be returned to the giver. Rather, it meant that giving temporal goods to the poor would result in eternal life being given to the almsgiver through the prayers of God's poor. Hugues maintained that this was not an exchange between relatively equal, horizontal relations but an asymmetrical, vertical relationship between man and God, between the material and the spiritual, and between this world and the world to come.[70]

The Sanctification of Charity

Emmanuel Bain has observed a significant shift in thirteenth-century biblical exegesis, with mendicant theologians like Alexander of Hales, Hugues de Saint-Cher, Jean de la Rochelle, Nicolas de Gorran, and Albert the Great paying far more attention to the corporal works of mercy as opposed to the biblical injunction to perform the spiritual works of mercy (to instruct the ignorant, counsel the doubtful, admonish sinners, and so forth), which had been the focus of earlier exegetes.[71] Charitable service through the performance of the corporal works of mercy emerged as part of the larger

---

68. Innocent III, *Libellus de eleemosyna*, in PL 217, col. 749d–750a.

69. See Innocent III, *Libellus de eleemosyna*, in PL 217, col. 754c.

70. Bain, *Église, richesse et pauvreté*, 313–14.

71. Bain, *Église, richesse et pauvreté*, 324–25. As Bain shows, this new emphasis on the corporal works is already evident in the slightly earlier writings of Peter the Chanter.

apostolic movement of the twelfth and thirteenth centuries, and one of the most prominent representations of charity "in action" from this period can be found in accounts of contemporary saints' lives. In chapter 5 we will examine some examples of ordinary lay women and men who dedicated their lives to caring for the sick poor in Champagne's hospitals. These hospital workers may have been inspired by what André Vauchez has called "a new category of saint," which developed as part of the apostolic movement, with sanctity increasingly tied to the practice of charity.[72] Saint Francis of Assisi did much to popularize this charity-driven spirituality: "To the Poverello, the love of God was indissociable from the love of men. It was not enough to imitate Jesus in gestures and conduct; it was also necessary to seek out and love him in the most wretched of his creatures."[73] Admittedly, the image of the charitable saint helping the beggar or leper had been a hagiographical topos stretching back to Saint Martin of Tours in the fourth century, to say nothing of earlier, foundational examples in the New Testament. Yet unlike most of the "contemplative" saints during the periods immediately before and after the twelfth and thirteenth centuries, many of the saints from the late twelfth and thirteenth centuries (or those regarded as having lived exemplary lives even if they were not formally canonized) were distinctly charitable—venerated for founding or working in hospitals—and a striking number were Franciscan tertiaries, reflecting the influence of Franciscan spirituality.[74]

---

72. Vauchez, *Sainthood in the Later Middle Ages*, 199.

73. Vauchez, *Sainthood in the Later Middle Ages*, 390. Admittedly, while Francis and some of the earliest brothers did work among the poor (and some brothers lived in hospitals with the poor), their primary occupation was not to improve the social and economic conditions of the poor. Still, Francis and the earliest friars displayed a radical commitment to living both as and among the poor, and they inspired later social agents of change, particularly among the tertiaries who worked in hospitals.

74. These included Margherita of Cortona (d. 1297), a Franciscan tertiary, who after her husband's death founded a hospital and charitable confraternity; Angela of Foligno (d. 1309), a wealthy widow and tertiary who cared for lepers in a hospital in Foligno; Agnes of Bohemia (d. ca. 1281), a tertiary who founded a hospital in Prague and also founded the Crosiers of the Red Star, a lay confraternity that served the sick and ran dozens of hospitals in eastern Europe; Douceline of Digne (d. 1274), a Franciscan tertiary and beguine who first cared for the poor her father took into his own home and, following his death, worked in the hospital of Hyères; Jutta of Huy, a wealthy married woman, who had close ties to the Cistercians and worked for eleven years caring for lepers; Aldobrandesca (d. ca. 1309), a Humiliati and widow who worked in a hospital in Siena; Saint Ubaldesca (d. 1206), a lay sister who served the sick in the hospital of Saint John of Jerusalem in Pisa; Raimondo Palmerio of Piacenza (d. 1200), a shoemaker and married father who founded a hospice for abandoned children and a hospital for poor women; Saint Omobon of Cremona (d. 1197), a tailor who founded a hospital; Saint Gerard Tintori of Monzo (d. 1207), who founded and worked in a hospital; Saint Walter of Lodi (d. 1224), who founded a hospital; Saint Andrew Gallerani, who founded the hospital of the Confraternity of Mercy in Siena; and Saint Gerardo Tintore, who established a hospital in Milan. See Vauchez, *Sainthood in the Later Middle Ages*, 200–201; Augustine Thompson, *Cities of God: The Religion of the Italian Communes, 1125–1325* (University Park: Pennsylvania State University

Moreover, even as the First Order shifted its attention away from the kind of caritative work that friars like Anthony of Padua, Gerard of Modena, and Henry of Milan had been engaged in during the late 1220s and 1230s to the clerical and pastoral work of preaching and hearing confession, the penitential spirituality of the Third Order, inspired as it was by Franciscan charism, became increasingly defined by caritative work.[75]

The close association between caregiving and spirituality is vividly illustrated by the life of the beguine Marie d'Oignies, who spent years with her husband serving lepers in the hospital of Willambrouk before retiring to a hermit's cell to lead a life of mystical contemplation. In writing about Marie's works of mercy, Jacques de Vitry not only underscored her spiritual powers, like the curative power of her prayers, but also called attention to the fact that Marie was more troubled by the suffering of others than her own travails.[76] In fact, while expressing compassion for the sufferings of others, she rejoiced in her own tribulations and wished that she could take on the afflictions of others. Marie regarded physical suffering as spiritually valuable in teaching patience and discipline. For Jacques, who believed that women were in some ways better suited than men for the holy work of caring for the *miserabiles*, probably due to women's association with the body, Marie's willingness to do revolting work, such as washing lepers' sores, rendered her a kind of holy martyr and an example of selfless service to others.[77]

Although many non-aristocratic lay women and men cared for the sick and poor in hospitals as a form of penitential piety, hagiographers tended to underscore the penitential humility of royal and aristocratic practitioners of the works of mercy, since, as Anne Lester has pointed out, "it was precisely

---

Press, 2005), 180–81, 196; Lori Pieper, "Saint Elizabeth of Hungary: The Voice of a Medieval Woman and Franciscan Penitent in the Sources for Her Life," (PhD dissertation, Fordham University, 2002), 205, 210, 218–19; Brodman, *Charity and Religion*, 182–83.

75. Some later Spiritual Franciscans, like Ubertino da Casale and Angelo Clareno, living outside the cities in hermitages, also displayed a genuine concern about the problem of material poverty for the involuntary poor. See Michael Cusato, O.F.M., "Where Are the Poor in the Writings of Angelo Clareno and the Spiritual Franciscans?" in *Angelo Clareno Francescano: Atti del XXXIV Convegno internazionale, Assisi, 5–7 ottobre 2006* (Spoleto, Italy: Centro Italiano Di Studi Sull'alto Medioevo, 2007), 123–65; Michael Cusato, O.F.M., "Two Uses of the *Vita Christi* Genre in Tuscany, c. 1300: John de Caulibus and Ubertino da Casale Compared. A Response to Daniel Lesnick, Ten Years Hence," *Franciscan Studies* 57 (1999): 131–48.

76. Jacques de Vitry, *The Life of Marie d'Oignes*, trans. Margot H. King, ed. Margot H. King and Miriam Marsolais (Toronto: Peregrina, 1993), 85, 100–101. Iacobus de Vitriaco, *Vita de Marie de Oignies, Supplementum*, ed. R. Huygens, *Corpus Christianorum, Continuatio Mediaevalis*, vol. 252 (Turnhout, Belgium: Brepols, 2012).

77. Jeanne Ancelet-Hustache, *Gold Tried by Fire: St. Elizabeth of Hungary* (Chicago: Franciscan Herald Press, 1963), 91–92, 183–84.

the inversion of social status that made their actions penitential."[78] A royal lay woman known for her compassion for the *miserabiles* was Elizabeth of Hungary, the daughter of King Andrew II of Hungary, about whom a great deal is known due to a number of hagiographical texts as well as the testimony that was part of several canonization inquests that occurred just after her death in 1231.[79] After the death of her husband, Louis IV of Thuringia, Elizabeth developed close ties to the Franciscans and may have become a Franciscan tertiary and beguine.[80] She distributed food to the poor and sick, washed their feet each year on Holy Thursday, made them clothes and habits for burying their dead, and used 2,000 marks from her dower to found a hospital for the poor dedicated to Saint Francis at Marburg in Thuringia.

Despite her elite upbringing, Elizabeth joined the hospital brothers and sisters in preparing and serving meals, dressing and undressing patients, bathing them, washing their linens, trimming their nails, untying their shoes, supporting them with her shoulders, and placing strips of cloth on the sores of sick patients. Nor was Elizabeth exclusively preoccupied with the sick, since she was also known to spend time entertaining poor children who were living at the hospital. What Conrad of Marburg and others most emphasized, however, was the way Elizabeth personally performed the most miserable tasks so that she might experience the misery of the sick herself. According to Conrad of Marburg's *Summa vitae*, "she cheerfully tended to [the sick] with her own hands and, using the veil from her own head, cleaned the saliva and mucus from the faces and the filth from the mouths and noses of the sick."[81] She kissed the sores of the leprous and washed the wounds of a beggar with an ulcerous head and would cut his hair while holding his head in her lap. Elizabeth was drawn to the sickest, most abject patients in her hospital. She not only endured sights and smells that her handmaids in the hospital could not begin to tolerate but took delight in doing so, often smiling

---

78. Lester, *Creating Cistercian Nuns*, 143.

79. Ancelet-Hustache, *Gold Tried by Fire*; Albert Huyskens, *Quellenstudien zur Geschichte der Hl. Elisabeth Landgräfin von Thüringen* (Marburg, Germany: Elwert, 1908); Christa Bertelsmeier-Kierst, ed., *Elisabeth von Thüringen und die neue Frömmigkeit in Europa* (Frankfurt: Peter Lang, 2008); Edith Pasztor, *Donne e sante: studi sulla religiosità femminile nel Medio Evo* (Rome: Edizioni Studium, 2000), 153–71.

80. There is debate about whether Elizabeth became a Franciscan tertiary. See André Vauchez, "Charité et pauvreté chez sainte Elisabeth de Thuringe d'après les actes du procès de canonisation," in *Etudes sur l'histoire de la pauvreté*, ed. Michel Mollat, vol. 1 (Paris: Publications de la Sorbonne, 1974), 171–72; Pieper, "Saint Elizabeth of Hungary," 44–45, 51–55.

81. Kenneth Baxter Wolf, ed. and trans., *The Life and Afterlife of St. Elizabeth of Hungary: Testimony from Her Canonization Hearings* (Oxford: Oxford University Press, 2010), 59.

and laughing. For a while Elizabeth cared for a paralyzed orphan boy who hemorrhaged blood, often cleaning his bloody (and soiled) clothes. When this child died, she adopted a malodorous leprous girl, who until that point had always been shunned. Elizabeth hid the sickly girl in her own house and cared for her until Elizabeth's harsh confessor, Conrad of Marburg, discovered the hidden child. He expelled the girl from Elizabeth's house, only to have Elizabeth adopt a new child, this one afflicted with ringworm. What Elizabeth's hagiographers underscored was the fervor and love with which she devoted herself to assisting the most helpless. Elizabeth's charity, which involved unpleasant, self-abnegating labor, carried as much meaning for her as it did for the recipient and required that she personally experience the sufferings of the afflicted, in short, that she experience *compassio*, which was the defining feature of her spirituality.[82]

Although hagiographers and witnesses who gave testimony about Elizabeth's sanctity as part of the canonization inquest were intent on promoting her sanctity as exceptional, their own accounts make clear that Elizabeth was not working alone but collaborating with a team of hospital workers at Marburg that was engaged in difficult and often unpleasant work. This group of hospital workers included the servants Irmingard, another Elizabeth, and Hildegunde, as well as the *custos* of the hospital, Hermann and his wife Irmentrude. Yet most of the people around Elizabeth, including her confessor, are depicted by witnesses as having been incapable of understanding the depth of her charity, such as her willingness to risk contracting contagious diseases or the pleasure she derived from giving away all of her wealth in the form of alms. In the face of the wretched, Elizabeth seemed to have none of the natural human feelings of revulsion. And whereas Elizabeth's confessor cast her charity in terms of her spiritual development—as an antidote to her pride and a way to obtain merit in the eyes of God—witnesses described Elizabeth as focused squarely on the recipients of her charity, not on the way her charity might benefit her.[83]

The Franciscans were quick to highlight their association with Elizabeth, whom they depicted as embodying the Franciscan virtues of poverty

---

82. Vauchez, "Charité et pauvreté chez sainte Elisabeth."

83. The *vita* of Yvette of Huy by Hugh of Floreffe, in contrast, largely ignores the lepers who were cared for by Yvette, focusing instead on how she embodied pious humility, dramatized by her efforts to contract leprosy (bathing with the lepers and even mixing her blood with theirs). See Anneke B. Mulder-Bakker, ed., *Living Saints of the Thirteenth Century: The Lives of Yvette, Anchoress of Huy; Juliana of Cornillon, Author of the Corpus Christi Feast; and Margaret the Lame, Anchoress of Magdeburg*, trans. Jo Ann McNamara (Turnhout, Belgium: Brepols, 2011), 93–95.

and love of the poor. In loving the poor as brothers and sisters in Christ rather than as mere instruments of her own salvation, Elizabeth was inspired, they argued, by the example of Saint Francis.[84] In the left lancet window in the cathedral of Strasbourg, erected in the mid-thirteenth century, Elizabeth is depicted engaged in each of the six corporal works of mercy. In the rose window at the apex, she is rewarded by being crowned by the Virgin Mary, taking her place among the Elect on Christ's right-hand side.[85]

There are also examples of the sanctification of charity in medieval Champagne, the region that will be the focus of subsequent chapters. Brief mention was made earlier of the knight Jean de Montmirail (d. 1217), who was never canonized but was beatified in 1250. The example of Jean de Montmirail has parallels with Elizabeth of Hungary in that he, too, came from the upper aristocracy. Jean had a lifelong friendship with King Philip II, with whom he went on crusade and in whose royal court he was raised, and Jean was also close to the count of Champagne. At least later in life, however, Jean's overriding preoccupation was in helping the poor and sick, particularly lepers. In 1203 he established a leprosarium in Montmirail, and five years later, he and his wife founded a *domus Dei* in the same town. Their eldest daughter, Elizabeth, took vows and became a professed sister at this hospital, devoting her life to serving the sick poor. In 1210, after twenty-five years of marriage, Jean left his wife and children to enter the Cistercian abbey of Langpont. A *vita* of Jean was written in ca. 1230 (thirteen years after his death) by a fellow monk, who described how Jean's charity even outdid that of the legendary Saint Martin, since Jean was known to give away *all* of his clothes to a pauper, not just half of a cloak like Saint Martin, and Jean even did this in the dead of winter![86] An *exemplum* recounted both by Jacques de Vitry and Étienne de Bourbon illustrated Jean de Montmirail's penitential piety as he devotedly cared for a pauper who was greatly afflicted with bleeding and dirty ulcers. Upon seeing the pauper, Jean reportedly went up to him and asked him why he did not go to a hospital to recover. When the poor man informed him that he was not able to get to a hospital, Jean lifted the man onto his shoulders and carried him to one. Once there, Jean washed the man's dirty feet as well as his legs, which were filled with blood. With Jean's heart paining for the poor

---

84. Pieper, "Saint Elizabeth," 171–79.

85. Joan A. Holladay, "The Education of Jeanne d'Evreux: Personal Piety and Dynastic Salvation in her Book of Hours at the Cloisters," *Art History* 17, no. 4 (December 1994): 593.

86. Touati, *Maladie et société*, 207.

man, he exclaimed, "O miserable and proud heart! Now will you be able to crack." Jean then drew from the water that he had used to bathe the poor man and drank it with his two hands.[87]

What also distinguished a number of the charitable saints from this period were their own experiences of suffering, which made them identify with the afflictions of others and led them to act compassionately. For example, representations of the adversities faced by the saintly King Louis IX of France—his frequent illnesses, his ascetic lifestyle, his crusading failures, and the loss of family members—embodied what Jacques Le Goff has termed the thirteenth-century "valorisation de la souffrance," a suffering that hagiographers linked to Louis's compassion for the downtrodden.[88] Guillaume de Saint-Pathus, who detailed the king's many acts of charity, including founding and patronizing hospitals, underscored that the king "had a marvelous tender compassion for people who were in a bad way."[89] A litany of anecdotes was invoked by Louis's hagiographers to illustrate his compassion: picking up the bodies and limbs of the Christians who were killed at Sidon or using his own fingers to wash away the grime between the toes of a poor man. When the newly expanded (and refounded) hospital at Compiègne was completed, the French king was said to have carried the first sick person, wrapped in a sack cloth, into the hospital with his son-in-law, Count Thibaut V of Champagne, where they placed him on a bed and, along with the king's son Philip, ministered to him.[90] Iconographic images of the humble and compassionate king performing each of the seven works of mercy, in some cases in a hospital setting, appeared in the Books of Hours of Jeanne d'Evreux and Marie de Navarre as well as in public spaces, such as the now-lost altar retable in the lower chapel of the Sainte Chapelle in Paris.[91] In representations of charitable saints, compassion

---

87. Lecoy de la Marche, ed., *Anecdotes historiques, légendes et apologues, tirés du recueil inédit d'Étienne de Bourbon, dominicain du XIIIe siècle* (Paris: Librairie Renouard, 1877), no. 156, p. 133. Guillaume d'Auvergne, the bishop of Paris, cited an *exemplum* involving Jean de Montmirail in five of his extant sermons. See Guillelmi Alverni, *Sermones de tempore*, ed. Franco Morenzoni, *Corpus Christianorum, Continuatio Mediaevalis*, vol. 230 (Turnhout, Belgium: Brepols, 2010), xix.

88. Jacques Le Goff, *Saint Louis*, trans. Gareth Evan Gollrad (South Bend: Notre Dame University Press, 2009), 703–4; Guillaume de Saint-Pathus, *Vie de Saint Louis*, ed. H. François-Delaborde (Paris: Alphonse Picard, 1899), 87–88, 97–99, 102.

89. Le Goff, *Saint Louis*, 718.

90. Guillaume de Saint-Pathus, *Vie de Saint Louis*, 99.

91. For the *vitae* by Geoffrey of Beaulieu and William of Chartres, see *The Sanctity of Louis IX: Early Lives of Saint Louis by Geoffrey of Beaulieu and William of Chartres*, ed. M. Cecilia Gaposchkin and Sean L. Field, trans. by Larry F. Field (Ithaca: Cornell University Press, 2013). See also Holladay, "The Education of Jeanne d'Evreux"; Guest, "A Discourse on the Poor"; M. Cecilia Gaposchkin, *The Making of Saint Louis: Kingship, Sanctity, and Crusade in the Later Middle Ages* (Ithaca: Cornell University Press, 2008), 201.

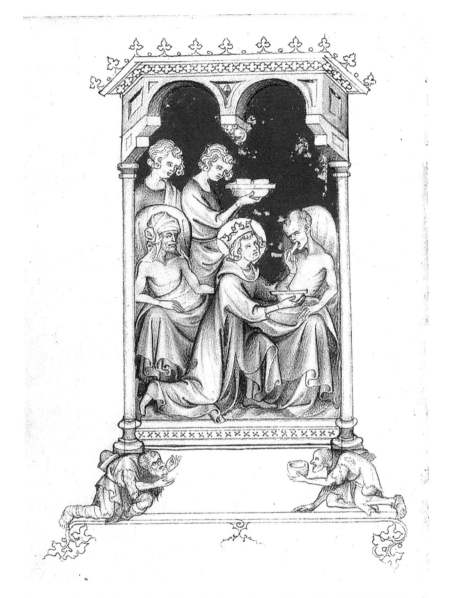

FIGURE 1.   St. Louis feeding the sick, from the Hours of Jeanne d'Evreux, Jean Pucelle (ca. 1324–28), fol. 142v. The Cloisters Collection.

was depicted as a central motivator for exemplary religious behavior. This sanctification of compassionate behavior may have helped inspire some lay women and men (and clergy) to provide support to hospitals, where such works of mercy were performed daily.

The Teaching of Charity and the Allure of Redemptive Almsgiving

In addition to saints' lives, models for teaching charity and hospitality abounded in the Middle Ages, including the Bible, books of hours, *exempla* in sermons, and visual representations. The late thirteenth-century *Miroir des bonnes femmes* was comprised of thirty *exempla* illustrating "good women," including female saints and women from the Bible, many of whom were notable because of their compassion and charitable activities.[92] Even in the *Enseignements* that King Louis IX composed for his children, he urged them to feel compassion for the poor and all those who were suffering.[93] Chivalric romances explored the theme of hospitality, which was regarded as an important courtly ideal. As Matilda Tomaryn Bruckner has argued, medieval romances distinguished between bourgeois or commercial hospitality on the one hand, in which a bourgeois host offered hospitality, in most cases, to a merchant, in exchange for payment, and courtly hospitality on the other hand, which was given freely rather than sold.[94] In Aimon de Varennes's romance *Florimont*, for example, the fact that commercial hospitality "is sold, [and] measured out, instead of freely given . . . makes of the host a 'vilain' unworthy of courtly consideration."[95] In seeking to codify what constituted proper "courtly" hospitality, romances such as *Florimont* enumerated what constituted genuine largesse, just as theologians and canon lawyers discussed different forms of charitable behavior, including those that were without merit. But according to these romances, even courtly hospitality involved "the principle of exchange that ties Hospitality into the circulation of courtly services," which involved "a system of debits and credits."[96] As we have seen, this tension between gift and reward was a central feature of theological discussions of the works of mercy, and it was prominent in the teaching of charity as well.

Visual representations of the works of mercy also served a didactic function and often carried a particular moral message. Federico Botana has established that beginning in the twelfth century there was a burgeoning imagery of the works of mercy, including mural panel paintings, manuscripts, sculptures, and stained glass.[97] Worshippers in the cathedral of Chartres would

---

92. Holladay, "Education of Jeanne d'Evreux," 602.

93. Le Goff, *Saint Louis*, 718.

94. Matilda Tomaryn Bruckner, *Narrative Invention in Twelfth-Century French Romance: The Convention of Hospitality (1160–1200)* (Lexington, KY: French Forum Publishers, 1980), 118–19.

95. Bruckner, *Narrative Invention*, 128.

96. Bruckner, *Narrative Invention*, 134, 118.

97. Botana, *Works of Mercy*, 7.

have been surrounded by windows and sculptures representing the saintly Bishop Lubin healing and anointing a bedridden Saint Calétric, Saint Martin healing a paralytic, the Good Samaritan dressing the wounds of a pilgrim, and Saint Pappolus visiting a bedridden Saint Laumer.[98] On the baptistery in Parma, constructed in 1196, six reliefs on the west portal, one for each of the works of mercy in Matthew 25:35–36, contained verses on their bases to help the viewer recognize and learn how to properly perform the work of mercy depicted: "this is an example of how you should open the door to pilgrims," "this one washes the legs of the sick with much care," and so forth.[99]

The salvific power of mercy was frequently emphasized by visually juxtaposing the works of mercy with the Last Judgment or the Heavenly City, thus suggesting that salvation could be attained by performing such good works; by implication, failure to do so would have a far less auspicious result.[100] Artistic renderings of the works of mercy also linked them to the Eucharistic sacrifice, this at a time of increasing Eucharistic fervor. Federico Botana has shown that besides the Crucifixion itself being described in medieval texts as a work of mercy in redeeming humanity, images depicting the performance of works of mercy were at times positioned in such a way as to create a "strong association between the works of mercy and the Eucharistic sacrifice."[101] Just as the Eucharist was thought to make Christ's presence real, so too was Christ believed to be present in the performance of works of mercy (at times even disguised as the afflicted), which like the Eucharist was cast as an expression of love. Moreover, an *exemplum* narrated by Jacques de Vitry described how a noble woman in a church felt such pity upon seeing a poor woman suffering from the cold that she decided that even though it would mean that she would miss the Mass, it was more important for her to offer the poor woman the warm wrap she was wearing. The noble woman led the poor woman up the church tower in order to give her the wrap, and upon her return to the church below, she learned from the priest that miraculously, he had been unable to say a word during her absence. The noble woman's charity had actually become the Mass, the ultimate sacrifice.[102] Christ had

---

98. Touati, *Yves de Chartres*, 14–15.

99. Botana, *Works of Mercy*, 30–31n63.

100. Botana, *Works of Mercy*, 47, 197.

101. Botana, *Works of Mercy*, 188.

102. Jacques de Vitry, *The Exempla*, ed. Crane, 42–43, no. 93; Bird, "Texts on Hospitals," 116; Sharon Farmer, "The Leper in the Master Bedroom: Thinking Through a Thirteenth-Century Exemplum," in *Framing the Family: Narrative and Representation in the Medieval and Early Modern Periods*, ed. Diane Wolfthal and Rosalynn Voaden (Tempe: Arizona Center for Medieval and Renaissance Studies, 2005), 96. Another version of this story is told by Étienne de Bourbon in his *Tractatus de diversis*, which can be found in *Anecdotes historiques*, ed. Lecoy de la Marche, 128.

been made present and real through the noble woman's charitable act. In that moment, she had supplanted the priest.

In trying to understand what might have made a hospital donor identify with the anonymous sick and poor staying in a hospital, it is worth recalling that it was common for visual representations of the works of mercy to depict the works being performed in hospitals, thereby strengthening the association of hospitals as sites of such acts of compassion.[103] Furthermore, Christ frequently appears in visual representations as one of the beneficiaries of the works of mercy, thereby linking Christ with the contemporary suffering stranger.[104] In a fourteenth-century fresco cycle in the baptistery of Parma depicting the seven works of mercy, Christ appears from a cloud in each scene, holding the Scriptures with one hand and pointing to the beneficiaries of the works of mercy with his other hand, thereby recalling the Prophecy of the Last Judgment in Matthew 25:40, "as long as you did it to one of these my least brethren, you did it to me."[105]

Medieval *exempla* also underscored the sacramental dimension of charity, the notion that to perform a work of mercy was a way of worshipping God. It was widely believed that one's best chance to meet the person of Christ—outside of Mass—was by showing mercy to a needy stranger, and this was corroborated by God's own words in the Greek translation of Hosea 6:6: "I desire mercy [toward your neighbor], not [just] sacrificial service."[106] An *exemplum* that Jacques de Vitry cited in a sermon (and that was repeated in later *exempla* collections) told the story of a charitable noblewoman permitting a male leper to rest in her absent husband's bed, thereby risking the anger of her husband, who hates lepers. When the husband returns home and enters the bedroom, the leper has miraculously disappeared, replaced by a magnificent aroma, symbolizing paradise and the fact that the leper had been Christ in disguise. When the wife tells her husband what happened and that the leper she cared for miraculously turned out to have been Christ, the husband, who until then has behaved like a lion, becomes contrite like a lamb and begins to lead a more religious life.[107] In the words of Jacques de

---

103. Botana, *Works of Mercy*, 44–46. On fourteenth-century iconographic representations of "caritas" in the *Liber regulae* for the hospital of Santo Spirito in Sassia, see Gisela Drossbach and Gerhard Wolf, eds., *Caritas im Schatten von Sankt Peter: Der Liber Regulae des Hospitals Santo Spirito in Sassia: Eine Prachthandscrift des 14. Jahrhunderts* (Regensburg, Germany: Verlag Friedrich Pustet, 2015).

104. Botana, *Works of Mercy*, 158n31.

105. Botana, *Works of Mercy*, 86–88.

106. Gary A. Anderson, *Charity: The Place of the Poor in the Biblical Tradition* (New Haven: Yale University Press, 2013), 105.

107. Farmer, "Leper in the Master Bedroom." There were numerous variations on this *exemplum* of Jacques de Vitry (including a different version cited by Étienne de Bourbon about a poor man

Vitry, citing Matthew 25:35, "Whoever therefore through these works shows charity to his neighbor applies that charity to God . . . as the Lord said, 'I was hungry and you gave me food.'"[108]

During the thirteenth and early fourteenth centuries, a number of vernacular texts on the Christian virtues and vices were written, and these texts showed a particular concern with teaching the works of mercy. We often think of the *later* Middle Ages as having produced a plethora of works of *moralia*, or moral instruction. Yet it was the Fourth Lateran Council in 1215 and the ecclesiastical reform movement that spurred lay catechism, including the teaching of the seven deadly sins, the seven cardinal virtues, and the need for the laity to regularly examine themselves in preparation for confession. As a result of the Fourth Lateran Council, the longstanding system of penitential tariffs, whereby a specific penance was stipulated for each possible offense, was gradually phased out; the imposition of penance was instead increasingly left up to the individual confessor, not that penitential tariffs were ever rigidly adhered to even before the Fourth Lateran Council. As part of this transformation in the way that penance was imposed, the thirteenth century saw the production of a number of *summae casuum*, or Latin confession manuals, which described various sins and the methods of satisfaction for each. As the confession manuals of Raymond of Peñafort and others show, the works of mercy represented an increasingly popular form of penance, particularly as an antidote to the sin of avarice.[109] The thirteenth-century bishop and theologian Robert Grosseteste even defined avarice as a sin against charity.[110] Moreover, avarice and mercy were often paired up as corresponding vice and virtue.[111] By the late thirteenth century, several vernacular works were being produced that built on the Latin penitential tradition in addressing the works of mercy. These vernacular works also translated contemporary scholastic ideas about charity and the works of mercy into a more accessible, popular medium, one that could reach members of the laity, either directly (including through the use of accompanying

---

instead of a leper). See Stephani de Borbone, *Tractatus de diversis materiis praedicabilibus*, no. 863, p. 567. See also an *exemplum* used by the Dominican, Henri de Provins, in a sermon he preached in 1273 at Saint-Gervais in Paris, in Nicole Bériou, *L'avènement des maîtres de la Parole: La prédication à Paris au XIIIe siècle* (Paris: Institut d'Études Augustiniennes, 1998), 1:824. On earlier examples (going back to Jerome and Gregory the Great) of Christ being found among lepers, see Rawcliffe, *Leprosy*, 60–64.

108. Jacques de Vitry, *The Exempla or Illustrative Stories*, ed. Crane, no. 95, 44–45; Farmer, "Leper in the Master Bedroom."

109. Botana, *Works of Mercy*, 69.

110. Odd Langholm, *The Merchant in the Confessional: Trade and Price in the Pre-Reformation Penitential Handbooks* (Leiden: Brill, 2003), 235.

111. Newhauser, "Justice and Liberality."

visual representations) or as adapted by friars and parish priests in the context of preaching, hearing confession, and catechism. The production of these vernacular works of moral instruction roughly coincided with the increasing democratization of Christian charity, as large numbers of not only aristocrats but also ordinary townspeople across Europe made voluntary charitable bequests to hospitals, leprosaria, and charitable confraternities and as increasing numbers of lay men and particularly lay women devoted their lives to charitable work in the spirit of apostolic piety.

An example of this can be seen in *La somme le roi*, written in 1279 by Laurent d'Orléans, a Dominican friar, papal inquisitor, and royal confessor to King Philip III of France. Friar Laurent wrote *La somme* at King Philip's request, and the text was to become one of the most widely diffused works of the late thirteenth century. Almost one hundred French manuscript copies from the late thirteenth and fourteenth centuries are extant, placing it in the same "bestseller" category as Froissart's *Chronicles* and Guiart des Moulins's *Bible historiale*.[112] In addition, *La somme* was translated into many vernacular languages. A moral treatise on the virtues and vices, Friar Laurent's work was written for the edification of the laity.[113] In fact, twice in the text, he declares, "This text is for the laity, and not for clerics who have books."[114] At the same time, *La somme* reflected its author's erudition and scholastic background at Paris, where he had been prior of the Dominican school at Saint-Jacques. The text contains almost seven hundred citations and examples, mostly from the Bible but also from classical texts, the works of various Christian writers, and accounts of saints' lives. It is written in a highly ordered form, with numbered subdivisions and sub-subdivisions, which was typical of late thirteenth-century scholastic texts. It would have been easy for preachers in need of preaching material to cull Friar Laurent's text for examples and citations on a particular vice or virtue such as mercy.[115]

Friar Laurent defined the virtue of mercy as feeling "sorrow and compassion for the misfortunes and needs of others."[116] By stressing God's inherent liberality, having impoverished himself in the incarnation, Laurent framed

---

112. On the diffusion of the text, see Anne-Françoise Leurquin-Labie, "La *Somme le roi*: De la commande royale de Philippe III à la diffusion sous Philippe IV et au-delà," in *La moisson des lettres: l'invention littéraire autour de 1300*, ed. Hélène Bellon-Méguelle et al. (Turnhout, Belgium: Brepols, 2011), 195–212.

113. Leurquin-Labie, "La *Somme le roi*," 210–12.

114. Frère Laurent, *La somme le roi*, ed. Edith Brayer and Anne-Françoise Leurquin-Labie (Paris: Société des Textes Français Modernes, 2008), 48, 142, 146.

115. A number of the extant manuscripts belonged to friars or friaries, and some were even accompanied by an alphabetical, thematic index. See Leurquin-Labie, "La *Somme le roi*," 206–7.

116. Frère Laurent, *La somme le roi*, 300.

the doing of works of mercy both as the quintessential "imitatio Christi" and the most direct way to help God. Laurent enumerated the seven spiritual works of mercy and the seven corporal works of mercy, giving examples and citations for each. For instance, in his discussion of the fourth corporal work, visiting the sick, he cited the almost contemporary charitable example of Marie d'Oignies and her work with lepers as embodying perfect virtue. Laurent also invoked as exemplary those who went to the crusader states to serve sick and wounded crusaders in hospitals. He then gave practical advice about what one should talk about while visiting a sick person; he recommended, for instance, comforting the sick with good words, reminding them of the Passion and Jesus' suffering for humanity.

Following his discussion of the spiritual and corporal works of mercy, Laurent launched into the proper form of almsgiving, echoing many of the same points that were raised by scholastics and preachers, including Peter the Chanter, Jacques de Vitry, and Étienne de Bourbon.[117] Laurent argued, for instance, that for alms to be pleasing to God, they must come from a pure source. Alms derived from theft, rapine, or usury are not meritorious.[118] *La somme* distilled this idea about the importance of the source of alms and transmitted it to a wider lay audience. We have already observed that theologians and canonists were developing a hierarchy of which classes of people should receive priority in the provision of charity, and Friar Laurent, likewise, asked whether one should first give alms to one's family, friends, or strangers in need.[119] Finally, *La somme* addressed the ideal manner of almsgiving (just as Étienne de Bourbon did in his collection of preaching material), saying that it should be done voluntarily, with a glad heart (and with devotion, that is, not for vain glory) and that almsgiving should be done as soon as possible and during one's lifetime. These concrete, practical considerations were now distilled in a more accessible, vernacular, and illustrated form.[120]

In his lengthy discussion of the virtue of the works of mercy, Friar Laurent also expounded upon what it is that moves people to perform works of mercy, rhetorically making a case for the rewards that that the performance of mercy would bring to its practitioners. But Laurent also made an

---

117. Frère Laurent, *La somme le roi*, 316-17.

118. Baldwin, *Masters, Princes, Merchants*, 1:307–11; Peter the Chanter, *Verbum adbreviatum*, 661–63; Young, *Scholarly Community*, 137–39, 150–55.

119. Tierney, "Decretists and the 'Deserving Poor,'" 370.

120. During the 1390s, Friar Laurent's ideas about the proper forms of charity and the way it could counteract avarice were incorporated into a householder's book, *Le Ménagier de Paris*, which was written in the voice of a wealthy, older, Parisian husband, instructing his fifteen-year-old bride on her moral duties. See *The Good Wife's Guide (Le Ménagier de Paris): A Medieval Household Book*, trans. and ed. Gina L. Breco and Christine M. Rose (Ithaca: Cornell University Press, 2009), 82–83.

argument that was likely to appeal to those who were competitive and ambitious, whether merchants, townspeople, or lords, suggesting that "mercy is a good merchant who wins everywhere and never loses."[121]

Other texts from this period allegorically describe the Christian almsgiver as a merchant or banker engaged in spiritual commerce both with the needy recipients of alms and with God. In a manuscript containing a Tuscan translation of *La somme le roi*, for example, the *Esposizione del Paternostro*, an illustrative program depicts a banker, described in the accompanying textual commentary as "a man of honest appearance, who deals money at a *banco* and has two angels above his shoulders who communicate to him holy counsel, that is, to spend his money on the poor for the love of Jesus Christ."[122] He is seated behind a *banco*, holding a pair of scales, as two angels above him provide him with "the gift of good counsel" (the title of the section) about the virtue of mercy by pointing to four paupers, one of whom is on crutches. The commentary explains, "He has good counsel who in this world spends his time and wealth giving alms to the poor, so that he can acquire the glory of eternal life, in which the good deeds that each person has done will be credited to them and, as it is said in the gospel, our Lord Jesus Christ will pay you back a hundredfold of merit in his glory for each good deed that you will have done in this life."[123] The illuminator of this manuscript chose the figure of the good banker or moneychanger as the one who receives the counsel to perform the works of mercy in part, as Federico Botana has argued, to suggest that the works of mercy could function as a form of penance for the sin of avarice, which was closely associated with banking and was discussed at some length in an earlier section of the *Esposizione del Paternostro*.[124] But the image of the banker as practitioner of mercy may have also been an allusion to the notion of the works of mercy as interest-bearing loans to

---

121. Frère Laurent, *La somme le roi*, 305. Some Franciscan sermons also described Christ as a "good merchant." See Bériou, "L'esprit de lucre," 279n46.

122. Botana, *Works of Mercy*, 66. The Tuscan translation of *La somme le roi* was executed ca. 1300 by the Florentine notary Zucchero Bencivenni. According to Botana, the manuscript with the miniatures (Florence, Biblioteca Nazionale Centrale di Firenze, MS II.VI.16) can be dated ca. 1340 and was likely intended for a lay confraternity connected to Santa Maria Novella, Florence. See Botana, *Works of Mercy*, 61–62n54, 64. For the text of the Tuscan translation, see Luigi Rigoli, ed., *Volgarizzamento dell'Esposizione del Paternostro fatto da Zucchero Bencivenni* (Florence: Academia della Crusca, 1828). A distinction was often drawn during the thirteenth century between good bankers or moneychangers (who may also have provided some credit functions) and their evil counterparts, the usurers ("usurarii"). On this distinction, see Todeschini, *Les marchands et le temple*; Giovanni Ceccarelli, "'Whatever' Economics: Economic Thought in Quodlibeta," in *Theological Quodlibeta in the Middle Ages: The Thirteenth Century*, ed. Christopher Schabel (Leiden: Brill, 2006), 1:497.

123. Botana, *Works of Mercy*, 66.

124. Botana, *Works of Mercy*, 69–70.

God, converting money into spiritual capital, which, as we shall see, was a concept frequently invoked. The virtue of mercy was, in the words of the *Esposizione*, "good business."[125] In subsequent scenes, what appears to be the same banker is shown lodging the poor by guiding some poor people, one of whom is on crutches, into a building, possibly a hospital run by a confraternity, giving alms, visiting the sick, visiting prisoners, and so on.[126]

La voie de paradis, written by an anonymous Frenchman in the early fourteenth century, has much in common with Friar Laurent's *La somme*. *La voie* is a Middle French adaptation of a Latin treatise, the *Tractatus de tribus dietis*, which is itself a longer adaptation of one of the redactions of Robert de Sorbon's treatise on confession, *De tribus dietis*, written during the 1260s and intended as a preaching tool.[127] *La voie de paradis* treats many of the same subjects as the scholastic treatises on which it is partially based, and it retains a highly subdivided format. As F. N. M. Diekstra has shown, however, *La voie* seems targeted to a less lettered (or even unlettered) audience, and it shows far less concern with scholastic argumentation and proof.[128] In the prologue, the author several times alludes to the fact that readers may be listening to the book as it is read aloud.[129] *La voie* ended up serving as the basis for the Middle English *Weye of Paradys*, a penitential manual intended for laymen. Over the course of the thirteenth century, technical Latin treatises on specialized topics had given way to more general Latin pastoral manuals for priests (and confessors) to help them with the *cura animarum*, and by the end of the century, written religious instruction was targeting the penitent himself or herself, either directly or indirectly, with manuals being written in the vernacular and focused more on interior (as opposed to exterior) penance and the virtues, including the works of mercy. *La voie de paradis*, for example, has a much more expansive discussion of the corporal and spiritual works of mercy than Robert of Sorbon's treatise on confession, on which *La voie* was based.[130] And *La voie* was frequently illustrated with miniatures that show the reader how to perform the various works of mercy, such as lodging the stranger or clothing the naked. *La voie* also has a meditation on the Passion for each of the canonical hours, suggestive of the possible links between the works of mercy and affective meditation.

---

125. Botana, *Works of Mercy*, 72.
126. Botana, *Works of Mercy*, 64–79.
127. *The Middle English "Weye of Paradys" and the Middle French "Voie de Paradis": A Parallel-Text Edition*, ed. F. N. M. Diekstra (Leiden: Brill, 1991), 29–34.
128. *Middle English "Weye of Paradys,"* 35.
129. *Middle English "Weye of Paradys,"* 107–08.
130. *Middle English "Weye of Paradys,"* 34.

La voie de paradis evoked the image of the "cross of compassion" with its four arms, one arm for the compassion felt for Christ's Passion, another arm for the dead in Purgatory (who, according to the author, once they reach Paradise, will repay all those who prayed for them), the third arm of compassion representing those tormented in this world with illness or poverty, and the final arm devoted to those persisting in sin.[131] One can imagine how this image might have served as an object of meditation and a way of linking affective meditation on Christ's Passion with performing works of mercy. According to *La voie*, the works of mercy are the ideal way to make satisfaction for sin. On Judgment Day, those who didn't perform works of mercy will sit on the left side of the Lord, whereas those who did will sit to the Lord's right. The only thing of value that one can take to the grave are the works of mercy performed in one's life. But according to the author, the works of mercy, including almsgiving, begin with feeling pity and showing mercy for oneself through true contrition; only then will one be able to have compassion for others. The author of *La voie* described those who voluntarily helped the poor as usurers to God; their loan, a work of mercy, would be handsomely repaid later by God.

Giacomo Todeschini has shown that the friars' moralization of the market drew on a long tradition, stretching back to St. Augustine, who had described Christ as a heavenly merchant. But according to Augustine, God also wanted Augustine's listeners to be merchants by investing what they had in almsgiving, thereby transferring their earthly treasures to heaven, with the assurance of a significant future return on their investment.[132] During the twelfth century, theologians such as Richard of St. Victor argued that wealth and profits were not inherently bad; only the failure to distribute this wealth—accumulating and then hoarding it—was seen as a vice. The system of exchange and profits, he and other theologians argued, could be virtuous if it led to distributive charity.[133] As Odd Langholm has shown, medieval penitential handbooks, which were explicitly directed at the pursuit of salvation, were also brimming with commercial metaphors, describing the Christian penitent as a merchant in need of refilling his purse with virtues.[134] These handbooks instructed merchants and others to fight their avaricious impulses by investing some of their profits in charity.[135] In their sermons,

---

131. *Middle English "Weye of Paradys,"* 314.

132. Brown, *Ransom of the Soul*, 91–92.

133. Todeschini, *Les marchands et le temple*, 184–85.

134. Pope Innocent III compared the church as a whole to a "good merchant." See Todeschini, *Franciscan Wealth: From Voluntary Poverty to Market Society* (New York: Franciscan Institute, St. Bonaventure University, 2009), 15, 30.

135. Langholm, *Merchant in the Confessional*, 235.

friars frequently employed a vocabulary and imagery replete with references to money, credit, and commercial transactions, including in their discussions of almsgiving and the works of mercy.[136] While condemning usury and the love of riches more broadly, the friars defended "virtuous wealth" and the pious purposes to which this wealth could be put, including its contribution to the social welfare, the "bonum commune."[137] Friars cast merchants' fairs in a positive light, even arguing that good Christians must follow the example of merchants, by carefully accumulating greater capital as a way of enriching themselves, although in this case, the capital was that of virtues.[138] Likewise, in his *Summa* on the "art of preaching," the English theologian Thomas of Chobham figuratively described the virtues with which one can buy eternal life as the money given to the merchant by God "to buy certain precious goods at the market."[139]

During the thirteenth century, it became increasingly common for preachers to describe almsgiving as a loan to God, citing the verse from Proverbs 19:17 ("He who has mercy on the poor, lends to the Lord"). Usury served as a useful metaphor for conveying the sense not only that God was the ultimate recipient of alms given to the poor but also that God would repay the almsgiver with interest. Thomas of Chobham, for example, used the moral denunciation of usury as an opportunity to exalt almsgiving and argue that it provided far greater reward (or interest), with a greater guarantee of being repaid, than any usurious loan made to another human: "Let us not seek interest for the principal of a loan from anyone but Him." Invoking the "centuplum accepturus," or the hundredfold reward, referenced, in a different context, in Matthew 19:29, Thomas continued, "everything whatsoever that we do for Him will be paid back to us with the greatest interest" ("cum usura maxima").[140] "There are even good usurers" ("Sunt

---

136. Bériou, "L'esprit de lucre," 283; Bériou, "Le vocabulaire de la vie économique dans les textes pastoraux des frères mendiants au XIIIe siècle," in *L'économia dei conventi dei frati minori e predicatori fino alla metà del Trecento: atti del XXXI Convegno internazioinale, Assisi, 9–11 ottobre 2003* (Spoleto, Italy: Centro italiano di studi sull'alto Medioevo, 2004), 151–86; Bériou, *L'avènement*, 1:552–55.

137. Bériou, "L'esprit de lucre," 267–87. For specific textual examples, see Bériou, "L'esprit de lucre," 283n62. See also Longère, "Pauvreté et richesse chez quelques prédicateurs," 1:255–73. On the complex relationship between the mendicant orders and economic matters, see Nicole Bériou and Jacques Chiffoleau, eds., *Économie et religion: L'expérience des ordres mendiants (XIIIe–XVe siècle)* (Lyon: Presses Universitaires de Lyon, 2009); Todeschini, *Franciscan Wealth*.

138. Bériou, "L'esprit de lucre," 283–84 and note 66.

139. Langholm, *Merchant in the Confessional*, 4.

140. Thomas of Chobham, *Summa de commendatio virtutum*, 223; Sophie Delmas, "La Summa de abstinentia attribuée à Nicolas de Biard: circulation et réception," in *Entre stabilité et itinérance: Livres et culture des ordres mendiants, XIIIe–XVe siècle* (Turnhout, Belgium: Brepols, 2014), 303–27; Bériou, "L'esprit de lucre," 284–85 and note 68.

etiam boni usuarii"), Guillaume d'Auvergne declared in one of his sermons. The bishop of Paris, who had close ties to the friars, then quoted from Proverbs 19:17. According to Guillaume, these "good usurers" were those who gave alms, those who let go of grudges, and the like, and these individuals would be recompensed with the ultimate payment at the last of the fairs ("fine nundinarum").[141] In a different sermon, Guillaume quoted from the same verse from Proverbs, while making clear that the "spiritual riches" of the hundredfold reward—"the graces and virtues with which the elect are enriched" in this world—which were superior to any material wealth, would be promised in this life to those who abandoned temporal things and followed the Lord. Giving one's property to the poor, Guillaume cautioned, should not be understood as abandoning it but sowing it in the fields of the Lord so as to be deemed worthy to receive the "centuplum" here and eternal life in the future.[142]

In the same vein, the most famous thirteenth-century Franciscan theologian, Bonaventure, suggested in a sermon based on the theme of Luke 6:36 ("Be merciful just as your Father is merciful") that mercy enriches its practitioners with merit and spiritual riches just as usury enriches the moneylender with temporal riches.[143] Bonaventure then quoted from Proverbs 19:17, a verse that seems to have had particular resonance among thirteenth-century friars.[144] The analogy between almsgiving and lending at interest to God was in some ways a surprising one for a Franciscan to make, since usury was often cast as the antithesis to, and even a crime against, *caritas*. Indeed, usury was often blamed for causing poverty, thereby creating the need for almsgiving.[145] Yet the mendicants often tended to establish their foundations right in the heart of a city's commercial district as a way to weigh in on

141. Guillelmus Alvernus, *Sermones de communi sanctorum et de occasionibus*, ed. Franco Morenzoni, *Corpus Christianorum. Continuatio Mediaevalis*, vol. 230C (Turnhout, Belgium: Brepols, 2013), sermon 82, p. 281.

142. Guillelmus Alvernus, *Sermones de communi sanctorum*, sermon 18, p. 64.

143. Saint Bonaventure, *Sermones dominicales*, ed. Jacques-Guy Bougerol (Grottaferrata, 1977), sermon 28, p. 331; Bériou, "L'esprit de lucre," 285.

144. The *Summa de abstinentia*, a collection of "distinctiones" that served as a preaching tool and that was probably authored by the Dominican, Nicolas de Biard, also compared almsgiving to moneylending. See Delmas, "La Summa de abstinentia." In his commentary on Proverbs 19:17, the Franciscan biblical exegete Nicholas of Lyra also linked humans' lending to God through almsgiving to God's hundredfold repayment. Nicolaus de Lyra, *Postilla super totam Bibliam* (Strasbourg, 1492; repr. Munich, 1971), note e.

145. Todeschini, *Les marchands et le temple*, 187. In a sermon that the Paris chancellor Jean d'Orléans preached for the fourth Sunday of Lent, he accused usurers of being plunderers of the poor and suggested that usurers' clothes were red from the dried up blood of the poor. See Bériou, "L'esprit de lucre," 279–80.

and help shape the morality of market practices.[146] The mendicants at the University of Paris were deeply engaged in thinking about how charging for credit might be morally justified. Mendicant theologians and preachers frequently used economic terms and concepts, particularly in seeking to rechannel those terms toward the highest spiritual ideals.[147] By comparing the charitable behavior of one person toward another to God's relationship with humanity, Bonaventure reaffirmed that genuine Christian charity was the opposite of a vulgar economic transaction, that it was in essence a divine gift distributed by grace, reflecting God's love of humanity. In endowing humans with the capacity for charitable service and giving, God made it possible for creatures to imitate the incarnated image of Christ and mystically reunite with their Creator. Viewing the charitable dynamic between humans from this mystical standpoint, Bonaventure cast charity both as a form of *imitatio Christi*—"the spiritual reiteration of divine charity"—as well as a vehicle for an individual's mystical reunion with God.[148]

Like Bonaventure, the Franciscan Guillaume de Lanicea (d. 1310) compared the almsgiver to the hardworking moneylender in his treatise on the virtues and vices, *Dieta salutis*. But Guillaume used the analogy of the moneylender to draw attention to the importance of giving alms to deserving recipients who could actually intercede spiritually on behalf of the almsgiver. In that sense, almsgiving really was very much like other economic transactions, since it too was based on an expectation of reciprocity. "Just as moneylenders do not give their money to those who are not able to pay it back, or to those who will not come to the fairs," Guillaume declared, "so too the prudent man does not give alms to stage-players who have nothing, namely from the grace of God and who will not come to the fairs of paradise."[149] As we have seen, thirteenth-century theologians and canonists were developing hierarchies of those they regarded as most or least deserving of alms. But apart from the question of the recipient's deservedness, Guillaume de Lanicea underscored that the almsgiver should be alert to the degree to which the potential recipient of alms could spiritually help repay the almsgiver, and this was clearly tied to the recipient's deservedness in the eyes of God. The almsgiver would only receive a spiritual reward at the "fairs of paradise" if

---

146. James M. Murray, *Bruges, Cradle of Capitalism, 1280–1390* (Cambridge: Cambridge University Press, 2005), 119.

147. On how the spirituality and language of the friars were influenced by the very marketplace which they sought to reject, see Barbara H. Rosenwein and Lester K. Little, "Social Meaning in the Monastic and Mendicant Spiritualities," *Past and Present* 63 (1974): 23–32.

148. Todeschini, *Les marchands et le temple*, 181.

149. Bériou, "L'esprit de lucre," 284n66.

the recipient of the alms was empowered to repay him there. In that sense, almsgiving was just as much a reciprocal exchange as moneylending.

The Dominican theologian Hugues de Saint-Cher, in his commentary on Luke 6:35, in which Jesus exhorted his listeners to lend to their enemies without expecting anything in return, even went so far as to suggest that showing mercy toward the poor would render God one's slave: "He who accepts a loan is a slave of the usurer, therefore he who shows mercy on the poor makes God his slave."[150] Although in the Christian tradition humanity was generally cast as being indebted to God, insofar as Christ was believed to have made the ultimate sacrifice on behalf of humanity, here, in a stunning reversal, Hugues de Saint-Cher suggested that human almsgiving rendered Christ a slave or debtor to the almsgiver. Almsgiving represented a way for humans to transform themselves into God's creditors, rather than passively remaining forever in God's debt. The longstanding notion that almsgiving was redemptive had taken on a wholly new meaning in the highly commercial context of thirteenth-century Europe. And as we have seen, it was largely the friars who were responsible for reconceptualizing in plainly commercial terms how the human act of giving alms could transform the human-divine relationship.

Although most discussions of the recompense given to almsgivers made clear that this reward came in the form of spiritual redemption, often underscoring the contrast between material and spiritual recompense (and the superiority of the latter), some thirteenth-century preachers and moralists suggested that almsgiving would also result in material recompense for the giver.[151] Rhetorically, this was clearly a way of convincing readers or listeners of an additional reason to give generously to the poor.[152] Sermon *exempla* frequently addressed the fear of potential almsgivers that their giving might result in their impoverishment in this life. Étienne de Bourbon's preaching *exempla* included numerous cases that, invoking Proverbs 28:27 ("He who gives to the poor will lack nothing"), reassuringly illustrated that the very thing that was given in alms would be restored or replenished.[153] In one *exemplum* based on a story in the *Lives of the Desert Fathers*, two friends are living together during a famine, one who is generous and always receiving all who came to him with needs, and another who refuses to give up anything and eventually goes off on his own. But the latter one gradually

---

150. Bériou, "L'esprit de lucre," 285.
151. Bériou, "L'esprit de lucre," 287.
152. Bériou, "L'esprit de lucre," 287.
153. De la Marche, ed., *Anecdotes historiques*, 121–28.

becomes impoverished and is forced by need to return to his generous friend. One day, when it appears that both men no longer have anything to live off of, the generous friend insists that his miserly friend go and see if any food remains. To his great surprise, he discovers that their reserves are suddenly and miraculously replenished, which leads the tightfisted friend to become merciful and generous.[154]

Other *exempla* went even further in suggesting that almsgiving might improve one's material security and prosperity in this life. The frequent invocation of Jesus' promise of the hundredfold reward in Matthew 19:29 was used to remind listeners of the assurance of worldly recompense, not just spiritual rewards in the world to come. Thomas of Chobham was quite explicit in one of his sermons that the hundredfold reward would be received in this life, quite separate from the promise of eternal life in the future.[155] Innocent III asserted that giving alms had value for three reasons besides charity: first, for the capacity of receiving grace; second, for reducing eternal punishment; and third, for obtaining temporal wealth.[156] Almsgiving was thus both a short-term and long-term investment that was thought to pay material and spiritual dividends. Likewise, in his collection of preaching material, Étienne de Bourbon made clear that one reason to give alms was that doing so would increase one's wealth ("bona multiplicat"). Quoting from Proverbs 28:27: "he who gives to the poor will not be poor" and Luke 6:38: "give and it will be given to you," Étienne provided a litany of historical examples in which almsdoers received material rewards during their lifetimes.[157] In several cases, the central point of the example was that the material reward was or would have been even greater had the gift been larger. Étienne repeated, for example, a story from the *vita* of John the Almoner, in which a man discovers that the more charitable he is, the greater the profits he makes.[158] In this story there was a direct, quantitative correlation between gift and material reward. In another *exemplum*, after a married couple hears their priest preach about the hundredfold reward, they decide to give the

---

154. Stephani de Borbone, *Tractatus de diversis materiis praedicabilibus*, 311–12.

155. Thomas de Chobham, *Sermones*, ed. Franco Morenzoni, *Corpus Christianorum, Continuatio Mediaevalis*, vol. 82A (Turnhout, Belgium: Brepols, 1993), sermon 6, p. 64.

156. Innocent III, *Libellus de eleemosyna*, in PL 217, col. 753d–754a.

157. Stephani de Borbone, *Tractatus de diversis materiis praedicabilibus*, 307–14, 318–20, 339–40.

158. The man, who once had been miserly, begins telling his servant to steal a certain number of coins each week in order to give them to the poor, and each week the servant steals twice as much as instructed and gives it all away to the poor, with the result being that his master makes even more money. When the servant finally reveals what he has been doing to his master, the master realizes that his servant's additional generosity is the reason for his own growing prosperity. See Stephani de Borbone, *Tractatus de diversis materiis praedicabilibus*, 311.

priest their cow with the expectation that they will receive the hundredfold reward. After waiting a long time and receiving nothing, the couple becomes increasingly impoverished and angry, and decides to kill the priest. On his way to do so, however, the husband comes across a lump of gold on the road and thus discovers the priest's words to be true after all.[159] In *La somme le roi*, discussed earlier, Friar Laurent copied the historical examples cited in Étienne de Bourbon's collection of preaching material to illustrate the point that "mercy is a good merchant because it multiplies temporal goods."[160] After citing Proverbs 3:9–10 (that by honoring God with one's wealth and giving one's goods to the poor, God will fill storehouses with wheat and cellars with wine), Laurent cited historical examples to demonstrate that performing works of mercy would result in the almsdoer's receiving temporal as well as spiritual and perdurable gains.[161] In one of his other *exempla* illustrating the same point, Étienne first quoted Ambrose: "to give alms isn't to lose but to sow"; and second, Gregory the Great, from one of his letters (10.8): "that which is given to the poor, isn't given but loaned, because that which is given is received with manifold profit."[162]

Interestingly, one finds the idea that almsgiving represented a kind of loan to God in a thirteenth-century Jewish text from northern France as well. Jews and Christians had long shared a belief in the power of redemptive almsgiving. In the Book of Daniel (Daniel 4:27), the Prophet Daniel tells King Nebuchadnezzar, "Redeem your sins with alms and your injustices by compassion on the poor."[163] Some Jewish beggars in late antiquity even pleaded with those who passed them by, "acquire a merit through me" ("zeki bi").[164] Moreover, as Alyssa Gray has shown, redemptive almsgiving—the notion that almsgiving can serve as atonement for sin and that the prayers of the recipient of alms can rescue the donor from death or a severe divine decree—was an idea that not only originated in Jewish sources but was also a prominent feature of both Palestinian (although, interestingly, not Babylonian) rabbinical

159. Stephani de Borbone, *Tractatus de diversis materiis praedicabilibus*, 313. A version of this story was also included in the *Speculum morale* formerly attributed to Vincent of Beauvais. See Vincent de Beauvais, *Speculum quadruplex*, 1474–75; Bériou, "L'esprit de lucre," 286. Addressing the possible fear that almsgiving might not result in a recompense for the giver, Matfre Ermengaud, in his *Breviari d'amor*, stated, "One can truly hope that if one does good, one will receive good. And even if it is late in coming, it will not fail to come." Nelli, "L'aumone dans la littérature occitane," 54.

160. Frère Laurent, *La somme le roi*, 305–7.

161. Frère Laurent, *La somme le roi*, 305.

162. Stephani de Borbone, *Tractatus de diversis materiis praedicabilibus*, 314.

163. Brown, *Ransom of the Soul*, 96.

164. Anderson, *Charity*, 25.

sources and late antique Christian sources.[165] The Book of Ecclesiasticus suggested that alms can extinguish sin just as water can put out fire.[166] The Talmud, meanwhile, called someone who gives *tzedakah* in order to inherit the world to come ("olam ha'ba") a "tzaddik gamur" (a completely righteous person).[167] Like Christians, medieval Jews believed that charity removed sin and thereby protected them from the judgment of Hell.[168] In his study of medieval Jewish charitable bequests, Judah Galinsky found that both Hebrew and Jewish Latinate wills contained the same *pro anima* formulas as Christian wills.[169] Admittedly, unlike Jewish wills, Christian wills reflected a belief in the intercessory power of the clergy and the saints. However, just as Christian charitable bequests earned the donor prayers that were said on his or her behalf, so too was German Jews' charity tied to a liturgical commemoration of souls, including the souls of the dead ("hazkarat neshamot"), since like Christians, German Jews believed that public prayers could sway the destiny of the dead. Thus, it was common practice in Germany for a memorial Yizkor prayer to be recited every Shabbat, Yom Kippur, and the second day of festival days in order to ask God to show mercy toward the souls of the deceased on whose behalf *tzedaka* had been given.[170]

Beyond a common belief in the spiritually redemptive power of almsgiving, however, during the twelfth and thirteenth centuries both Christians and Jews living in northern France and Germany showed a heightened concern that charity be given properly, that is, to the right kind of recipients, for the right reasons (and voluntarily), and from legitimate sources. In medieval eyes, not only could religious charity be discriminating, but part of what made charity a pious act was precisely its insistence on discriminating between worthy and unworthy recipients. Were these parallel conceptions of what constituted pious charity due to what Galinsky has termed "charity's nondenominational character"?[171] Or were these similar ideas about charity due to a high level of Jewish assimilation with the dominant Christian culture? As

165. Alyssa M. Gray, "Redemptive Almsgiving and the Rabbis of Late Antiquity," *Jewish Studies Quarterly* 18, no. 2 (2011): 144–84.

166. Brown, *Ransom of the Soul*, 97; *The Wisdom of Ben Sirach (Ecclesiasticus)* 3:30.

167. Judah Galinsky, "'Hazkarat Nishamot' (i.e. 'Yizkor'), 'Poskim al ha-Zeddaka,' and the Funding of Communal Activities in Medieval Ashkenaz," unpublished paper. I am grateful to Professor Galinsky for permitting me to quote from his unpublished paper.

168. Jonathan A. Seif, "Charity and Poor Law in Northern Europe in the High Middle Ages: Jewish and Christian Approaches," (PhD dissertation, University of Pennsylvania, 2013).

169. Judah Galinsky, "Jewish Charitable Bequests and the Hekdesh Trust in Thirteenth-Century Spain," *Journal of Interdisciplinary History* 35, no. 3 (2005): 423–40.

170. Galinsky, "'Hazkarat Nishamot' (i.e. 'Yizkor')."

171. Galinsky, "Jewish Charitable Bequests," 440.

Ephraim Shoham-Steiner has suggested, perhaps Jews were eager to emulate the dominant Christian culture's charitable practices and ideas about charity so that Jews were viewed as being as compassionate and charitable as Christians.[172] Another explanation, however, relates to the increasingly urbanized, populous, and profit-oriented world of thirteenth-century northern Europe, where it was increasingly common to see beggars, migrants, and itinerants of various kinds wandering around cities and towns, and where there were a multitude of new outlets for giving charity. As we have seen, the commercial nature of thirteenth-century society reshaped Christian understandings of almsgiving as in some ways being like other commercial transactions that involved exchange.

Peter Brown has demonstrated, however, that Christians and Jews living in late antiquity also shared the belief "that heaven and earth could be joined by money," or as Proverbs 13:8 put it, "the ransom of the soul of a man is his wealth."[173] That one could transfer one's own "treasure" from earth to heaven by giving one's wealth to the poor, as Jesus enjoined the rich young man to do in Matthew 19:21, became inextricably tied to the idea of the soul's need for expiation. Sin was increasingly understood in financial terms as a debt that could be repaid through almsgiving.[174] Indeed, as Brown shows, in late antiquity God increasingly acquired the image of being the "debt manager" for believers: "He could set the terms for the repayment of the debts of sin. Better yet, He could remit those debts—canceling the arrears of a lifetime in a splendid moment of forgiveness. He could also repay good deeds like any other creditor who had received a loan. But He did so at rates of interest far above those current in the real world. To say that 'he who is kind to the poor lends to the Lord' was to be certain of a repayment whose generosity broke all the rules of a zero-sum economy."[175]

While drawing on a long intellectual tradition, the commercialization of charity in the religious imagination of thirteenth-century Christians and Jews also reflected the commercial and monetized economy of their own day. Medieval Jewish ideas about wealth and charity reflected the long-standing idea that all wealth belonged to God and was placed in trustworthy human hands merely as a temporary loan to be distributed according to God's wishes. A section of R. Jacob ben Asher's compilation of *halakha*, for

---

172. Ephraim Shoham-Steiner, *On the Margins of a Minority: Leprosy, Madness, and Disability Among the Jews of Medieval Europe*, trans. Haim Watzman (Detroit: Wayne State University Press, 2014), 186.

173. Brown, *Ransom of the Soul*, ix.

174. Brown, *Ransom of the Soul*, 96–98.

175. Brown, *Ransom of the Soul*, 97–98. See also Anderson, *Charity*.

example, the *Arba'ah Turim* (from ca. 1300), warned that a person's money is not his own but rather a "deposit with him to do with it according to the will of the depositor [God], whose will is that he should distribute his money to the poor. This is the best portion he can have of it, as it is written: 'your charity goes before you.' Also, it is a tried and tested fact that a person will not lack as a result of giving charity. On the contrary, it will increase his wealth and honor."[176]

What was novel in the thirteenth century in the Jewish context, however, was the notion not only that humans were obligated to give charity (from money that was, in a sense, loaned to them from God) but that the act of giving charity also obligated God to repay a loan to the almsgiver. The clearest development of this idea is found in a tale in the *Sefer ha-Ma'assim*, written in late thirteenth-century northern France, possibly northern Champagne, that invoked the same verse from Proverbs 19:17, "He who shows kindness to the poor lendeth unto the Lord," that Bonaventure and others drew on as a way of suggesting that a person's charitable giving earned him or her credit with God.[177] The Talmud had shown ambivalence toward this verse, which was seen as theologically problematic, since it implied that God could be in a subservient position, like a poor person, obligated to anyone who gave charity: "R. Johanan taught: 'What is the meaning of the verse, "He who shows kindness to the poor lendeth unto the Lord (Prov. 19.17)?" Were it not written in the Scripture, one would not dare to say it: as it were, "the borrower is a servant to the lender."'"[178] In the thirteenth-century tale found in the *Sefer ha-Ma'assim*, however, the earlier Talmudic ambivalence about this verse in Proverbs had entirely disappeared. The tale recounted how Elijah the Prophet came to tell an exceedingly poor man that God would grant him seven good years of bounty; Elijah gives the poor man the choice of whether to accept these seven good years now or wait until his old age. Although this story was based on an Elijah legend from the rabbinic period, there were distinctive features to the medieval version.[179] One of these features was the

---

176. Jacob ben Asher, *Arba'ah turim ha-shalem, Yore Deah* (Jerusalem: Mosdot shirat Devorah, Mekhon Yerushalayim, 1993), 247 (siman). I am indebted to Professor Judah Galinsky for sharing a translation of this text.

177. Rella Kushelevsky, *Tales in Context: Sefer ha-ma'asim in Medieval Northern France* (Detroit: Wayne State University Press, 2017), no. 29, pp. 210–13.

178. Talmud Bava Batra 10a; Anderson, *Charity*, 67. As Anderson points out, Protestants were later troubled by the Jewish and Catholic "doctrine of rewards," which in Protestant eyes not only rendered charity a selfish act that was motivated by the promise of rewards but also implied that "the believer dictates to God the terms of his salvation."

179. On earlier versions of this tale, see Yaffa Berlovitz, "Seven Good Years," in *Sippur Okev Sippur, Encyclopedia of the Jewish Story*, vol. 1, ed. Yoav Elstein, Avidov Lipsker, and Rella Kushelevsky

prominent role of the poor man's wife in the story. The poor man is initially inclined to delay accepting Elijah's offer until his old age, when he will not be able to work. But he tells Elijah that before deciding on when to accept the seven good years, he will need to consult with his wife and the members of his household. The man's wife is adamant that he accept the seven good years right away so that they can give away their newfound wealth to the poor and thereby earn an even greater, eternal reward. The wife also insists that a scribe be present to record each and every gift that they make. She tells her husband, "You may not benefit at all [from this wealth] until you bring me a scribe who will write down everything I give to the poor."[180] Once the scribe has been summoned, the wife tells him, "And write everything down, as it says: 'He who shows kindness to the poor lends to the Lord [and that which he has given he shall be repaid].'"[181] Earlier versions of this legend did not include this verse from Proverbs, which explicitly appears four times in this thirteenth-century French version. Each time, it is the wife who cites this verse, and she clearly envisions charity as an investment in the ultimate reward, salvation. But the wife also assumes that their charity will assure them of sufficient resources for the rest of their earthly lives; she and her husband are horrified when, at the end of their seven years of bounty, they find that they are once again poverty-stricken. Outraged, the wife goes storming to the rabbi to ask how it could be that she and her husband gave so much charity (300 camels loaded with documentation of their gifts, she says), only to be impoverished. The scene recalls Étienne de Bourbon's *exemplum* about the couple that give their cow to a priest, expecting a one hundredfold reward. "Doesn't it say," the wife asks the rabbi, quoting the verse from Proverbs, "'He that has pity on the poor lends to the Almighty?' and I have done a great deal of charity and lent to the Almighty, and now I and my household are dying of starvation."[182] The rabbi tells her to take all of the written records of her charity and spread them out on the roof of the study hall, and first thing in the morning, stand on the roof and remind God of

(Ramat-Gan, Israel: Bar Ilan University, 2004); Eli Yassif, *Ninety-Nine Tales: The Jerusalem Manuscript Cycle of Legends in Medieval Jewish Folklore* (Tel Aviv, 2013), tale 79 (Hebrew); *Mimekor Yisrael: Selected Classical Jewish Folktales: Abridged and Annotated Edition*, collected by Micha Joseph bin Gorion, ed. Dan Ben Amos and Emanuel bin Gorion, trans. I. M. Lask, intro. Dan Ben Amos (Bloomington: Indiana University Press, 1990), nos. 219, 427. Professor Galinsky has called my attention to two earlier examples of this legend: Midrash Zuta—Ruth (Buber) Parsha 4 on the "seven good years" (10th century) and R. Nissim (11th century). See also Kristen H. Lindbeck, *Elijah and the Rabbis: Story and Theology* (New York: Columbia University Press, 2010).

180. Kushelevsky, ed. and trans., *Tales in Context*, 210.
181. Kushelevsky, ed. and trans., *Tales in Context*, 210.
182. Kushelevsky, ed. and trans., *Tales in Context*, 212.

the verse from Proverbs and all the charity she and her husband have done. As soon as she does this, according to the tale, God says to Elijah, "Go and support them all their days in this world."[183]

One finds in the *Sefer ha-Ma'assim* tale not only an increasingly assertive medieval Jewish insistence upon the power and redemptive promise of charity but also a desire to quantify and record charitable giving, just as one would any other commercial transaction, including the lending of money. In this tale, God is no longer cast as a creditor, depositing wealth to trustworthy humans so that they can give charity, as God usually was depicted in rabbinic literature; rather, God becomes the ultimate debtor to those who gave charity. None of this would have surprised a thirteenth-century Christian, and the story in the *Sefer ha-Ma'assim* may well reflect a Jewish cultural appropriation of mainstream Christian thought (although the notion of God as debtor within medieval rabbinic circles continued to be rare). As we have seen, popular Christian vernacular texts and sermons cast charity much the way *Sefer ha-Ma'assim* did, as a kind of loan to God, with the divine debtor bound to repay his charitable creditors.

The metaphor of almsgiving as a kind of money loan may also reflect the belief that some cases of moneylending could serve as a form of charity. As we shall see in later chapters, some hospitals engaged in moneylending, and those who ran these hospitals may well have considered this lending as part of their charitable mission. The central point, however, is that for both Christians and Jews in medieval Europe, almsgiving was in some respects another economic transaction that involved exchange, like buying, selling, exchanging, or lending property or money, a point made by a number of thirteenth-century theologians. What differentiated almsgiving from these other economic transactions, however, was the possibility of its being spiritually redemptive. Spiritual or even material redemption was by no means believed to be guaranteed as a result of almsgiving or the performance of the works of mercy more generally. There were risks involved, including the possibility that there would be no ultimate reward. From a theological standpoint, the risks inherent in charitable giving somewhat mitigated the charge that charity was purely motivated by the self-interested desire for reward.[184] The potential redemptive reward nonetheless played a crucial factor in fostering charitable behavior, whether for medieval Christians or Jews, as the textual examples we have examined show.

---

183. Kushelevsky, ed. and trans., *Tales in Context*, 212.
184. Anderson, *Charity*, 106–9.

Conclusion

The way that acts of mercy were represented in thirteenth-century sermons, saints' lives, vernacular literature, and art—in short, the way that charity figured in the medieval *mentalité*—helps explain the reasons for the birth of the "hospital movement" and the larger charitable revolution. As Jacques Le Goff put it, "Caritas was the essential social link between medieval man and God, and between all men in the Middle Ages."[185] The texts we have been examining provide a window into how scholastic discussions about the ideal form of almsgiving were disseminated to the laity. Preaching surely represented one of the most direct ways that the laity were exposed to scholastic ideas about almsgiving. Nicole Bériou and others have shown that charity and the works of mercy were a common theme in thirteenth-century sermons, as preachers exhorted their listeners to perform works of mercy. Penitential and confessional texts such as *La somme le roi* and *La voie de paradis* were well suited to be used by preachers looking for material on the vices and virtues. The lives of charitable saints, such as Elizabeth of Hungary, also served as models of piety to be emulated. And the imagery of the works of mercy exhorted viewers to perform such works, conveying their salvific power and ability to foster social cohesion; like the didactic texts we have been examining, these images sought to teach viewers the right way to perform charity. Through images, sermons, and various kinds of scholastic, vernacular, and hagiographical texts, medieval culture was saturated with a discourse about the social and spiritual meaning of the works of mercy. These religious and cultural forms were meant to teach people how to perform the works of mercy, ultimately propelling them to action. We should not assume, however, that lay charitable practices were necessarily responses to scholastic and clerical ideals. In fact, the clerical discussions about the importance of charity may have been a response to a burgeoning of lay charity, an attempt on the part of the clergy to "play catch-up" with a lay movement already well underway.

With the rise of a confessional society and the growing preoccupation with Purgatory as a place, charity was increasingly regarded as the most powerful form of penance, one that was equally accessible to the laity and clergy.[186] In a time of growing anxiety about how one's conduct on earth might affect one's experience in the world to come, the words from Matthew 5:7 ("Blessed are the merciful, for God shall have mercy on them"),

---

185. Le Goff, *Money and the Middle Ages*, 144–45.
186. Young, *Scholarly Community*, 157–62.

which were invoked often, brought a sense of reassurance that divine mercy might be earned in the next world by showing mercy toward one's helpless neighbors in the earthly world. Furthermore, in the context of the expanding profit economy, the works of mercy were understood as the virtuous antidote to the vice of avarice. It was the friars, whose moral and religious reputations were partly built on their commitment to voluntary poverty and their denunciation of greed, who took the lead in arguing that wealth could be rendered virtuous if it was used for the needs of the poor. Yet Christian moralists and preachers, particularly those associated with Peter the Chanter's circle, also placed a great deal of emphasis on the way that charity was practiced. The intentions and gladness with which alms were given, the source of those alms, the deservedness of the recipient—all of these moral-religious questions mattered a great deal, in their eyes, in determining whether the almsgiver would receive a recompense.

As we have seen, almsgiving was increasingly conceived and described in commercial terms, with God even cast as a debtor and the almsgiver as a virtuous moneylender. Charitable service, such as working in a hospital, it should be added, was considered just as much an act of renunciation and generosity as almsgiving and was also regarded as a form of penance and a way to build up credit with God. Since churchmen were deeply engaged in thinking through the moral and religious dimensions of the commercial profession, including how to determine the just price and what exactly did and did not constitute usury, it was in some ways not surprising that they would apply commercial language to describe almsgiving, which involved the interplay between the material and spiritual, the human and divine. While almsgiving was generally differentiated from other kinds of economic transactions in that it involved the exchange of material goods for spiritual redemption, some thirteenth-century moralists and preachers, as we have seen, like Étienne de Bourbon, Thomas of Chobham, and Frère Laurent, insisted that the performance of the works of mercy would also be repaid with a material recompense in this world. These churchmen sought to reassure potential donors who might have been reluctant to give away some of their wealth to the poor that they were making the wisest kind of investment by earning credit with God, credit that would both fund a heavenly treasure and result in a hundredfold reward in the form of material recompense in this world.

The growing Eucharistic piety, such a hallmark of thirteenth-century devotion, may also have contributed to the performance of the works of mercy. The works had long been linked to the foundational sacrifice of Christ, and a plethora of visual images were produced during this period that associated the Eucharist with the corporal works of mercy. As Gary A. Anderson has put it, "Christ's merciful self-donation was continually re-presented in the sacrifice of the Mass," and this may have served as a reminder of humanity's obligation to repay its debt through its own sacrifices in the form of acts of compassion.[187] The association between Christ's suffering and the suffering of one's earthly neighbors became stronger with the increasing humanization of Jesus and the emphasis on God's voluntary self-impoverishment through the Incarnation. Performing the works of mercy was cast not only as *imitatio Christi* but also as a way to help Christ. As John Chrysostom told his congregation in one of his sermons a millennium earlier, Christ's Real Presence could be encountered not only at the altar during the celebration of the Mass but in the face of the beggar or leper at the "many altars" on the street corners of Antioch.[188] In a very real sense, the hospitals or "houses of God" (*domus Dei*) that were founded across Europe during the twelfth and thirteenth centuries were designed to house "many altars" for encountering Christ's Real Presence among the sick and the poor. Let us now turn to the building of these "houses of God" and the creation of a charitable landscape in Champagne.

---

187. Anderson, *Charity*, 186.
188. Anderson, *Charity*, 67.

❧ CHAPTER 2

The Creation of a Charitable Landscape

Although a caritative movement swept across all of western Europe during the twelfth and thirteenth centuries, resulting in, among other things, the foundation of many hospitals, there were regional differences in the kinds of charitable institutions that developed, the people who founded and patronized them, and even the meaning of gifting in a particular locale. Why, for example, did "poor tables" or "tables of the Holy Spirit" emerge in the Low Countries but not elsewhere?[1] Why was the constitutional form of English hospitals less "monastic" (with relatively few English hospitals under the Augustinian Rule) than hospitals on the continent?[2] How did the prominent role that confraternities and parishes played in the provision of charity in northern Italy affect the nature of hospitals there?[3]

To understand the rise of the hospital in twelfth- and thirteenth-century Champagne, there is a need to examine the role of the counts and countesses in the provision of charity. While the counts' patronage of religious

---

1. Brodman, *Charity and Religion*, 212–13; on Liège, see de Spiegeler, *Les hôpitaux et l'assistance à Liège*; on Arras, see Bernard Delmaire, *Le diocèse d'Arras de 1093 au milieu du XIVe siècle: Recherches sur la vie religieuse dans le nord de la France au moyen age* (Arras, 1994).

2. Sethina Watson, "Fundatio, Ordinatio, and Statuta: The Statutes and Constitutional Documents of English Hospitals to 1300," doctoral thesis, St Hilda's College, Oxford University, 2003.

3. Henderson, *Renaissance Hospital*.

institutions has been studied, far less attention has been paid to their patronage of hospitals. Did they regard hospitals as simply another religious institution in need of support, or were there distinctive elements in their relationship to these charitable institutions, a number of which the counts had founded and which remained under their jurisdiction? The same question can be asked of Champagne's aristocracy, known for its benefaction of monastic houses, but which also showed a "compulsion for provisioning the poor and sick."[4] Champagne's increasingly influential urban bourgeoisie also played a prominent role in bequests to hospitals and in other economic transactions with these institutions. Did different social classes patronize different hospitals, perhaps in part due to the neighborhood in which a particular hospital was located? Did they make different kinds of gifts? Were the motivations underlying the benefaction of aristocrats and townspeople different? Finally, what was the relationship between Champagne's hospitals and other ecclesiastical institutions, such as monasteries, chapters, and cathedrals? Given that the county was such an important center for monastic life, particularly reformed monasticism, we need to consider the impact that monasteries may have had in supporting or eclipsing the provision of charity in hospitals. Scholars of medieval religious institutions have not examined the central role that these charitable institutions played, both in the larger religious and institutional landscape and in the urban economy. As this and later chapters will show, the creation and functioning of Champagne's hospitals was a product of broader religious, political, and economic developments.

Commerce and Charity

In many ways, the county of Champagne exemplified the commercial prosperity of the twelfth and thirteenth centuries. With its six principal fairs (two in Provins, two in Troyes, and one each in Lagny and Bar-sur-Aube) and numerous secondary fairs, Champagne was a year-round commercial hub that attracted merchants from Italy, Languedoc, Provence, Germany, Flanders, and the north of France.[5]

Some foreign merchants ended up staying in Champagne permanently. The Cahorsin merchant Bernard de Montcuc married a woman from a

---

4. Lester, *Creating Cistercian Nuns*, xiii.

5. The standard studies of Champagne's fairs are Bourquelot, *Études sur les foires de Champagne*; Chapin, *Les villes de foires de Champagne*; Bautier, "Les foires de Champagne."

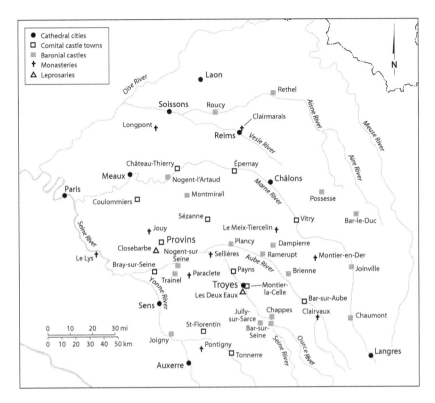

FIGURE 2.   Map of Champagne

prominent Troyen family and ended up serving three times as mayor of
Troyes.[6] The fair towns were also centers of industry, with woolens made
in Provins and linens made in Troyes exported to Italy.[7] A large percentage
of the households in thirteenth-century Provins were involved in woolen
and linen clothmaking. A *censier* or landbook for the hospital of Provins,
which lists the names of individuals who owed the hospital a seigneurial
rent, or *cens*, conveys the wide range of Provinois occupations, from money
lenders ("le useriers," "prestat"), blacksmiths ("faber"), millers ("munerius"),
and winesellers ("forravin") to those involved in the production or sale of
lace products ("li buriers"), wood ("charpentier"), textiles ("le tainturier"),

6. David Nicholas, *The Growth of the Medieval City: From Late Antiquity to the Early Fourteenth Century* (London: Longman, 1997), 192.

7. Theodore Evergates, *Henry the Liberal* (Philadelphia: University of Pennsylvania Press, 2016), 174.

and leather ("li peletiés").[8] A cartulary for the city of Provins contains 670 records in old French from 1271 to 1311 that provide a sense of the prosperity of the bourgeois class in the city. Of particular interest are the many dozens of records of individuals' emancipation from guardianship, which often included an inventory of a family's property (furniture, buildings, lands) that was "restored" to a minor once he or she was of an age that no longer required guardianship. These records provide a fascinating picture of the property holdings of middle-class families in Provins, large numbers of whom were involved in the woolen cloth trade (carders, dyers, fullers, weavers, and the like), while others worked as innkeepers, upholsterers, and saddlers. Many of these bourgeois families owned modest amounts of land, houses, and furniture, as evidenced by the bequests made to children (and in some cases, siblings) as part of the process of freeing them from guardianship, and these are many of the same bourgeois families that made bequests to the hospitals of Provins.[9]

During the two principal fairs that took place in Troyes (the "hot" fair ran from mid-July until September 14, while the "cold" fair of Saint Rémi lasted from November 2 until the week before Christmas) the city's population swelled, creating both economic opportunities and placing a strain on the city in various ways.[10] One of the paradoxes about the urbanization and commercial growth of this period across Europe is that profound economic and social transformations were accompanied by what at least appeared to be a rise in poverty. According to contemporary chronicles, the streets of European towns and cities were frequently clogged with poor beggars. When Denis de Champguyon, the dean of the cathedral chapter in Troyes, drew up his testament in 1299, he allocated 20 *l. t.* to be distributed to the poor of Troyes on the day of his burial. If, as was typical of these kinds of funeral pittances, each poor person was meant to receive 1 *d.*, Pierre had left enough to distribute to some 4,800 poor people in a city of—at most—20,000 people, and his testament even instructed his executors to distribute more

---

8. Michel Veissière, "Provins et ses environs à la fin du XIIIe siècle: A propos d'une publication récente (Censier de l'hôtel-Dieu de Provins)," *Provins et sa region: Bulletin de la Société d'histoire et d'archéologie de Provins* 131 (1977): 31–34. For an edition of the *censier*, see M. T. Morlet and M. Mulon, eds., "Le censier de l'Hôtel-Dieu de Provins," *Bibliothèque de l'École des Chartes*," 134 (1976): 5–84. The manuscripts for the *censiers* are found in AD: Seine-et-Marne, 11Hdt B177–B182.

9. Véronique Terrasse, *Provins: Une commune du comté de Champagne et de Brie (1152–1355)* (Paris: L'Harmattan, 2005). For a critical edition of the cartulary, see *Actes et comptes de la commune de Provins de l'an 1271 à l'an 1330*, ed. Maurice Prou and Jules d'Auriac (Provins, France: Briard, 1933).

10. On the influence of the fairs on the growth of the urban population, see Chapin, *Les villes de foires de Champagne*, 29–52.

coins if more poor people than expected were to show up.[11] Yet the reasons for an increase in charitable activity and the emergence of new institutional forms of charity are complex and cannot be explained merely as a response to an increase in poverty. Spiritual anxiety about the profits being made in the new economy, for example, may have contributed to an increase in alms-giving as much as a perceived rise in material poverty.[12] More generally, the intensely commercial nature of the county and the resulting prosperity are vital for understanding the proliferation of hospitals during the twelfth and thirteenth centuries.

As Theodore Evergates has shown, while Count Thibaut was the "pri-mary architect" of the county's trade fairs, it was his son, Count Henri "the Liberal," who "transformed them from regional exchanges into interna-tional centers of commerce and finance," making the fairs "the engine of his principality's prosperity and the primary source of his own revenues."[13] The counts continued to play a vital role not only in promoting the fairs but also in overseeing a system of public law courts that ensured that contracts were enforced and merchants' security and property rights safeguarded, regard-less of where the merchant was from.[14] The economic prosperity generated by Champagne's fairs was also a vital source of revenue for the county's hospitals, just as it was for its monastic houses, and this was true in other regions as well.[15] Apart from the six major annual fairs at Troyes, Provins, Bar-sur-Aube, and Lagny, there were also twelve smaller comital fairs.[16] In addition, a number of lords hosted their own fairs in places like Nogent-sur-Seine, Nogent-l'Artaud, Bar-sur-Seine, Merrey, Plancy, and Perthes. These non-comital, seigneurial fairs, while smaller, were nonetheless important sources of revenue for monasteries, especially during the twelfth century, while during the early thirteenth century the revenues from these fairs

---

11. AD: Aube G2633 (1299).

12. Little, *Religious Poverty*.

13. Evergates, *Henry the Liberal*, 78, 174.

14. In addition to the princely court system, municipal courts and ecclesiastical tribunals also played a role at the fairs. See Edwards and Ogilvie, "What Lessons for Economic Development," 132–35.

15. The fair of Guibray, for example, which was the largest in lower Normandy, generated signif-icant revenues for both the hospital of Saint-Michel de Falaise and the leprosary of Falaise. Together, these two hospitals possessed a majority of the fair's stalls outside the permanent walls. See Arnoux, *Des clercs au service de la réforme*, 121 and note 27, 124.

16. See Bourquelot, *Études sur les foires*, 75–108. See also Michel Bur, "Remarques sur les plus anciens documents concernant les foires de Champagne," in *La Champagne médiévale: Recueil d'articles*, ed. Michel Bur (Langres, France: Dominique Guéniot, 2005), 463–84; Bur, "Note sur quelque petites foires comtales de Champagne," in *La Champagne médiévale*, 485–97.

were increasingly redirected from monasteries to hospitals located in these areas.[17] For instance, Count Milon added a second fair at Bar-sur-Seine in 1210 to support the hospital of Saint-Jean-Baptiste, which he had recently founded in the town.[18] The fair was to be held in June on the vigil and feast day of Saint John the Baptist. In addition to the seigneurial and comital fairs, Champagne also hosted fairs in the episcopal cities of Langres, Châlons-sur-Marne, and Reims. Most importantly, many of the rents that Champagne's hospitals and religious houses received came from the fairs. Recent work by economic historians has shown that Champagne's trade fairs flourished for longer than previously thought and only began to decline after 1296.[19] This corresponds with the continued prosperity of the county's largest hospitals, which saw a surge in the number of bequests they received during the second half of the thirteenth century, unlike many monasteries, which experienced a decline in pious gifts.

Champagne's economic prosperity was vital for its charitable institutions, and a central feature of the county's economy was the active market in fiefs, in which hospitals and monasteries participated and from which they benefited. The fief served as a significant income-producing investment. Just as monasteries purchased the *mouvance* or lordship of fiefs, so too did some hospitals, as we shall have occasion to observe in greater detail in chapter 4. But in addition to directly profiting from fiefs over which they exercised lordship, hospitals were also the beneficiaries of a wide range of gifts from other fiefholders. Champagne's aristocracy played a critical role in fueling the rise of hospitals. As important as the counts were in founding many hospitals and endowing them with properties, the subsequent gifts made by aristocratic families like the Garlandes, Plessis-aux-Tournelles, Dampierres, and Saint-Sépulchres were equally vital. A competitive culture among the aristocracy of making charitable bequests helped propel members of these families to outdo their rivals (whether other families or relatives) in the scale and frequency of their charitable giving. And by the late twelfth and early thirteenth centuries, giving to hospitals was very much in vogue, even threatening to eclipse giving to monastic houses.

---

17. Michel Bur, "Les 'autres' foires de Champagne," in *La Champagne médiévale: Recueil d'articles*, ed. Michel Bur (Langres, France: Dominique Guéniot, 2005), 512–13. Bur notes that the Champenois aristocracy experienced financial constraints during the 1250s and 1260s that led them to re-appropriate revenues from the fairs that they had been directing to hospitals and monasteries.

18. Bur, "Les 'autres' foires de Champagne," 510. See Alphonse Roserot, *Dictionnaire historique de la Champagne méridionale, Aube: des origines à 1790* (Angers, France: Edition de l'Ouest, 1948), 1:128.

19. Edwards and Ogilvie, "What Lessons for Economic Development."

By this time, however, fiefholding in Champagne was no longer domi-nated by the aristocracy.[20] Moreover, many people who did not have knightly status, such as squires ("armigeri"), who were non-noble, non-knightly members of the lower aristocracy, owned fiefs, and many of them shared their profits with hospitals. Women represented a powerful subset of Cham-pagne's property holders, since partible inheritance meant that women were regularly the heirs of property. Some 20 percent of the count's fiefs were held by women.[21] As we shall see in the next chapter, women who were act-ing on their own were frequent donors to Champagne's hospitals, but even in the case of donations by a man, the consent of his wife or sister was often required.

The Largesse of the Counts and Countesses

Champagne's counts served as significant patrons, protectors, and founders of the county's hospitals, and this was true in other regions of northern France as well.[22] The most famously generous of Champagne's counts was Henri I "the Liberal," who was to have a profound impact on the county's charitable and religious institutions.[23] But even his father Count Thibaut II (r. 1125–1152) was known to show unusual compassion toward the poor and sick. A story that was included by Caesarius of Heisterbach, Jacques de Vitry, Étienne de Bourbon, and Thomas of Cantimpré in their *exempla* col-lections and then repeated by thirteenth-century preachers in their sermons recounted Thibaut's close relationship with a certain leper who lived near Sézanne. The count was known to frequently visit the leper, wash his feet, give him alms, and give him the kiss of peace. According to the *exemplum*, after Thibaut once visited the leper, he was told that the leper had actually died and been buried some time earlier, leading the count to conclude that the leprous man he had just visited was in fact Christ disguised as a leper.[24] This anecdote, which would have had particular meaning in Champagne since it took place there and involved Count Thibaut, was meant to illustrate

---

20. Theodore Evergates, *The Aristocracy in the County of Champagne* (Philadelphia: University of Pennsylvania Press, 2007), 52–53.

21. Evergates, *Aristocracy*, 28.

22. Bernard Delmaire, "Hôpitaux urbains et hôpitaux ruraux en Artois entre le XIIe et XIVe siècle," *Histoire médiévale et archéologie* 17 (2004): 221–40.

23. See Evergates, *Henry the Liberal*.

24. Caesarius of Heisterbach, *Dialogus miraculorum*, dist. 8, ch. 31, p. 105; Jacques de Vitry, *The Exempla*, no. 94, pp. 43–44; Stephani de Borbone, *Tractatus de diversis materiis praedicabilibus*, 351–52; See also Touati, *Maladie et société*, 210–15; Lester, *Creating Cistercian Nuns*, 137 and note 74.

the powerful count's humble service to a disfigured leper and dramatize the potential spiritual rewards for performing this kind of charitable service. The count's interest in helping the downtrodden was credited as being one of the reasons that Bernard of Clairvaux developed such a special rapport with him. According to the *First Life of Saint Bernard*, "There wasn't a work of charity that Thibaut didn't practice; his house was a port where all castaways found a refuge."[25] Bernard reportedly urged the count to personally visit the sick and poor in hospitals, and Thibaut followed this advice. He was also known to appoint two Premonstratensian canons to ensure that wherever the count traveled, the sick and leprous would be fed at the count's table. These canons were also expected to travel around the county during the winter with sacks, distributing clothes, skins, bonnets, shoes, and lard to all the poor.[26] Writing in the 1190s, some forty years after Thibaut's death, the Premonstratensian chronicler, Robert of Auxerre, remembered him as having been "father of orphans and protector of widows, eyes of the blind, feet of the deformed; singularly generous in supporting the poor, in fostering the monastic life, and in exhibiting an incomparable largess toward religious of all kinds."[27]

As Sethina Watson has shown, it was common for the political emergence of medieval towns to foster new institutional forms of charity.[28] Charity could itself serve as an expression of political order, with even a hospital's location generating political meaning.[29] As soon as Philip Augustus retook Normandy in 1204, for example, he began providing for Normandy's hospitals as a way to ingratiate himself with the Norman urban elite.[30] Theodore Evergates has demonstrated that "the rise of Champagne as one of the more important princely states of twelfth-century France . . . can be attributed largely to the interests, vision, and policies of Henry the Liberal," Count Thibaut's son.[31] It was Henri who transformed the city of Troyes from an episcopal city to a comital capital, with a new administrative and residential palace located in the St. Denis suburb. Indeed, as important as the trade fairs of Troyes and Provins were to the growth of these cities, their role as the administrative

25. Henri d'Arbois de Jubainville, *Histoire des ducs et des comtes de Champagne*, vol. 2 (Paris: Aug Durand, 1860), 340–41.

26. Henri d'Arbois de Jubainville, *Histoire des ducs*.

27. Evergates, *Henry the Liberal*, 32.

28. Watson, "City as Charter: Charity and the Lordship of English Towns, 1170–1250," in *Cities, Texts, and Social Networks, 400–1500: Experiences and Perceptions of Medieval Urban Space*, ed. Caroline Goodson, Anne E. Lester, and Carol Symes (Farnham, U.K.: Ashgate, 2010).

29. Watson, "City as Charter."

30. Touati, "La géographie hospitalière," 17.

31. Evergates, *Henry the Liberal*, viii.

centers and residences of the counts was equally vital to the expansion and increasing economic vitality of these cities.[32] Perhaps inspired by his father's generosity, Henri went even further in patronizing chapters of secular canons, monastic houses, hospitals, and leprosaria. Apart from his patronage of religious and charitable houses, however, Henri oversaw the economic and cultural development of the city. He initiated the building of a network of secondary canals that helped irrigate the city and led to the establishment of tanners and butchers and the erection of a number of mills around the city, some of them owned by hospitals. The count and countess surrounded themselves at the comital court with writers, poets, and theologians.

Henri's reputation for being generous earned him the nickname "the Liberal" ("le Large"). At Henri's funeral, the dean of the comital chapel of Saint-Étienne distributed the staggering sum of 4,000 *l.* to the poor, as if, in the words of Evergates, "to seal Henry's reputation for generosity."[33] The secular cleric, Walter Map, who served the English king, Henry II (a contemporary of Count Henri of Champagne's and a hospital founder and patron in his French domains in his own right), and was once hosted by the count in Troyes, called him "the most generous ["largissimus"] of men, so much so that to many he seemed prodigal, for to all who asked, he gave."[34] Yet according to Map, the count also recognized the necessary limits of generosity, "for if you seek to give ill-begotten gains, you become miserly in order to seem generous."[35] The well-known story recounted by Jean de Joinville, who hailed from the Champagne region, about Henri and his treasurer, Artaud of Nogent-l'Artaud, was, as Evergates has put it, primarily "a cautionary tale about the presumptions of a nouveau riche," in this case represented by Artaud himself.[36] The story also revealed the contemporary perception that the count's generosity knew no limits. According to the story, a poor knight approaches the count, just as he is entering the church of Saint-Étienne in Troyes to hear Mass, to ask him for dowries for his two daughters. Artaud reprimands the knight for his lack of courtesy toward the count, saying that

---

32. Nicholas, *Growth of the Medieval City*, 89.

33. Evergates, *Henry the Liberal*, 164.

34. Evergates, *Henry the Liberal*, 157. On King Henry II of England as a patron and founder of hospitals, see Lindy Grant, "Royal and Aristocratic Hospital Patronage in Northern France in the Twelfth and Early Thirteenth Centuries," in *Laienadel und Armenfürsorge im Mittelalter*, ed. Lukas Clemens, Katrin Dort, and Felix Schumacher (Trier, Germany: Kliomedia, 2015), 105–14.

35. Evergates, *Henry the Liberal*, 157.

36. Evergates, *Aristocracy*, 182. On the different versions of this story, see Evergates, *Henry the Liberal*, 180–81; Stephani de Borbone, *Tractatus de diversis materiis praedicabilibus*, 327; Goswin Frenken, ed., *Die Exempla des Jacob von Vitry: Ein Beitrag zur Geschichte der Erzählungsliteratur des Mittelalters* (Munich, 1914), 106–7.

Henri has given away so much of his wealth that he had nothing more to give.[37] Henri then severely scolds Artaud for saying this, and to Artaud's horror, the count gives him to the poor knight as charity. Artaud is only able to regain his freedom after paying the poor knight a ransom of 500 *l*. Apart from conveying the count's suspicion of the *nouveau riche*, the story also illustrated the great lengths the count was willing to go to help those in need. Perhaps Artaud learned from the count's spirit of generosity, since Artaud's name appears in the martyrological obituary for the hospital of Provins as having funded the building of a separate dormitory and refectory for the hospital sisters.[38]

Among the *exempla* in Jacques de Vitry's collection was a second story involving Count Henri that was intended to illustrate the potential material benefit of investing or giving as opposed to hoarding.[39] When the count is confronted with a naked, nine-year-old beggar who has nothing in which to keep the money that he has been given, the count gives him a penny and tells him to buy a purse with it and then to return. But the boy ends up buying a small purse with a halfpenny so that he can keep the other halfpenny for himself. When the count discovers what the boy has done, he explains to him that if he had used the whole penny to buy a larger purse, the count would have been able to fill it with twice as many pennies, and the boy would have ended up with far more. The moral of the story—that the more one invests and gives away, the more one will acquire—bears a strong resemblance to some of the *exempla* discussed in the previous chapter about the material benefits of almsgiving, but in this story it was the famously generous count of Champagne who served as the moral instructor.

Among the hospitals that Count Henri founded were the hôtel-Dieu-le-Comte in Troyes, the hospital of Saint-Abraham in Troyes, the hospital of Provins, the hôtel-Dieu Saint-Esprit in Provins, and the hospital of Sézanne.[40] Henri's wife, Marie de France, initiated the rebuilding of the hospital of Lagny in 1194. Due to the counts' patronage of hospitals, relatively few twelfth-century, non-comital, seigneurial hospitals were founded in Champagne, especially in the dioceses of Troyes, Châlons, and Sens, where the counts

---

37. Jean de Joinville, *Vie de Saint Louis*, ed. Jacques Monfrin (Paris: Dunod, 1995), nos. 90–91, p. 47.

38. *Recueil des historiens de la France: Obituaires de la province de Sens*, ed. Auguste Molinier, vol. 1, part 2 (Paris: Imprimerie Nationale, 1906), 965.

39. Frenken, ed., *Die Exempla des Jacob von Vitry*, 107.

40. The counts of Bar-sur-Seine were also active in founding hospitals. Count Milon IV founded the hospital of Bar-sur-Seine in 1210 with the consent of his wife and their son. See Roserot, *Diction-naire*.

made their power felt.[41] But during the thirteenth century this changed, especially in the northwest and southeast, where comital power was weaker, and
a number of seigneurial hospitals were founded in towns such as Rethel,
Porcien, Roucy, Coucy, Tonnerre, Ligny, Noyers, Grancey, and Châteauvil-
lain.[42] These seigneurial hospital foundations, however, tended to be poorer
than the comital and urban hospitals of Troyes, Provins, Bar-sur-Aube, and
Meaux. Even in a diocese like Meaux, however, there were hospitals founded
by lords, like the hospital in Crécy-en-Brie, founded before 1209 by Gaucher de Châtillon, who was lord of Crécy and count of Saint-Pol. Gaucher
endowed this hospital with land, vineyards, a tithe, a house, and rents from
the toll and commercial halls of Crécy. Gaucher's son, Hugues, continued to
patronize his father's hospital foundation even while founding an abbey of
his own at Pont-Notre Dame.[43]

The counts and countesses also showed a deep concern with supporting
the religious life inside hospitals. In 1208, for example, Countess Blanche of
Navarre, who was the mother of Thibaut IV, gave the hôtel-Dieu-le-Comte
some land at Bray that she had just purchased to fund the hospital's hiring of
a priest to serve its chapel of Sainte Marguerite.[44] Just a year later, the countess founded a daily mass for the dead at the hospital for the late Clarembaud
de Chappes, and she gave a rent of 10 l. from the entrances to the fairs of
Troyes to pay for the priest's prebend.[45] She also made a donation of forty
arpents of land to the hospital of Château-Thierry in 1203.[46] A second hospital, La Barre, was established in Château-Thierry in 1211 by Guy de la Barre,
a canon at the comital chapel of Château-Thierry.[47] Within a year, Countess
Blanche had taken over the hospital, had put up the funds to build a chapel
there, and was referring to the hospital as her foundation.[48] In 1235–36 Count

---

41. There were certainly examples already in the twelfth century of non-comital, seigneurial
hospital foundations, especially some distance from Troyes and Provins. In 1165, shortly before he
entered Clairvaux as a monk, the castle lord Jean de Possesse, with the assent of his brother Hugh,
established a hospital for pilgrims and the poor in Possesse, on the northeast periphery of Champagne. See John Benton and Michel Bur, eds., *Recueil des actes d'Henri le Libéral, comte de Champagne
(1152–1181)* (Paris, 2009), no. 231, p. 304. On Jean de Possesse, see Evergates, *Henry the Liberal*, 112–14.

42. Bur, "Les 'autres' foires de Champagne," 499–512.

43. Henri Stein, "Cartulaire de l'hôtel-Dieu de Crecy-en-Brie," *Bulletin de la conference d'histoire et
d'archéologie du diocèse de Meaux* 2 (1899): 136–45.

44. Arbois de Jubainville, *Histoire des ducs*, vol. 5 (Paris: A. Durand, 1863), no. 629, p. 40.

45. Arbois de Jubainville, *Histoire des ducs*, vol. 5, no. 714, p. 54.

46. AD: Aisne H-dépot 19, non côté (25 March 1203).

47. These two thirteenth-century hospitals in Château-Thierry are often confused or conflated
with each other.

48. Theodore Evergates, *Feudal Society in Medieval France: Documents from the County of Champagne* (Philadelphia: University of Pennsylvania Press, 1993), 140–42.

Thibaud IV converted the hospital of La Barre into a female Cistercian house that continued to oversee the hospital.[49] When Jeanne of Navarre, the countess of Champagne, queen regent of Navarre, and queen consort of France, drew up her testament in March of 1305, just weeks before her death, she, too, founded a hospital in Château-Thierry.[50]

In order for a fief to be alienated, the lord had to grant a license, also called an amortization, which was usually accompanied by a fee. Historians of monasticism in Champagne have observed that by the second half of the thirteenth century, the counts who earlier had been quite lax in granting amortizations to religious institutions had become increasingly restrictive in alienating their fiefs, now charging monasteries for grants of amortization.[51] For the most part, however, the counts continued to grant free amortizations to hospitals, perhaps reflecting that they viewed hospitals differently than monasteries, whether as more charitable and thus more deserving of their support or simply as being in greater financial need.[52] But thirteenth-century counts also lent significant financial support to hospitals in other forms. In his testament of 1257, Count Thibaut V left 200 *l.* for the hospitals of Provins, 100 *l.* for the hospitals of Vitry, 100 *l.* for the hospital of Château-Thierry, 100 *l.* for the hospital of Montmirail, 200 *l.* for the hospitals of Troyes, 60 *l.* for the hospital of Sézanne, and 50 *l.* for the hospital of Meaux. Thibaut also allocated 20 *l.* for hospitals in his castles, indicating that well into the thirteenth century, counts were continuing to oversee the provision of charity directly from their residences. And like other aristocrats who allocated funds to be distributed to the poor at their funerals, Thibaut left a staggering 1,000 *l.* to poor commoners for purchasing clothing and shoes on the feast of Saint Rémi after his death.[53] Thibaut's charity may have been influenced by the

---

49. See Lester, *Creating Cistercian Nuns*, 41–42, 65; Evergates, *Aristocracy*, 75; C. Nusse, "Charte de fondation d'un Hôtel-Dieu à Barre," *Annales de la Société historique et archéologique de Château-Thierry* 48 (1874): 191–92.

50. Elizabeth A. R. Brown, "La mort, les testaments et les fondations de Jeanne de Navarre, reine de France (1273–1305)," in *Une histoire pour un royaume (XIIe–XVe siècle). Actes du colloque Corpus Regni organisé en hommage à Colette Beaune*, ed. Anne-Hélène Allirot (Paris: Perrin, 2010), 124–41.

51. See, for example, Lester, *Creating Cistercian Nuns*, 195–99.

52. In 1269, Count Thibaut V gave general charters of amortization to the hôtel-Dieu-le-Comte of Troyes, the hospital of Provins, and the hospital of Meaux. See Arbois de Jubainville, *Histoire des ducs*, vol. 6, nos. 3567 (p. 51), 3572 (p. 52), 3592 (p. 55). In his general grant of amortization to the hospital of Provins in 1269, Thibaut made clear that he was acting "for the sake of piety and on account of the salvation of our soul and that of our predecessors." See Dupraz, no. 59; AD: Seine-et-Marne 11Hdt A12, fol. 26. In 1273 Count Henri III made another free grant of amortization of specific properties acquired by the hospital, and he indicated that he considered the hospital his own ("nostre Meson Dieu"). See Dupraz, no. 60 AD: Seine-et-Marne 11Hdt A12, fol. 26–26v.

53. Alexandre Teulet, et al., eds., *Layettes du trésor des chartes* (Paris, 1863–1909), 3:391–92. An English translation of this testament can be found in Evergates, *Feudal Society*, 70–72.

example of his father-in-law, King Louis IX (the two were together for the opening of the new hospital the king founded at Compiègne), and Thibaut also had the examples of his own ancestors and comital predecessors.[54] Among the many other ways that the counts supported hospitals was giving them prebends over which they had collation: the hôtel-Dieu-le-Comte was given prebends in the chapter of Saint-Étienne, the hospital of Provins was given a prebend in the chapel of the comital palace for one year whenever a canon died, and likewise, the hospital of Bar-sur-Aube collected the prebend for one year when a canon died from the chapter of Saint-Georges of Bar.[55]

Although we usually think about Champagne's counts and countesses as the patrons of religious and charitable institutions, they could also turn to these institutions for assistance. Faced with significant indebtedness in 1226, Count Thibaut IV (whose debts by 1228 had amounted to 23,340 *l. t.*) turned to the abbey of Saint-Denis outside Paris for a loan of 2,000 *l. parisis*.[56] The count already had a dependent relationship with the royal abbey in that he had sworn homage to it for his possessions at Nogent-sur-Seine. In order to secure this loan from the abbey, he turned to yet another religious institution, namely his own comital chapter of secular canons at Saint-Étienne in Troyes to ask that it provide him with two precious liturgical objects—a gold altar table and a large gold cross—to give to Saint-Denis as collateral for the loan. The most powerful patrons of religious and charitable institutions, in other words, relied upon these institutions for credit in times of need.

The Hospitals of Troyes

By the mid-thirteenth century, the city of Troyes had an increasingly diverse set of religious communities, with six parishes; several abbeys (including the recently established Augustinian abbey of Notre-Dame-en-Isle, the Cistercian abbey of Notre-Dame-des-Près); Dominican and Franciscan convents (founded in 1232 and 1236, respectively); several chapters of secular canons, including the cathedral of Saint-Pierre, the comital chapter of Saint-Étienne, and the chapter of Saint-Urbain; five hospitals; as well as several commanderies belonging to hospital-military orders, some of which were managing

---

54. On royal and aristocratic hospital patronage, see Grant, "Royal and Aristocratic Hospital Patronage."

55. Arbois de Jubainville, *Histoire des ducs*, vol. 4.2, p. 626.

56. Thomas Lacomme, "Gager sa dette avec le mobilier liturgique: Thibaud IV de Champagne, l'abbaye de Saint-Denis et la collégiale Saint-Étienne de Troyes (XIIIe siècle)," *Éditions du CRINI* 9 (2017).

their own hospitals (the Templars, the Antonines, and the Trinitarians).[57] The leprosary of Les Deux Eaux, which had been founded by 1123, was located just three kilometers south of Troyes. A number of aristocratic families placed young family members there, and some older aristocrats, particularly widows, chose to spend their final years wearing the religious habit at this leprosary.[58] By 1300, it was the wealthiest of the twenty-eight leprosaries in the diocese of Troyes, with an annual revenue of 700 *l. t.* and extensive properties, including granges, houses, land, vineyards, tithes, rents, and a mill.[59] Much of the support these various religious institutions received came from revenue generated by a robust market in fiefs as well as the commerce that flourished at Troyes's three annual fairs and various markets. But religious institutions, including hospitals, also participated directly in these fairs and markets, and they frequently purchased fiefs as income-producing investments. The chapter of Saint-Étienne in Troyes had its own market at Clos for two weeks each January, and the leprosary of Les Deux Eaux also had its own one-day fair, as did the abbey of Notre-Dame-aux-Nonnains.[60]

By far the largest, wealthiest, and most prestigious hospital in Troyes was the hôtel-Dieu-le-Comte, which by 1300 had an annual revenue of 2,000 *l.*

---

57. During the twelfth and early thirteenth centuries, the Templars had a significant presence in the area around Troyes, with commanderies in Troyes, Avaleur, Bonlieu, Fresnoy, Mesnil-Saint-Loup, Payns, Perchois, Resson, Sancey, Serre near Montceaux, Thors, and Villiers. The Templars of Troyes even had the financial resources to spend the staggering sum of 10,000 *l.* in 1229 for the repurchase of a right in the count's forest. It is difficult to know, however, just how active the Templars were in the management of hospitals. Damien Carraz has argued that they were far less active in managing hospitals in Provence, for example, than in Champagne or Italy. The Templars were overseeing the hospital of Saint-Nicolas in Langres (dep. Haute-Marne), the hospital at Chappes (dep. Aube), and the hospital of Possesse (dep. Marne). See Carraz, *L'ordre du Temple*, 508–9. See also Joseph Roserot de Melin, *Le diocèse de Troyes des origines à nos jours* (Troyes, France: Imprimerie de la Renaissance, 1957), 104, 107; Arnaud Baudin, Ghislain Brunel, and Nicolas Dohrmann, eds., *L'économie templière en Occident: Patrimoines, commerce, finances: Actes du colloque international (Troyes—Abbaye de Clairvaux, 24–26 octobre 2012* (Langres, 2013). By the mid-thirteenth century, the Trinitarians and Antonines had both established foundations in the city of Troyes, and the Hospitallers were managing several hospitals in the diocese of Troyes. See Jean Murard, "L'ordre des Trinitaires ou des Mathurins à Troyes, Bar-sur-Seine et la Gloire-Dieu," *Mémoires de la Société Académique de l'Aube* 129 (1995): 37–56; de Melin, *Le diocèse de Troyes*, 103–4, 106. On the Antonines, see Adalbert Mischlewski, *Un ordre hospitalier au moyen âge: Les chanoines réguliers de Saint-Antoine-en-Viennois* (Grenoble: Presses Universitaires de Grenoble, 1995).

58. Touati, *Maladie et société*, 337–38; Auguste Harmand, "Notice historique sur la léproserie de la ville de Troyes," *Mémoires de la Société Académique de l'Aube* 14 (1848): 429–669.

59. Touati, *Archives de la lèpre*, 44, 65, 380–81.

60. Roserot de Melin, *Le diocèse de Troyes*, 111–12; Boutiot, *Histoire de la ville de Troyes et de la Champagne méridionale* (Troyes, France: Dufey-Robert, 1870), 1:355. Countess Marie established the fair at Les Deux Eaux in 1181 and lent her protection to all merchants (and to their merchandise) coming to and going from the fair. See Harmand, *Notice historique*, 30.

and granges in Chapelle-Saint-Luc, Verdumel, Poivres, and Donnement.[61] The hospital was founded by Count Henri the Liberal around 1157, the year he founded the chapter of Saint-Étienne, which was attached to the new comital palace and served as the count's chapel.[62] Long after its founding, the hospital continued to receive a wide range of privileges and exemptions from the counts, and it also enjoyed papal protection, beginning with Pope Celestine III in 1197. The hospital originally bore the same name as the chapter of Saint-Étienne and was administered by its canons. Both the chapter and the hospital were located in the "new town" of Troyes (beyond the old walled city), the bustling commercial and industrial center that had been developed by Count Henri the Liberal and was under his jurisdiction. The church of Saint-Étienne, the first Gothic church in southern Champagne, was actually the largest church in Troyes until the cathedral was rebuilt in the 1220s (following the devastating fire of 1188), and the church rivaled the cathedral in beauty and size.[63]

Poor relief could serve as a divisive force, sometimes giving rise to jurisdictional conflicts among elites, as was true in twelfth-century Troyes, where the two largest hospitals served as surrogates in a political struggle between their respective patrons, the bishop of Troyes and the count of Champagne. Tensions between Count Henri I and the bishop of Troyes and his cathedral canons had already flared in 1152, and these kinds of tensions and rivalries extended to relations between the hospital of Saint-Nicolas, which was under the authority of the cathedral, and the hôtel-Dieu-le-Comte, under the jurisdiction of the count and Saint-Étienne.[64] Although at its founding, the chapter of Saint-Étienne was exempt from episcopal control, much to the consternation of Count Henri, in 1169 the pope confirmed that the chapter was part of the bishop's possessions.[65] Faced with protests from the count, the pope briefly reversed himself, giving the chapter a seven-year exemption from episcopal control, only to then confirm in 1171 that Saint-Étienne was

---

61. Auguste Lognon, ed., *Documents relatifs au comté de Champagne et de Brie, 1172–1361* (Paris: Imprimerie Nationale, 1914), 3:131.

62. Roserot, *Dictionnaire*, 3:1563; Evergates, *Henry the Liberal*, 49 and note 63. The foundation charter for the hospital was destroyed in the fire of 1188. The earliest mention of the hospital comes from 1174; see Benton and Bur, eds., *Recueil des actes*, no. 371, pp. 464–65. The hospital's cartulary refers to a later "magna carta" from 1189 in which Henri II confirmed his father's various gifts to the hospital. See Aube: 40H1 (1189, charter from Henri II); 40H189, fol. 97 (copy in the cartulary). On the site of the hôtel-Dieu-le-Comte and the Gallo-Roman parts of its structure, see Michel Lenoble, "Le site de l'ancien hôtel-Dieu de Troyes," *La vie en Champagne* 38, no. 414 (November 1990): 3–18.

63. Evergates, *Henry the Liberal*, 46.

64. Evergates, *Henry the Liberal*, 36–37.

65. Evergates, *Henry the Liberal*, 127.

in fact under the authority of the bishop.[66] In the event, however, no bishop seems to have exercised this right, leaving the comital chapter and canons to manage their own affairs.[67]

When the cathedral chapter of Saint-Pierre in 1222 sought to lower the water level of the Trévois Canal, the hôtel-Dieu-le-Comte, which possessed three mills there, immediately opposed the proposed change.[68] The chapter of Saint-Pierre had been unhappy ever since Count Henri I helped establish the Trévois Canal (using water from the preexisting Moline Canal), which, while useful in bringing much-needed water to the comital palace, the hôtel-Dieu-le-Comte, and the center of the city more generally, also resulted in the lowering of the water on the Moline Canal, where Saint-Pierre had its own mills. The cathedral appealed to the pope, who delegated two judges to arbitrate the conflict. But the hospital was supported by the chapter of Saint-Étienne and the count, who moved to undercut the judges appointed by the pope, suggesting they were incompetent to judge the case. In addition, the provost and townspeople of Troyes also wrote a letter to the judges, laying out the vital functions that the canal served for the city and arguing that they would not tolerate any changes being made to the canal.[69] With its central location in Troyes, its ownership of significant property and rights, and its close association with the count, it was easy for a hospital like the hôtel-Dieu-le-Comte to get embroiled in urban politics, including the power struggles between the count and the bishop.

In the years immediately following the founding of the hôtel-Dieu-le-Comte, its *magister* was a canon from the chapter of Saint-Étienne. But the hospital gradually sought to assert greater autonomy from the chapter, and one way it did so was to align itself even more closely to its principal patron and founder, the count of Champagne, who considered the hospital his own. In a charter from 1199, Count Henri II referred to the hospital as "the hospital which is my own" ("domus Dei que mea est propria").[70] Moreover, by 1214 the hospital began to be referred to in many documents as the "count's hospital" rather than as the "hospital of Saint-Étienne" (that is, belonging to the comital chapter) but the hospital and chapter continued to be interconnected in various ways. One of Henri II's significant grants to the hospital was the right to collect "an *annualia*, or the first-year's income, from each

---

66. Evergates, *Henry the Liberal*, 128.

67. Evergates, *Henry the Liberal*, 130.

68. Arbois de Jubainville, *Histoire des ducs*, 3:257–60.

69. Arbois de Jubainville, *Histoire des ducs*, 3:258–59. On the count's opposition to the judges delegate, see no. 1504.

70. AD Aube 40H1, layette 1, cotte A, no. 22 (September 1199).

new prebendary of St-Étienne," which, as Evergates has suggested, signaled the hospital's "importance as a highly visible social service funded by the count."[71] Tensions grew, however, between the chapter and the hospital, which increasingly sought to exercise greater independence, culminating in Countess Blanche's intervention and imposition of a new rule in 1212.[72] From then on, the hospital's master was named or revoked by the count or countess, not the chapter, although the count was expected to consult the chapter's dean along with two or three canons in selecting a hospital master. Already in 1199, however, it was Countess Marie who appointed Master Herbert, a canon at Saint-Étienne and a doctor ("medicus"), to be the "procurator pauperum" of the hôtel-Dieu, and in 1223 he resigned his office to Thibaut IV.[73] Upon Herbert's becoming magister, the count ordered that his prebend at Saint-Étienne become the property of the hôtel-Dieu. It was also the count, not the dean, who had the authority to receive new brothers and sisters in the hospital. The hospital's financial accounts were reviewed by a commission of two canons from Saint-Étienne, one or two townspeople chosen by the count, the count's almoner, and the hospital's magister, again reflecting that the hospital was not simply under the control of Saint-Étienne.[74] By 1263, when new hospital statutes were drawn up by the count's almoner, the hospital began exerting even greater autonomy, since it was now up to the magister and the hospital's religious community to make their own decisions about whom to receive as members of the community without receiving any input from the count.[75]

Whereas the counts and countesses were deeply invested in the hôtel-Dieu-le-Comte, which was, after all, a comital foundation, they showed little interest in the nearby hospital of Saint-Nicolas, which was under the jurisdiction of the cathedral chapter of Saint-Pierre. Indeed, one of the few comital charters mentioning the hospital of Saint-Nicolas came from Count Thibaut IV,

---

71. Evergates, *Henry the Liberal*, 49.

72. Arbois de Jubainville, *Histoire des ducs*, vol. 5, no. 812, p. 71; Nicholaus Camuzat, *Promptuarium sacrarum antiquitatum Tricassinae diocesis* (V. Moreau, 1610), fol. 401v–402v.

73. AD Aube 40H1, cotte 2; Arbois de Jubainville, *Histoire des ducs*, vol. 5, no. 1581, p. 206.

74. Arbois de Jubainville, *Histoire des ducs*, IV.2, p. 746; Arbois de Jubainville, *Histoire des ducs*, vol. 5, no. 812, p. 71; Camuzat, *Promptuarium*, fol. 402.

75. Philippe Guignard, ed., *Les anciens statuts de l'Hôtel-Dieu-le-Comte de Troyes* (Troyes, 1853), xiii. It was not uncommon for hospitals connected to cathedral chapters to assert some degree of autonomy from the chapter over issues such as the choice of a hospital *magister*. Long-simmering tensions between the reform-minded cathedral canons of Paris and the nearby hôtel-Dieu erupted into violent conflict in 1497, when the canons accused the hospital's *magister* of fraudulent accounting and placed him in prison. The hospital's brothers and sisters were enraged by what they viewed as a violation of their autonomy, and the cathedral was ultimately forced to reinstate the hospital's *magister*. See Christine Jéhanno, "Entre le chapitre cathédral et l'hôtel-Dieu de Paris: les enjeux du conflit de la fin du moyen âge," *Revue Historique*, 313, no. 3 (2011): 527–60.

who austerely demanded that the hospital recognize that it could not acquire anything in Champagne without his consent and the payment of an amortization fee.[76] This was in marked contrast with the many free licenses that he and the other counts granted comital hospital foundations. Because the hospital of Saint-Nicolas grew out of the cathedral's hospital, eventually acquiring its own building while remaining a dependent of the cathedral chapter, there is no clear foundation date.[77] The hospital was housed in close proximity to the cathedral, along Le Meldançon, a tributary of the Seine, in the Saint-Jacques neighborhood. Not surprisingly, a significant percentage of the donors to Saint-Nicolas were clerics, especially canons. However, the hospital was supported by far more townspeople than the more aristocratic hôtel-Dieu-le-Comte, perhaps because many of the donors to the latter wished to associate with what they regarded as the count's hospital.[78] More-over, the rise of Champagne's burgher merchant-artisan class was criti-cal for a hospital like Saint-Nicolas, since it was the townspeople of various occupations—cobblers, roof repairers, launderers, lawyers, and notaries—on whom this hospital largely depended for bequests.[79]

In the high and later Middle Ages, the creation of new religious insti-tutions, such as hospitals with chapels and cemeteries, often sparked juris-dictional disputes, with the defenders of traditional parish rights invariably feeling threatened. From 1245 until 1276, the hospital of Saint-Nicolas was embroiled in a conflict with the curate of Saint-Nizier, who accused the hospital of stealing his parishioners and (unknowingly) administering sacra-ments to excommunicates. The curate tried to force the hospital chapel to cease ringing its bells to signal the start of Mass, which he viewed as violat-ing his prerogatives as curate, and he tried to have the hospital stop burying his parishioners in the hospital cemetery, which he also believed violated his prerogatives and despoiled him of burial fees.[80]

---

76. Arbois de Jubainville, *Histoire des ducs*, IV.2, p. 753; vol. 5, no. 3053, p. 467.

77. See Benton and Bur, eds., *Recueil des actes*, p. 114 on the errors made by Roserot and Lalore in thinking that a charter from 1156 is the earliest to refer to the canons or brothers of the hôtel-Dieu Saint-Nicolas in Troyes; the charter in question actually refers to the monks from the priory of Saint Nicolas-la-Chapelle in Nogent-sur-Seine.

78. The one prominent noble family that did associate with the hospital of Saint-Nicolas was the Saint-Sépulchres, lords of Villacerf and Froiderive.

79. It is possible that the urban franchises of Thibaut IV in 1230–31 may have had an impact on charitable institutions by creating the new social category of the free residents of comital towns like Troyes, Provins, and Bar-sur-Aube. However, in the case of Troyes, by 1240 the count's men had lost their commune. See Theodore Evergates, *Feudal Society in the Bailliage of Troyes Under the Counts of Champagne, 1152–1284* (Baltimore: Johns Hopkins University Press, 1975), 47–55.

80. AD: Aube 43H4, layette 35, no. 1. These kinds of disputes between hospitals and churches were quite common. For another example, see the conflict between the hospital of Nemours and the

The hospital of Saint-Abraham in Troyes was founded as a result of a gift from Count Henri I in 1179, while in Jerusalem, to the bishop and canons of Hebron. This gift included a rent of 60 *l.* and a house in Troyes, which was located just outside the city walls, near the church of Saint-Antoine.[81] It would appear that the bishop of Hebron sent some religious to occupy this house in Troyes, which for a short time continued to be a dependent of the chapter in Hebron. By the thirteenth century, a community of women and men were living in this house, now referred to as a *domus Dei,* and they followed the Augustinian Rule. By 1201, however, Thibaut III had entrusted the hospital to the abbot and convent of Saint-Martin de Troyes.[82] Another hospital within Troyes was the hospital of Saint-Bernard, which was founded by 1123. Unlike the other hospitals in the city, Saint-Bernard had an exclusively male religious community.[83] Charters identified the hospital as being near the wheat or millstone market ("domus Dei molarum" or "in foro situm est"), another reminder of the close association between the provision of charity and commerce.[84] In 1158, with the consent of the bishop of Troyes, Count Henry I made the hospital a dependent of the Great Saint Bernard Hospice of Montjoux, in Switzerland (founded in the eleventh century by St. Bernard of Montjoux), a facility for travelers that was overseen by regular canons.[85] The site of this hospice, high in the Pennine Alps, was the mountain pass used by Italian merchants when they traveled to and from Champagne's fairs. In 1174 Count Henri I gave the hospital of Saint-Bernard in Troyes the privilege of using the hôtel-Dieu-le-Comte's mills each week,

---

church of Saint-Jean de Nemours, both founded in the 1170s by the French royal chamberlain and lord of Nemours, Gauthier I de Villebéon. The church challenged the hospital's right to have a bell, to administer sacraments, to raise orphans, to baptize children, to conduct religious processions on feast days, to collect certain tithes, to celebrate Mass at certain times of the day, and so forth. See E. Richemond, *Recherche généalogiques sur la famille des seigneurs de Nemours du XIIe au XVe siècles* (Fontainebleau, France: Maurice Bourges, 1907), vol. 1, xvi–xviii.

81. Arbois de Jubainville, *Histoire des ducs,* vol. 2, no. 314, p. 381.

82. Arbois de Jubainville, *Histoire des ducs,* vol. 5, no. 534, p. 24. Theodore Evergates, ed., *The Cartulary of Countess Blanche of Champagne* (Toronto: University of Toronto Press, 2010), no. 228, p. 214.

83. The hospital of Saint-Bernard had already been founded by the time of Count Hugues, as is made clear in a charter of Count Henri I in 1158. See Benton and Bur, eds., *Recueil des actes,* no. 117, pp. 159–60. See also Boutiot, *Histoire de la ville de Troyes,* 1:179.

84. See the charter (1158) of Henri the Liberal in Benton and Bur, eds., *Recueil des actes,* no. 117, p. 160. Albert Babeau, "L'hôtel-Dieu Saint-Bernard de Troyes," *Annuaire administratif, statistique et commercial du département de l'Aube* 80 (1906): 33; Roserot de Melin, *Le diocèse de Troyes,* 107.

85. The hospital of Diu-li-Mire (or "Deo Medico") in Reims was also affiliated with the regular canons of Montjoux. See Desportes, *Reims et les Rémois,* 306; Prosper Tarbé, *Reims: Essais historique sur les rues et ses monuments* (Reims: Librairie de Quentin-Dailly, 1844), 375.

free of charge, to grind a certain amount of grain.[86] A hospital affiliated with
the hospital order of Saint Esprit, which had been founded in Montpellier
around 1180, was established just outside Troyes, near the gate of Croncels,
at some point before 1203.[87] Although this hospital order was associated with
the care of abandoned children, it also cared for the poor and the sick, and
there is a record from 1229 of an "infirmarius" assisting the *magister* of the
hospital of Saint-Esprit in Troyes.[88] In the diocese of Troyes as a whole, it has
been estimated that during the twelfth and thirteenth centuries there were
more than fifty hospitals, many of them rural.[89]

The Hospitals of Provins

During the thirteenth century, Champagne's second comital capital, Provins,
had a growing population that may even have reached twenty thousand, and
like Troyes, Meaux, and many other cities had had to expand its walls to
encompass new neighborhoods.[90] The counts and countesses exerted strong
influence on religious institutions in Provins, even stronger in some ways
than in Troyes since there was no local bishop with whom to compete. Nor
was the status of Provins as a commune nearly as brief as it was in Troyes.
The city continued to function as a commune well beyond 1285, when the
county became part of the royal domain, yet given the continued strength of
the comital administration, Provins was never autonomous like some other
communes in northern France and the Low Countries.[91] The city developed
as a major commercial city quite a bit earlier than Troyes. By the late twelfth
century, Provins had developed an international reputation for its production
of woolen fabric, and this flourishing industry helped attract moneychangers,
financiers, and townspeople of various occupations. The mint of Provins,
paradoxically located right next to the city's main hospital for the poor and
sick, produced the *denier provinois*, the standard coinage for all of Champagne's fairs and the dominant coin of eastern France. A significant percentage of the profits from the coins went to the counts and countesses.[92] Provins
also had its own measures and weights. The city hosted two major annual

86. Benton and Bur, eds., *Recueil des actes*, no. 371, pp. 464–65; Boutiot, *Histoire de la ville de Troyes*,
1:219; Arbois de Jubainville, *Histoire des ducs*, vol. 3, no. 220, p. 365.

87. Boutiot, *Histoire de la ville de Troyes*, 1:292.

88. François-Olivier Touati, "Un dossier à rouvrir: L'assistance au moyen âge," in *Fondations et
oeuvres charitables au moyen âge*, ed. Jean DuFour and Henri Platelle (Paris: Éditions du CTHS, 1999), 36.

89. De Melin, *Le diocèse de Troyes*, 108.

90. Terrasse, *Provins*, 94–100.

91. Terrasse, *Provins*.

92. Bourquelot, *Histoire de Provins*, 160.

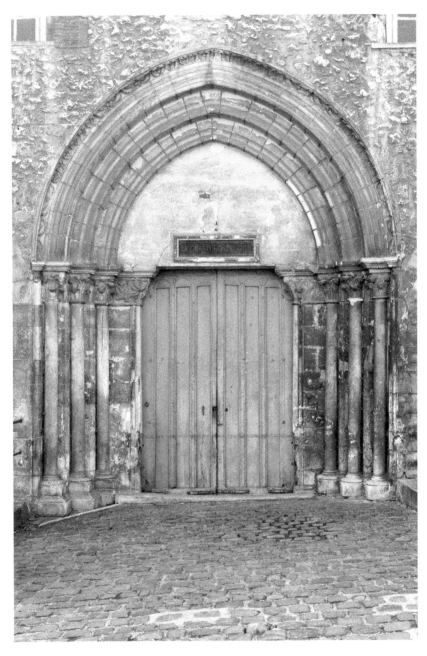

FIGURE 3. The hôtel-Dieu of Provins. Coyau / Wikimedia Commons / CC BY-SA 3.0.

fairs: the May fair, which lasted for forty-six days in the spring, and the fair of Saint-Ayoul, which ran from September 14 until All Saints.[93] In addition to these fairs, the city hosted the fair of Saint Martin, running from November 30 until January 1, and the upper village hosted a weekly market on Tuesdays.[94] As was the case for Troyes, Provins's religious and charitable institutions were themselves key players in the ethos of exchange that marked an increasingly commercial economy. These institutions were engaged in their own profit-making so that they had the resources to carry out their religious and charitable functions. During the thirteenth century, both the chapter of Saint-Quiriace and the city's largest hospital rented houses to merchants who came to Provins for the fairs.[95]

The origins of the largest hospital in Provins, the "grand hôtel-Dieu," so-called to distinguish it from the "petit hôtel-Dieu," about which there is virtually no information, are somewhat obscure, since there is no foundation charter extant.[96] The erudite seventeenth-century Provinois Eustache Grillon believed that the hospital was founded ca. 1050 by Count Thibaut I.[97] The hospital must have already been well known during the mid-twelfth century, since the abbot of Saint-Marian d'Auxerre, a certain Régnier, lived out the end of his life at the Provinois hospital and was often visited there by Count Thibaut. In 1146 the abbot was buried at the hospital, "a poor of Christ among the poor," as a chronicle put it.[98] The earliest act for this hospital is from ca. 1141–1145, whereby Count Thibaut II confirmed that Anseau le Gras and his father, Garnier, gave the *domus Dei* of Saint Jacques (before it was moved, around 1157) a house in Provins and a rent of 40 *sous* on the fair of May.[99] Once again, we see a case of a hospital's revenue tied to the fairs,

---

93. Bourquelot, *Études sur les foires*, 81–82.

94. Bourquelot, *Études sur les foires*, 102–4; Victor Carrière, *Histoire et cartulaire des Templiers de Provins* (Paris: Librairie Ancienne Honoré Champion, 1919), lxxxv.

95. Veissière, *Une communauté*, 156.

96. According to an eighteenth-century source, the "petit hôtel-Dieu" of Provins was located on the rue de Troyes in the lower village, east of Saint-Ayoul and its cemetery, and west of the river. Chanoine Nicholas Billate, "Histoire de l'hôtel-Dieu de Provins," BM Provins, mss 266, 267, 298. I am indebted to Monsieur Duchamp, director of the archives of the municipal library of Provins, for providing me with this information.

97. Bourquelot, *Histoire de Provins*, 96–97.

98. Bourquelot, *Histoire de Provins*, 105n2; Arbois de Jubainville, *Histoire des ducs*, 2:392.

99. While I have not been able to locate the original charter from 1141, which at one time was found in the manuscript (BM Provins, ms. 268) containing the hospital's landbook or "censier," I did consult BM Provins, ms. 85, no. 1, from ca. 1145, from the archbishop of Sens, which refers to the earlier gift made to the hospital by Anseau le Gras ("Ansellus Pinguis") and his father, Garnier. See François Verdier, *L'aristocratie de Provins à la fin du XIIe siècle* (Provins, France: Société d'Histoire et d'Archéologie de l'Arrondissement de Provins, 2016), 63. Chapin, *Les villes de foires de Champagne*, 39.

and this same act also included a provision from the count, authorizing the hospital to build houses in its enclosure and lodge foreigners during the May fairs to come. Thus, from a very early date the hospital's function extended to serving essentially as an inn for merchants.[100] With the count's own significant interests in the fairs, it is not surprising that he was content to see the hospital carrying out this role. In addition, however, Thibaut conceded another significant privilege to the hospital by granting it immunity from the comital exaction of one-half of all rental income on houses located in the area of the May fair while it was being held. Clearly, by the mid-twelfth century the hospital already owned houses and was renting them out during the fairs. The count, meanwhile, was willing to share his profits from the fair with the hospital, a privilege that Count Henri I renewed in 1164.[101] In 1211, Countess Blanche gave the hospital a rent of 30 s. on a house that was rented during the May fairs.[102] In a charter from 1213, Blanche indicated that drapery and belts were being sold in houses belonging to the hospital.[103] In 1230, Count Thibaut IV encouraged the hospital of Provins to build a market hall in Provins, and the count henceforth required all merchants selling cloth, woolen fabric, and silk to sell their goods in this hall when a fair was not taking place. The revenue from the feudal tax and rental fee collected from the merchants would be equally shared by the count and the brothers of the hospital.[104]

As he did with other secular chapters, Count Thibaut sought to convert the canons of Saint-Quiriace, whose chapter and church were located next to the comital residence in Provins, to regular status.[105] The result was a mixed chapter of secular and regular canons. However, Thibaut's son, Count Henri I, did not share his father's hostility to secular canons, and seeking to take advantage of the new count's more sympathetic ear, the secular canons of Saint-Quiriace agitated to have their chapter's former secular status restored.[106] After the archbishop of Sens and a papal committee delegate intervened, the regular canons were transferred to the building that had been "the house of the communal poor" of Saint-Jacques (Saint Jacques being a

100. Arbois de Jubainville, *Histoire des ducs*, 2:338.

101. Bourquelot, *Histoire de Provins*, 2:386–89. The chapter of Saint-Quiriace also rented houses to merchants who traveled to Provins to sell their wares.

102. Arbois de Jubainville, *Histoire des ducs*, vol. 5, no. 782, p. 66.

103. Verdier, *L'aristocratie*, 232 and notes 243 and 244.

104. Arbois de Jubainville, *Histoire des ducs*, vol. 5, no. 2096, p. 298.

105. Evergates, *Henry the Liberal*, 64.

106. Evergates, *Henry the Liberal*, 62–63.

popular name for hospitals, since Jacques was the patron saint of pilgrims).[107] This hospital was then reestablished in a new building at the bottom of the slope leading to Provins's upper village, in what may have been the former palace of the countesses, where the hospital still stands today.[108] Whereas in its earlier location the hospital was somewhat on the periphery, its new location was far more central, located right beside the newly enlarged comital residence and the chapter of Saint-Quiriace, just below the city's mint, on the main east-west thoroughfare that connected the upper and lower villages and that crossed the two main commercial centers. Even if the hospital was already functioning in its new location during the reign of Henri I, his son, Count Henri II, would claim in two charters, dated 1189 and 1190, that he, Henri II, had founded the hospital with his own hands.[109] It is possible that the formal foundation of the hospital in its new building only happened after 1181, under Count Henri II, even though Henri I oversaw the transplantation of the old hospital of Saint-Jacques in the upper village to its new location by the Durteint River.[110] In another sign of just how closely intertwined the count and the Provinois hospital were to the city's commercial interests,

---

107. Henri I's charter from 1159 appears in Benton and Bur, eds., *Recueil des actes*, no. 128, pp. 170–72.

108. This assertion, which has often been unquestioningly repeated, was made by Eustache Grillon, the erudite doctor at the hospital of Provins and chronicler of its history. M. Amédée Aufauvre and Charles Fichot, *Les monuments de Seine-et-Marne: Description historique et archéologique et reproduction des édifices religieux, militaires et civils du département* (Paris, 1858). It is quite possible that Countess Mathilda had a separate house in Provins, which was in her dower. After the comital residence in Vitry burned down in 1142, there was a greater need for an additional place to stay, and this was particularly true for Mathilda, whose husband was such an itinerant count. If there was in fact a palace for the countess in Provins, it might not be so surprising that it was after Mathilda's death in 1160 that Thibaut gave it to the hospital in return for the hospital's surrender of Saint-Jacques to the regular canons who were leaving Saint-Quiriace. The date of the hospital's transfer is not known, although 1160 is often reported (with no evidence) as the year of the transfer. The earliest possible date would be 1157, when the regular canons were moved into Saint-Jacques, and the latest possible date would be 1177, the date of the earliest charter in the hospital's cartulary. Charters dated 1177 and 1191 still refer to the hospital as being "the newly transplanted house" ("domus novelle plantacionis"). See Dupraz, nos. 1 and 22; AD: Seine-et-Marne 11Hdt A12, fol.1, 16. I thank Ted Evergates for sharing his expert knowledge on these issues.

109. Dupraz, nos. 38 and 237; AD: Seine-et-Marne 11Hdt A12, fol. 23, 72v. This second foundation of the hospital of Provins took place during roughly the same period as the foundations of the hôtel-Dieu-Saint-Esprit and the leprosary of Closebarbe, the latter having been founded by lords and townspeople by 1165, and located just a few kilometers south of Provins.

110. References to the hospital of Provins in charters almost always identify it with a topographic label, perhaps to differentiate it from other hospitals in the city. Charters from the late twelfth century, for example, tend to identify the hospital in terms of its being located either just below the church of Saint-Pierre or near the bridge, since the Durteint River passed nearby. Almost every charter from the thirteenth century that mentions the hospital of Provins describes it as being in front of a fountain.

an account from 1258–59, following the reign of Count Thibaut IV, shows that a large percentage of the comital properties and revenues in the greater Provins region were concentrated near the Durteint bridge, right near the hospital, in the heart of the commercial textile neighborhood.

Among thirteenth-century ecclesiastical reformers, the grand hôtel-Dieu of Provins had a reputation for being an exemplary hospital. Moreover, Jacques de Vitry singled it out along with the hospitals of Paris, Noyon, Tournai, Liège, and Brussels as exemplifying religious discipline, unlike the majority of hospitals, which he suggested were lax and corrupt.[111] During the mid-thirteenth century, the hospital of Provins had as many as thirty-eight members, with twenty-five sisters, eight lay brothers, four priests, and one other cleric. The central ward of the hospital, which can still be seen today, was over 100 feet long and 35 feet wide, and there may have been as many as three separate chapels, each on a different floor.[112] We know from a charter dated 1198, for instance, that a chaplain was celebrating Mass at an altar in the lower crypt for the souls of a donor couple.[113] In 1250 the archbishop of Sens consecrated a new chapel on the ground floor, dedicated to Saint Denis.[114] As was true in many hospitals, the buildings of the hospital of Provins continued to be expanded during the thirteenth century.

The Provinois *magister* seems to generally have been elected by the hospital's chapter and confirmed jointly by the archbishop of Sens and the count, but this right of election and the process by which it was done at times led to conflict. Even at hospitals in which the count reserved the right to nominate the *magister*, the local bishop reserved the right to reject a nomination or revoke the spiritual powers of a wayward master.[115] There is no evidence,

---

111. Bird, "Texts on Hospitals," 110–13.

112. Bourquelot, *Histoire de Provins*, 384, 387. On the architectural features of the hospital, see Aufauvre and Fichot, *Les monuments de Seine-et-Marne*, 127–29.

113. Dupraz, no. 121; AD: Seine-et-Marne 11Hdt A12, fol. 35v. This crypt was probably located in the subterranean floor, where one can still today see a cavernous space, forty meters in length, with vaults supported by rows of columns.

114. Dupraz, no. 23; AD: Seine-et-Marne 11Hdt A12, fol. 19v.

115. See, for example, the case of the hospital of Chaumont-en-Bassigny. See Arbois de Jubainville, *Histoire des ducs*, IV.2, 744. As part of an arbitrated judgment to resolve a conflict between the count of Champagne and the bishop of Meaux over the nomination of masters to the hospital of Meaux, for example, Count Thibaut IV acknowledged that the bishop retained some limited rights over the master of the hospital of Meaux. Indeed, if the master was found to be mismanaging the hospital, the bishop could give the count forty days to revoke the master, or the bishop would do so himself. The accounts of the hospital of Meaux were to be examined four times a year both by the count's almoner and the bishop's official. See Arbois de Jubainville, *Histoire des ducs*, IV.2, p. 744 and IV.2, pp. 746–47. On the history of Meaux and the episcopal-comital tensions there, see Michel Bur, "Meaux dans l'histoire de la Champagne du Xe au XIIe siècle," in *La Champagne médiévale: Recueil d'articles*, ed. Michel Bur (Langres, France: Dominique Guéniot, 2005), 443–51.

however, that the archbishop of Sens ever challenged the authority of the count or the hospital's chapter in this regard. In the early 1220s, however, the nearby chapter of Saint-Quiriace, the preeminent church in Provins and the largest Gothic church in Champagne, which, while not technically a comital chapter, nonetheless received significant patronage from the counts, tried unsuccessfully to claim the right to participate in the election of a new master of the hospital.[116] The chapter made this claim on the grounds that the hospital's master held one of its prebends. As part of an arbitrated settlement in 1223–24, Saint-Quiriace renounced all claims to the right to participate in the hospital's elections.[117] Yet the counts and countesses were no longer willing to let the hospital simply elect its own masters. When it was discovered in 1221 that the hospital chapter had elected a new master without receiving Countess Blanche's authorization, the hospital community quickly found that it was in trouble with its principal patron and protector. In retroactively requesting the countess's authorization, the community begged her forgiveness for its transgression, rhetorically using the sick and poor and its mission of performing works of mercy to placate her anger: "kneeling at your feet with our poor and our sick, we ask for your mercy and not judgment. We are ready to make all the reparations and give all the satisfaction that you desire."[118] Just twenty years later, however, the community again failed to secure Count Thibaut IV's blessing before electing a new master, and the count was not pleased.[119] The counts of Champagne were equally insistent upon their right to confirm the election of abbots and abbesses in Benedictine and Augustinian abbeys, so their active involvement in the administration of hospitals was not unusual.[120]

There were also moments of friction between the Provinois hospital and the municipal government, which in some cases appears to have been an outgrowth of ongoing tensions between the commune and the count (or even the church) as they vied for political authority. The cartulary for the city of Provins lists the expenses incurred when an official from the commune had to travel to Paris due to litigation. One such trip from 1320 involved complaints against a certain "Adenin de la Meson Dieu" for vile, contemptuous behavior ("villenie") against Billon, the cleric of the commune.[121] Another

---

116. Evergates, *Henry the Liberal*, 63–64.

117. Dupraz, no. 16; AD: Seine-et-Marne 11Hdt A12, fol. 18–18v.

118. Arbois de Jubainville, *Histoire des ducs*, IV.2, p. 745.

119. Arbois de Jubainville, *Histoire des ducs*, IV.2, p. 745; vol. 5, no. 2579, p. 383.

120. Arbois de Jubainville, *Histoire des ducs*, IV.2, p. 616.

121. Maurice Prou et Jules d'Auriac, eds., *Actes et comptes de la commune de Provins de l'an 1271 à l'an 1330* (Provins, France: Briard, 1933), 255.

record in the city's cartulary for 1309–10 indicates that the brothers of the leprosary of Crolebarbe, just south of Provins, paid the city of Provins 20 *l.* for coming to their legal defense (working in tandem with the French crown) when the archdeacon of Provins sought to have brother Gile of the "Meson Dieu" serve as their new master.[122] In working to protect the autonomy of the leprosary from what was seen as an encroachment from the hospital, the city (and crown) may have viewed the hospital as a proxy for ecclesiastical or comital power, since the hospital was so closely associated with the counts. In other respects, however, the hospital of Provins seems to have been an important and well-respected institution in the eyes of the leaders of the commune. One of the most influential leaders of the commune during the early fourteenth century, Jehan de la Noe, a bourgeois who from 1308 to 1328 frequently served as a counsellor to the commune and appeared before the Parlement de Paris on behalf of the city, left one-third of his fief and landholdings at Montenglost to the hospital of Provins at his death in 1331.[123]

A papal bull from 1177 is the first extant record to mention the hôtel-Dieu Saint-Esprit of Provins. The hospital was not initially called Saint-Esprit, and unlike the hôtel-Dieu Saint-Esprit in Troyes, there is no evidence that it was ever affiliated with the Order of Saint-Esprit.[124] In fact, by 1177 it was served by the regular canons of Saint-Bernard of Montjoux in Switzerland. The Provinois hospital paid an annual tribute to the Swiss mother house, although there are no references to the brothers from Montjoux in the hospital's records after 1241.[125] Neither the sick nor the leprous were accepted in the hôtel-Dieu Saint-Esprit, and the hospital seems to have primarily housed pilgrims coming to visit the relics of Saint-Ayoul as well as housing the poor, the elderly, and abandoned children.[126] A comital foundation, the hospital may have been established by Henri I due to a lack of space in the city's principal hospital after it moved.[127] The new hôtel-Dieu Saint-Esprit was located in the upper village, in the new market, where by 1200 the counts possessed seventy-two commercial houses.[128] For a time, the hôtel-Dieu Saint-Esprit

---

122. Prou and d'Auriac, eds., *Actes et comptes*, 218–19; Terrasse, *Provins*, 219.

123. Terrasse, *Provins*, 246.

124. Michel Veissière, "L'hôpital provinois," *Bulletin philologique et historique* (1963, année 1961), 589. It was very common for hospitals named Saint-Esprit not to be affiliated with the hospital order of the same name. See Touati, "Les groupes des laïcs," 137–62.

125. Veissière, "L'hôpital provinois," 581–84, 589.

126. Veissière, "L'hôpital provinois," 586–87.

127. Veissière, "L'hôpital provinois," 586–87.

128. Verdier, *L'aristocratie*, 67.

collected one-half of the count's sales tax on all linen cloth sold in Provins, but this right was ultimately challenged.[129]

There seem to have been plans to build a *domus Dei* in Provins for poor students. The testament from 1219 for Jacques de Hongrie, Countess Blanche's sergeant, included bequests for various religious and charitable houses, including the hospital of Provins, the brothers of Saint John of Jerusalem, and the "*domus Dei scolarum*" of Provins, "if it will be built."[130] By the second half of the thirteenth century, there was a house of "bons enfants" in Provins to provide for the city's needy students.[131] It is also possible that during the thirteenth century Provins, which had a fairly large Jewish community, had a house for Jewish lepers.[132] Two separate charters refer to the place in the city where Jewish lepers lived.[133] Provins also had two or three hospitals under the direction of the Templars, who had established themselves in the city as early as 1130.[134]

The Hospital of Bar-sur-Aube

The origins of the hospital of Bar-sur-Aube are also obscure, since no foundation charter is extant, but the hospital had clearly been established at some point between 1130 and 1136. On the orders of Pope Innocent II, Guillenc, the bishop of Langres, consecrated the hospital's cemetery by 1136.[135] A papal bull from Eugenius III in 1147, which extended papal protection to the hospital, makes clear that it was managed by a *magister* and included

---

129. Benton and Bur, eds., *Recueil des actes*, vol. 2, no. 239 bis, p. 15; Verdier, *L'aristocratie*, 76. The hospital's right to collect this sales tax was later challenged by the chapter of Saint-Quiriace, which owned the land on which the hospital had been built. The chapter claimed that it had long collected the sales tax. In 1202 a commission appointed by Innocent III found that the hospital had no legal claim to the tax. See Veissière, "L'hôpital provinois," 581–84, 588.

130. Dupraz, no. 446; AD: Seine-et-Marne 11Hdt A12, fol. 129v–130.

131. The *censier* for the hospital of Provins referred to three houses owned by the hospital near "la meson au Bons Anfanz." See Morlet and Mulon, "Le censier," 32. A testament from 1267, found in the hospital's cartulary, makes bequests to the "Bons Enfants" of Provins and Sens. See Dupraz, no. 426; AD: Seine-et-Marne 11Hdt A12, fol. 124–124v. On the "Bons Enfants," see J. M. Reitzel, "The Medieval Houses of Bons-Enfants," *Viator* 11 (1980): 179–207.

132. On the Jews of Provins, see Verdier, *L'aristocratie*, 47–50.

133. François-Olivier Touati, "Domus judaeorum leprosorum: Une léproserie pour les Juifs à Provins au XIIIe siècle," in *Fondations et oeuvres charitables au moyen âge*, ed. Jean Dufour and Henri Platelle (Paris: Éditions du CTHS, 1999), 97–106. On Jewish lepers more generally, see Shoham-Steiner, *On the Margins of a Minority*.

134. Carraz, *L'ordre du Temple*, 508–9; Carraz, "Templars and Hospitallers," 104; Carrière, *Histoire et cartulaire*; Bourquelot, *Histoire de Provins*, 139–40, 392–93.

135. Roserot, *Dictionnaire historique*, 1:101; Henri d'Arbois de Jubainville, *Histoire de Bar-sur-Aube sous les comtes de Champagne, 1077–1284* (Paris: Auguste Durand, 1859), 75.

communities of both men and women.[136] A charter of notice from a few years later recorded by Count Thibaut II and his son, Henri I "the Liberal," shows the hospital being given various pieces of land, woods, a mill, and rents in money and kind.[137] Bernard of Clairvaux, the famous Cistercian abbot, even appears as a witness to one of the donations to the hospital.[138] The hospital must have been considered a fairly prominent institution during this period, since beginning in 1172 the *magister* was charged with overseeing the hospital of Vitry-en-Perthois, and the hospital was also given the churches of Colombé-la-Fosse (1172), Lignol (1176), and Fuligny (1180).[139] Thus, like some other hospitals, the religious community of the hospital at Bar-sur-Aube was not only charged with the physical and spiritual care of its own sick poor but also the administrative and spiritual care of the souls of several parishes. Pastoral responsibilities well outside the hospital's walls had become an accepted part of its charitable mission, just as many monasteries were increasingly involved in the patronage of parish churches.

A number of the *acta* for the hospital of Saint-Nicolas refer to the female *conversae* of the house. As early as 1170, the record of a donation by Simon Le Bègue de Laferté, mentions that his daughter had entered the hospital as a *conversa*.[140] Some later donations were specifically directed to the hospital's female *conversae*, such as Count Thibaut's granting them, in 1222, the use of his forest at Lignol for the purpose of obtaining the firewood needed to heat their own *conversae* residence.[141] In short, these women appear to have occupied their own space and perhaps building, and they may also have had their own institutional property. An act from 1198 records the master and hospital brothers ceding a vineyard in the valley of Thors to the community of *conversae* in exchange for their payment of 10 *l.* that the hospital owed.[142]

The hospital profited in various ways from the annual fair held in the city. In 1169, for example, Count Henri gave the hospital of Saint-Nicolas an annual rent of 100 *sous* on the right to display goods in his stall at the fair of Bar-sur-Aube.[143] By the early thirteenth century, however, the hospital's

136. AD: Haute-Marne 55H1; Roserot, *Dictionnaire historique*, 1:101; Arbois de Jubainville, *Histoire de Bar-sur-Aube*, 76.

137. Arbois de Jubainville, *Histoire de Bar-sur-Aube*, 76.

138. E.–A. Blampignon, *Bar-sur-Aube* (Paris: Picard, 1900), no. 15, pp. 390–92.

139. For Vitry, see AD: Aube HD33/50, no. 6; Arbois de Jubainville, *Histoire des ducs*, vol. 3, no. 206, p. 363; for Colombé-la-Fosse, see AD Aube, HD 33/126; for Fuligny, see AD: Aube, HD 33/145; for Lignol, see AD: Aube, HD 33/168. Also see Arbois de Jubainville, *Histoire de Bar-sur-Aube*, 77–78.

140. Arbois de Jubainville, *Histoire de Bar-sur-Aube*, 77.

141. Arbois de Jubainville, *Histoire de Bar-sur-Aube*, 80.

142. Arbois de Jubainville, *Histoire de Bar-sur-Aube*, 79.

143. Benton and Bur, eds., *Recueil des actes*, no. 283, pp. 362–63.

financial fortunes had taken a turn for the worse, and in 1239 Count Thibaut IV and the bishop of Langres turned the hospital's management over to a certain sister, Alix de Boulancourt and her female priory of Meix, near Alli-baudières, which belonged to the Order of Saint-Victor of Paris.[144] By the second half of the thirteenth century, there was a female monastic commu-nity overseeing the hospital, but this "monasterium" appears to have been in a separate building from the "domus hospitalis," and some bequests to the sisters of Saint-Nicolas make no reference to the hospital or the sisters' charitable activities.[145] Yet the convent sustained relationships with some of the same donors who just a few years earlier had supported the hospital. A charter from 1256 records a certain Beatrice and her husband, Guillaume Cleric, conceding a rent to the abbess and convent of Saint-Nicolas, as well as a vineyard that Beatrice and her first, now deceased, husband had donated in 1237 to the master and brothers of the *domus Dei* of Saint-Nicolas.[146]

Monastic Houses: Supporters of Hospitals or Competitors?

With its proximity to Burgundy, a center of monastic reform and renewal, and its own rich monastic landscape, including the famed Cistercian abbey of Clairvaux, Champagne played a formative role in the history of medieval monasticism. What was the relationship between Champagne's monastic institutions, particularly its Cistercian houses, and the rise of its hospitals? In his study of leprosaries in the province of Sens, François-Olivier Touati observed a strong monastic influence, especially that of Cistercian spiritual-ity, among those who joined the religious communities inside leprosaria. An

---

144. Roserot, *Dictionnaire*, 1:101. Arbois de Jubainville, *Histoire des ducs*, IV.2, p. 752; vol. 5, no. 2523, p. 374.

145. In even some early charters, donations are made to the church of Saint-Nicolas in Bar-sur-Aube, with no mention of the hospital. See, for example, the charter from 1229, with a donation from Humbert Chalviaus and his wife Evia de Courcelles: AD: Aube HD33/78. A donation charter from March 1262, in which the widow Ysabellis from Bar-sur-Aube, gave her house to the nuns of Saint-Nicolas, makes clear that her house was next to the "domus hospitalis" of the monastery: AD: Aube HD33/66. A testament from November 1286 from a canon from Saint-Machut in Bar-sur-Aube includes a bequest to the nuns of Saint-Nicolas, who were to celebrate the canon's anniversary and distribute pittances and wine to the poor of the hospital. The canon also made several bequests to the hospital of Saint-Esprit of Bar-sur-Aube. See AD: Aube 3H336. A testament from Jocelin de Lignol, however, who was a canon at Saint-Étienne de Troyes, includes no reference to any hospital or charitable activity, but simply a bequest to the nuns of Saint-Nicolas of Bar-sur-Aube: AD: Aube HD33/50, no. 11 (1261).

146. AD: Aube HD 33/78 (March 1256).

entrance charter from 1238, for example, recording Jacqueline de Louas-
ville's decision to join the leprosarium of Grand-Beaulieu at Chartres, indicated her preference "to serve God in religion rather than to enjoy the vain
glories of the world," "to pray among her sisters, to be a measure of help
by her aid and compassion to the most weak and sick."[147] As we shall have
occasion to examine in greater depth in chapter 5, these values of religious
communal life and humble, pious service to those living on the margins of
society were not only characteristic of the spiritual ideals of religious communities in northern French hospitals and leprosaria but were shared by
Cistercians and members of some of the other "newer" religious orders,
such as the beguines and mendicants. Indeed, rather than seeing Cistercian
influences on hospital religious communities, Anne Lester has argued that
the female Cistercian movement in Champagne was inexorably tied to the
plethora of charitable institutions that already existed in the county by the
early thirteenth century and that were often overseen by groups of religious
and quasi-religious penitential women. As Lester has shown, caregiving was
"a defining aspect of the women's religious movement, particularly as it
was manifest in Champagne," with over half of the Cistercian nunneries
established during the 1230s having their origins in hospitals or leprosaria.[148]
Hospitals at Appoigny, Château-Thierry, Couilly, Ramerupt, Mergey, Malay-
le-Roi, Troissy, and Vitry were all placed under the jurisdiction of Cistercian women during the 1220s and 1230s. In this sense, the female Cisterican
movement in Champagne grew out of a preexisting and vibrant hospital
movement.

Nor were Cistercian convents the only monastic houses to take over the
management of hospitals. In 1192, the hospital at Payns, founded earlier
than 1147, had been turned over to the Benedictine nuns of Notre-Dame-
aux-Nonnains.[149] In 1179, Henri I turned over the hospital of Épernay, along
with its lands and revenues, which had been built and acquired by a certain
Hugo "the blacksmith" ("faber"), to the canons of Saint-Martin of Épernay,
who were charged with managing the care of the poor and the guests.[150]
In 1210 the hospital of Chêne was ceded to the religious of the abbey of
Mores.[151] The hospitals of Brienne-le-Château and Chalette, both founded
by 1138 (with Brienne a dependent of Chalette), were both made subject to

---

147. Touati, *Maladie et société*, 407.
148. Lester, *Creating Cistercian Nuns*, 40.
149. Roserot, *Dictionnaire historique*, 2:1095.
150. Benton and Bur, eds., *Recueil des actes*, no. 496, pp. 615–16.
151. Roserot, *Dictionnaire historique*, 1:373.

the Benedictine abbey of Saint-Loup in Troyes in 1206. By 1224 the hospital of Brienne was no longer under the authority of Saint-Loup but was at least partially subject to the abbey of Montier-en-Der, and by 1230, the count of Brienne had given his rights over the hospital to the Teutonic Order.[152] In many of these instances, it is clear that the hospitals were burdened with significant financial and or managerial problems, and a bishop or count requested monastic oversight to address these problems.

Church reformers like Robert of Courson and Jacques de Vitry likewise argued for the need to make the religious communities inside hospitals more monastic. Intent on regularizing hospitals, reformers viewed the independence of hospitals (and the resulting variety of hospital forms) as problematic. Robert of Courson held legatine councils at Reims (1213), Paris (1213), and Rouen (1214) in which he issued decrees that sought to reform and regularize hospitals.[153] However, these conciliar decrees on hospitals (unlike the decrees touching on other subjects) were not picked up by the Fourth Lateran Council or subsequent councils; these hospital reform efforts were thus regional and failed to be incorporated into canon law. The promulgation of statutes for a number of northern French hospitals during the thirteenth century emerged even a bit earlier than Robert's legatine councils. These statutes reflected the same desire for greater discipline and regularity across hospitals.[154] This project of greater standardization among hospitals (based on a monastic model) is also evident in the records of episcopal visitations of hospitals in thirteenth-century Normandy and in and around Paris in the early fourteenth century.[155] In the case of hospitals taken over by monastic communities, the vision of reformers had in some sense been realized. However, in other instances, as we have seen, hospitals simply ceased to function as such, instead being turned into monastic houses. The increasing institutionalization of hospitals, including efforts to impose monastic discipline from outside, threatened their central charitable mission and sometimes led to their demise.

---

152. Roserot, *Dictionnaire historique,* 1:128–29, 292–93.

153. Sethina Watson has established a new chronology for Courson's legatine councils, which serves as a correction to Mansi and Le Grand. As she shows, a council in Reims in 1213 preceded the council held in Paris that same year. See Watson, *On Hospitals,* 272–81, 288–90.

154. Admittedly, there were some distinctive features to each hospital's statutes, but there was also a great deal of borrowing and mutual influence between hospitals. See Léon Le Grand, ed., *Statuts d'hôtels-Dieu et de léproseries: Recueil de textes du XIIe au XIVe siècle* (Paris: Picard, 1901).

155. Léon Le Grand, ed., "Les maisons-Dieu et les léproseries du diocèse de Paris au milieu du XIVe siècle, d'après le registre de visites du délégué de l'évêque (1351–69)," *Mémoires de la Société de l'Histoire de Paris et de l'Ile-de-France* 24 (1897): 61–365; Adam J. Davis, *The Holy Bureaucrat: Eudes Rigaud and Religious Reform in Thirteenth-Century Normandy* (Ithaca: Cornell University Press, 2006).

Still, relatively few of Champagne's hundreds of hospitals were subsumed by monastic houses, with the vast majority retaining their autonomy. Of those hospitals that were thought to be poorly administered, many were handed over to larger and better managed hospitals, not monasteries. In 1172, for example, the bishop of Châlons-sur-Marne made the hospital of Vitry-en-Perthois subject to the hospital of Bar-sur-Aube.[156] In 1196, Countess Marie and Garin, the bishop of Troyes, placed the hospital of Donnement under the authority of the hôtel-Dieu-le-Comte.[157] In 1244, Count Thibaut IV made the hospital of Meaux subject to the Trinitiarians of the same city.[158] In 1271, the bishop of Troyes found that the hospital of Meix-Tiercelin was so impoverished that it was neither offering hospitality to the poor nor observing the religious life; to correct this situation, the bishop made this hospital a dependency of the hospital of Saint-Nicolas in Troyes, with the hope that the "works of piety" ("opera pietatis") would be restored.[159] It was not uncommon in other regions for a larger hospital to have a number of smaller hospitals under its jurisdiction. By the mid-thirteenth century, the hospital of Sainte-Marie in Laon had as many as eleven dependent hospitals, including small, rural ones that functioned like a triage system; those who were gravely ill and in need of greater attention were sent from small, daughter hospitals to the mother hospital in Laon.[160] A hospital founded in Braux by the Champenois knight Renaud de Bar, which was intended "to receive and care for the infirm poor and even the sick," was originally to be overseen by the brothers of the hospital of Roncevalles in Navarre, known for serving pilgrims on the way to Santiago de Compostela. In 1297, however, the count of Bar sought to expel these brothers and replace them with brothers from the Order of St John of Jerusalem. This move was resisted by the prior of Roncevalles, who appealed to the *magister* of the hospital of Provins, arguing that the brothers of the Hospital of St. John were ignorant of and incapable of fulfilling this hospital's caritative mission.[161] The institutional provision of

---

156. Arbois de Jubainville, *Histoire des ducs*, vol. 3, no. 206, p. 363.

157. AD Aube, 40 H1, A3.

158. Arbois de Jubainville, *Histoire des ducs*, vol. 5, no. 2680, p. 401.

159. Henri d'Arbois de Jubainville, "Étude sur les documents antérieurs à l'année 1285, conservés dans les archives des quatre petits hôpitaux de la ville de Troyes," *Mémoires de la Société Académique de l'Aube*, vol. 21 (vol. 8, 2nd ser.) (1857), no. 8.

160. Alain Saint-Denis, "Medecins et medecine dans l'hôtel-Dieu de Laon aux XIIème et XIIIème siecles," *Colloque international d'histoire de la médecine médiévale: Orléans, 4 et 5 mai, 1985* (1985): 134.

161. BM: Provins, ms. 85, no. 107, dated October 4, 1297. Braux was located in the area of Ancerville (dep. Meuse), southeast of the founder's hometown of Bar-le-Duc. The hospital of Roncevalles had a number of dependent hospitals in France and England.

charity could be a site of power struggles, in this case between two competing hospital orders, neither of them local.

Hospitals by no means had a monopoly on institutional charity in Champagne. Rather, the hospitals founded during the twelfth and thirteenth centuries were part of an increasingly crowded field of charitable orders and institutions, with the more traditional Benedictine monks playing less and less of
a visible role in charitable activities. This was observed by contemporaries
as well, at least those who identified with the newer religious movements.
As Geoffroy de Vigeois, who belonged to the Order of Grandmont, put it,
"The charity of the first monks cooled off, from the moment when there
appeared the partisans of the various orders such as the Templars, Hospitallers, Grandmontains, Carthusians, Cistercians, the hospitals for the poor, the
convents of nuns, the groups of lepers and a congregation of certain new
canons. The custom also was established, with God's help, to make public
alms each year to the poor in the churches, castles, and towns."[162] In the
region around Troyes and Provins, there were multiple institutional channels
for the provision of charity, including parish churches (in 1237, for example,
the parish of Notre-Dame-du-Val in Provins established a confraternity for
the blind);[163] the bishop; the many hospitals that were independent in the
sense that they did not belong to a particular religious order, even if some of
them followed the Augustinian Rule; hospitals run by the Templars, the Hospitallers of Saint John of Jerusalem, the Order of the Holy Spirit, the Trinitarians, or the Antonines; the caregiving by groups of repentant, semi-religious
women, sometimes called the "Filles Dieu"; or the charity distributed by
various monastic houses, especially the caretaking activities of Cistercian
nuns. In Reims, there were several institutional options for poor clerical students by the late thirteenth century, including a house of Val-des-Écoliers; a
house of Bons Enfants ("Bonis Pueris"); the hospital of "Alberic le Creveit,"
which housed poor clerics; and the general hôtel-Dieu of Notre Dame, to
which one testator made a bequest specifically for the poor clerical students
who were living there.[164]

In addition, though, more traditional monastic houses also continued
to play a role in the provision of charity. In Reims, it is clear from testaments that the Benedictine abbeys of Saint-Rémi, Saint-Nicaise, and Saint-
Pierre-les-Dames and the Augustinian abbey of Saint-Denis each had its own

162. Touati, *Maladie et société*.
163. Bourquelot, *Histoire de Provins*, 193–94.
164. See the testaments from 1262 and 1285 in Pierre Varin, ed., *Archives administratives de la ville de Reims: Collection de pièces inédites*, vol. 1, part 2 (Paris: Crapelet, 1839), 810–11, 1000.

hospital for the poor during the later thirteenth century.[165] Gifts were some-times given to a monastery specifically for the provision of charity. Due to a significant gift of a tithe (worth 620 *l.*) from Elizabeth, the widow of the lord Hugues III of Broyes-Commercy, for example, the gatekeeper of Clair-vaux was charged with distributing clothes and shoes to eighty paupers each year.[166]

We know far less about non-institutional forms of charity, the kind of informal, familial or neighborly charitable practices that are so rarely recorded and are therefore difficult for the historian to reconstruct. Occasionally our sources permit us to catch a glimpse into other sources of support for the poor that existed, such as a "garden for the poor" in Plessis-aux-Tournelles, northwest of Provins, mentioned in passing in the cartulary for the hospital of Provins.[167] We do not know who owned or maintained this garden. Even with the scores of hospitals founded in Champagne during this period, there surely were not enough beds to accommodate all those in need of assistance, and the statutes for the hôtel-Dieu-le-Comte in Troyes and the hospital in Provins make clear that people with various physical ailments and conditions were regularly turned away. Some people in need of help also surely chose not to seek institutional support. What happened to the elderly widow who lived alone in Meaux and was unable to get dressed or undressed by herself? How did someone living in Bar-sur-Aube with a severe tremor manage to feed himself or hold a cup up to his mouth? Where did a poor, unattached, middle-aged woman in Provins turn for help? What kind of informal support networks did the poor and needy rely upon or even try to create as part of their strategies for basic survival? Were the donors to Champagne's hospitals as likely to give a *denier* to the beggars they encountered in their neighbor-hood? Or were the residents of Champagne who never made bequests to reli-gious and charitable institutions more likely to be the ones to give informal, spontaneous alms or, for that matter, to give physical assistance to a needy neighbor or friend?

Although the focus of this book is on the institutional provision of charity through hospitals, there was no stark divide between informal, neighborly, or familial forms of support and formal, institutional charity. Those in need of assistance often turned at various times both to institutions as well as to

---

165. See, for example, the testament from 1285 of Hugues le Large, the dean of Reims, in Varin, ed., *Archives administratives*, 1000.

166. Evergates, *Feudal Society*, 143–44.

167. Dupraz, no. 377; AD: Seine-et-Marne 11Hdt A12, fol. 112–112v.

family and friends. Moreover, the charitable institutions in one's town or city were generally not perceived as foreign, impersonal entities but places where a friend or relative lived or worked, where one went to hear Mass, or where one chose one day to be buried. Hospitals were familiar to those who paid a rent for land under a hospital's lordship or to those who bought items sold by a hospital at the market. Hospitals were not just the objects of charitable bequests but institutions with which people engaged in a range of different forms of economic exchange, including buying, selling, and renting property.

What was the relationship between the intensely commercial environment of Champagne and the "economy of salvation," which, as we have seen, was so central to the medieval understanding of charity? For some almsgivers, charitable giving represented both a form of penance for avarice and profit-making as well as a way to justify one's profit-making and transform one's surplus wealth into a virtue. For those who joined a community of caregivers in a hospital, a penitential life of serving the poor and sick embodied the apostolic life and seemed to offer a radical alternative to the bustling world of markets and fairs. The hospital worker who lived a life of self-renunciation and service also participated in the "economy of salvation," trying to save the sick and poor, frequently regarded as stand-ins for Christ, and thereby earn salvation. Working in a hospital was a way of building up credit with God for the ultimate reward. In short, medieval hospitals were enmeshed in a larger pattern of social and economic exchange. Let us now turn to the social networks involved in the giving and receiving of charitable support, which will help illuminate broader questions about the nature of social relationships and lived experiences.

🍂 CHAPTER 3

Hospital Patrons and Social Networks

The emergence of a vibrant commercial economy during the twelfth and thirteenth centuries is generally understood as marking a shift from a traditional gift economy to a profit economy, a development that not only had economic consequences but profound social and religious ramifications as well, including reshaping attitudes toward poverty and wealth.[1] For example, the rise of the profit economy may have contributed to the commodification of prayer, particularly during the later thirteenth and fourteenth centuries, as prayers and liturgical commemorations came to be viewed as desirable, calculable commodities that were worth paying for.[2] Donors to monasteries were no longer satisfied with simply being associated with a monastery; they wanted a specific liturgical service or reward for their benefaction beyond assurances that their gifts would have a redemptive or salvific effect.[3]

---

1. Little, *Religious Poverty*; Le Goff, *Money and the Middle Ages*.

2. Chiffoleau, *Comptabilité de l'au-delà*; Joel Rosenthal, *The Purchase of Paradise: Gift Giving and the Aristocracy, 1307–1485* (London: Routledge, 1972); Richard L. Keyser, "La transformation de l'échange des dons pieux: Montier-la-Celle, Champagne, 1100–1350," *Revue historique* 305, no. 4 (2003): 793–816; Richard L. Keyser, "Gift, Dispute, and Contract: Gift Exchange and Legalism in Monastic Property Dealings, Montier-la-Celle, France, 1100–1350," (PhD dissertation, Johns Hopkins University, 2001).

3. On the earlier model of associative gift exchange, see Megan McLaughlin, *Consorting with the Saints: Prayer for the Dead in Early Medieval France* (Ithaca: Cornell University Press, 1994).

Was the traditional gift economy, however, simply superseded by the medieval profit economy, as some historians have suggested?[4] This chapter argues instead that the highly commercial environment of thirteenth-century Champagne infused pious giving with even greater meaning, particularly bequests made to a charitable institution like a hospital, which had as its central mission the performance of the works of mercy. During the course of the thirteenth century, during which the number of bequests to traditional Benedictine monastic houses declined, the scale of giving to hospitals actually increased. The range of people from different social classes making charitable bequests also expanded, reflective of what one might term the growing democratization of charity. As compared with donors to monastic houses, however, lay donors to hospitals placed less emphasis on intercessory prayer and requested anniversary masses in exchange for donations less often than donors to monasteries. Instead, hospital donors focused on the performance of the works of mercy, which, in the economy of salvation, they viewed as the most efficacious form of currency. Donation charters were at times explicit in expressing the donors' hope that by showing mercy to those most in need, that same mercy would likewise one day be extended to them, whether from human hands or from God on the Day of Judgment. Whereas only a very small percentage of bequests to monastic houses during the second half of the thirteenth century contained the *pro anima* clause, indicating that the gift was given for the donor's soul, the phrase continued to be employed regularly in donations to hospitals, an indication of the continuing spiritual power ascribed to these donations. Although the inclusion of the *pro anima* clause was meant to distinguish a pious gift from an exchange or sale, the charters recording these gifts employed religious language that was transactional and based on an expectation of reward.

Those making bequests to hospitals were also frequently guided by pragmatic considerations. Some donors had a family connection to a hospital, with a relative working there whom they wished to help. Others made bequests as an entry gift to a hospital, or with the expectation that they might one day wish to join the hospital's religious community. Donors quite frequently indicated that they had already had interactions with the hospital, expressing gratitude for a service that the hospital had provided to them. And hospitals conferred a counter-gift on donors as a way of reaffirming the relationship and further fostering the cycle of gift and counter-gift. Charitable

---

4. Georges Duby, *L'économie rurale et la vie des campagnes dans l'Occident médiéval (France, Angleterre, Empire, IXe–XVe siècles). Essai de synthèse et perspectives de recherches* (Paris: Aubier, 1962); Little, *Religious Poverty*; Bijsterveld, "Medieval Gift."

giving clearly participated in a larger social, religious, and economic culture of exchange and reciprocity, which was itself an outgrowth of an increasingly commercialized society.

As Martha Howell has rightly observed, "commerce did not erode the power of the gift . . . rather, gifts took on a new significance in these commercial economies."[5] To be sure, some of the "new significance" of gifts was related to religious developments, such as a growing Eucharistic piety and preoccupation with Purgatory, both of which fueled a greater demand for the celebration of Masses, increasingly a condition for pious gifts. In this connection, Jacques Chiffoleau has described how late medieval testators in the Avignon region sought to calculate the precise cost of salvation and release from Purgatory, "calibrating their bequests to match the expected return."[6] Already during the thirteenth century, however, ideas and language about commerce and markets were redeployed in the spiritual realm, particularly within the context of the works of mercy. As we saw in chapter 1, there was a long tradition that stretched back to Late Antiquity of Christians (and Jews) giving charity to the poor to affect the fate of their own souls (and the souls of relatives) in the afterlife. Commercial metaphors were used to describe the relation between almsgiving and rewards.[7] Religious and social developments in thirteenth-century Europe, particularly the expanding market economy, gave new meaning to these ideas and metaphors, metaphors that once again became, as they had been in Late Antiquity, "metaphors to live by," in Peter Brown's words.[8]

This chapter examines the patrons of Champagne's hospitals—from the powerful counts, countesses, and aristocrats to the ordinary townsperson—and interrogates what these hospitals meant to them. Why did people make bequests to Champagne's hospitals during the twelfth and thirteenth centuries, and what was the nature of their interactions with these institutions? How was the experience of giving to a hospital different from (or similar to) giving to another kind of ecclesiastical institution, and how did hospitals compete for patronage in a landscape that was increasingly crowded with ecclesiastical and charitable institutions, from various kinds of monastic houses to friaries, parish churches, and the houses and hospitals of Templars, Hospitallers, and Filles Dieu? In probing what defined the symbiotic bonds

---

5. Martha C. Howell, *Commerce before Capitalism in Europe, 1300–1600* (Cambridge: Cambridge University Press, 2010), 47.

6. Chiffoleau, *La comptabilité de l'au-delà*; Howell, *Commerce Before Capitalism*, 190.

7. Brown, *Ransom of the Soul*, 98; Anderson, *Charity*.

8. Brown, *Ransom of the Soul*, 98.

between hospitals and a dense network of relations, we need to consider how the commercial environment of Champagne affected the character of pious gifts to hospitals. This chapter contends that pious gift-giving was in some ways becoming more commercialized, with pious gifts to hospitals becoming more like commercial exchanges, predicated on a systematic exchange of gifts for the salvation of one's soul or for various services a hospital might provide. There is even significance in the timetable specified by the numerous charters recording the donation of rents to hospitals. Very often the payment of these rents was timed to take place during one of Champagne's international trade fairs, reflective of what Jacques Le Goff long ago observed about the shift from "church time" to "merchant's time," with charity increasingly tied to the world of commerce.[9] At the same time that charity was becoming more commercialized, however, hospital donors were also intensely preoccupied with the spiritual value of the works of mercy, since they increasingly regarded these works as the wisest form of investment in the economy of salvation.

The Scale of Charitable Giving to Hospitals

The charters and cartularies for Champagne's hospitals indicate that these institutions acquired property through a wide range of different kinds of acquisitions, including gifts, quittances, amortizations, exchanges, and sales/purchases. Yet during the twelfth and thirteenth centuries, the largest number of acquisitions came in the form of donations and bequests. From 1210 until 1300, for example, there are extant records of 165 donations to the hospital of Provins, whereas during the same period, there are records of 51 purchases and 47 exchanges, over half of which involved monastic houses, churches, or priests. Furthermore, 54 additional donations to this hospital during this period appear in confirmation charters (recording the approval of a donation by a relative or lord if what was being donated was part of that person's lordship) and in records detailing disputes (accords, judgments, and arbitrations). Although these records frequently omit (or even change) crucial details and terms of the original gift, such as the date of the original act, they, too, provide valuable information about the scale and nature of the gifts received by hospitals and the identity of hospital donors. In addition, a thirteenth-century martyrological obituary for the hospital of Provins (with later additions) records the names of 510 hospital donors and their

---

9. Jacques Le Goff, "Temps de l'Église et temps du marchand," *Annales* 15, no. 3 (May-June 1960): 417–33.

gifts. Moreover, a treasure trove of data exists, particularly in the case of the hospital of Provins and the hôtel-Dieu-le-Comte in Troyes, for which there are extant cartularies as well as a significant number of original single-sheet charters.

With the influence of ideas disseminated from the Gregorian reform movement about the problems posed by lay lordship for the monastic and clerical world, the late eleventh century had also seen a sharp downturn in *pro anima* gifts from powerful aristocrats to Benedictine houses, only to see a brief renewal of expressions of friendship ("amicitia") between monastic houses and their longstanding aristocratic patrons during the middle decades of the twelfth century.[10] Another downturn in pious gifts to these monastic houses, however, followed during the thirteenth century, as the creation of new religious and charitable orders (mendicants, Templars, Hospitallers, hospitals, and leprosaria) created new outlets for pious giving.[11] Not only was there a decline in the number of donations to Benedictine monasteries in absolute terms, but donations also represented a smaller percentage of monasteries' acquisitions, with purchases and exchanges together constituting a larger and larger component of monastic acquisitions. During the first half of the twelfth century, donations to the Benedictine abbey of Saint-Nicaise in Rheims were 93 percent of its total acquisitions.[12] Like most monasteries of the time, this abbey's economy was almost exclusively based on its reception of gifts. By the second half of the twelfth century, however, donations had already fallen to 67 percent of its total acquisitions, and by the first half of the thirteenth century, gifts represented a mere 28 percent of the abbey's acquisitions. By this later period, the abbey's acquisitions were increasingly comprised of its purchases of properties and rents.[13] A similar pattern has been observed at the Cistercian abbey of Clairvaux, where gifts declined as a proportion of total acquisitions from over 90 percent in the period before 1193 to only 54 percent from 1193 until 1261.[14]

---

10. Florian Mazel, "Amitié et rupture de l'amitié: Moines et grands laïcs provençaux au temps de la crise grégorienne (milieu XIe–milieu XII siècle)," *Revue historique* 633, no. 1 (2005): 53–95.

11. On the steep decline in the number of pious gifts to monasteries in Burgundy and Champagne during the later thirteenth and fourteenth centuries, see Keyser, "Gift, Dispute, and Contract," 162–69; Jeannine Cossé-Durlin, ed., *Cartulaire de Saint-Nicaise de Reims* (Paris: CNRS, 1991), 114; Robert Fossier, "La puissance économique de l'abbaye de Clairvaux au XIIIe siècle," in *Histoire de Clairvaux, Actes du Colloque 1990* (Bar-sur-Aube, France: Association Renaissance de l'abbaye de Clairvaux, 1991): 73–83. Jochen Schenk has also observed a decline in donations to the Templars in Provins in the second half of the thirteenth century. See Schenk, *Templar Families*, 39–41.

12. Cossé-Durlin, ed., *Cartulaire de Saint-Nicaise de Reims*, 114.

13. Cossé-Durlin, ed., *Cartulaire de Saint-Nicaise de Reims*, 114.

14. Keyser, "Gift, Dispute, and Contract," 169; Fossier, "Puissance économique."

It is therefore significant that one finds the exact opposite trend with the hospitals of Champagne, reflective of a shift in the destinations of pious bequests. While bequests continued to be directed to monastic houses to support the contemplative life and intercessory prayer, by the thirteenth century increasing numbers of bequests were being made to religious orders engaged in an active pastoral ministry, like the mendicant orders, as well as orders and institutions associated with caritative roles, such as houses of Cistercian women, leprosaria, and hospitals. At the hospital of Provins, the number of donations peaked during the 1260s, 1270s, and 1280s, with almost thirty donations being given each decade, about the same number that the monastery of Montier-la-Celle, the richest ecclesiastical establishment in the prevoté of Troyes (with an estimated annual revenue of over 6,000 *l. t.*), was receiving during its peak period in the early thirteenth century.[15] Likewise, the number of donations received by the hospital of Saint-Nicolas in Troyes peaked during the 1270s.[16] As revealing as these bequests to hospitals are in terms of patterns of religious and charitable giving during the high Middle Ages, Carole Rawcliffe, writing about the hospitals of Norwich, rightly cautions that these bequests almost certainly represent a tiny fraction of what people actually gave to the sick and poor during this period: "There can be little doubt that the charitable bequests recorded in wills represent only a very small proportion of the alms which would have been dispensed each week or even every day. . . . In practice, most relief comprised spontaneous gifts of food, fuel, clothing or accommodation made, as the Church required, in response to particular circumstances."[17] Testaments and hospital records fail to capture the small gifts that were given directly to the street beggar or neighbor in need, that is, the informal, familial, or neighborly charity that we know addressed some of the most pressing needs of medieval Europe's poor, sick, and disabled.

Although many hundreds of hospitals and leprosaria were founded during the twelfth and thirteenth centuries, most of these institutions were small, containing only a few beds, and they simply could not begin to meet the enormous demands for care and assistance. Testaments from Saint-Quentin, northwest of Champagne, indicate that in addition to the seven hospitals that existed in the city by the fourteenth century, there were, as

---

15. Keyser, "Gift, Dispute, and Contract," 60, 160–64. Touati found that testamentary bequests to the leprosaries in the province of Sens also peaked during the second half of the thirteenth century. See Touati, *Maladie et société*, 503.

16. The hôtel-Dieu-le-Comte in Troyes differed from these two hospitals in that its donations did not increase during the latter half of the thirteenth century, but they did not decrease either.

17. Rawcliffe, *Hospitals of Medieval Norwich*, 158.

in Reims, parish societies ("cartriers" or "chartriers") of volunteers (or paid workers) who visited and helped the parish poor and oversaw the distribution of money, food, and clothing collected for the poor.[18] Among the many pious bequests found in a testament from 1248 of a bourgeois woman named Margue de Lens were gifts to poor beguines, poor students, leper houses, a large number of hospitals (both in Saint-Quentin and as far away as Troyes, Reims, Provins, and Noyon), parish charitable societies ("caritati"), and three confraternities as well as to "poor ladies lying in childbirth." In addition, Margue asked that at her death, her house be transformed into a hospice for the poor for a period of twenty years. The hospice was to have eight beds and receive a rent of ten measures of wheat and was to be managed by three women, chosen by her friends, who would be given 200 l. to maintain the house. After twenty years, the house was to be given to the heirs of Margue's friends and the contents of the house sold and distributed to the poor.[19] When a singularly wealthy beguine named Widle drew up her testament in Reims in 1275, leaving bequests totaling close to 400 l. par., she did not direct any of her bequests to the largest hôtel-Dieu of her city, which was under the purview of the cathedral chapter.[20] Although she made some bequests to relatives, friends (above all, to Rose, her "socia" or house and spiritual companion), and clerics as well as to the house of the Dominicans, where she chose to be buried, the majority of her bequests were directed to those in need of material assistance, whether orphaned or abandoned boys ("pueris inventis"), repentant prostitutes (Filles Dieu), poor adolescent boys serving the cathedral and learning Latin and chant (the Val-Écoles), lepers, the poor relief administrators of various parishes (to whom she bequeathed her portions of two houses), poor beguines, and the poor guests of various monasteries and other hospitals. One of her largest single gifts (80 l.) was simply left to the poor of Reims and neighboring villages, to be distributed by the executors of her will. As the testaments of Margue and Wilde show, a concern with helping the *miserabiles* did not necessarily mean supporting hospitals or even institutional forms of charitable provision.

---

18. Pierre Desportes, ed., *Testaments Saint-Quentinois du XIVe siècle* (Paris: CNRS Editions, 2003), xxxiii. The "carcerarii" could refer to those who were bedridden or otherwise unable to work, but the term could also refer to parish poor relief funds or administrators. See Gaston Robert, "Les chartreries paroissiales et l'assistance publique à Reims jusqu'en 1633," *Travaux de l'Académie nationale de Reims* 141 (1926–27), 166–68.

19. Desportes, ed., *Testaments*, 124–27.

20. Gaston Robert, "Les beguines de Reims et la maison de Saint-Agnès," *Travaux de l'Académie nationale de* Reims 137 (1922–1923), 261–66.

Nonetheless, hospitals were among the most popular recipients of charitable gifts in many parts of Europe during this period, and the social and religious utility of hospitals was clearly on the minds of testators. A study of testaments from thirteenth-century Flanders found that 44 percent of all Flemish testaments contained at least one bequest to a hospital.[21] Similarly, 40 percent of all testaments in thirteenth-century Barcelona included bequests to a hospital, as did 90 percent of testaments in Rodez in the south of France ca. 1300.[22] The Franciscans and Dominicans were the most popular recipients of testamentary bequests in thirteenth-century Liège, perhaps in part because the friars so frequently served as confessors and executors of testaments. However, bequests to hospitals were extremely common there as well. Out of forty-two extant testaments from Liège, thirty-three (79%) included at least one bequest to a hospital. Even in the fourteenth century, when bequests to religious and charitable institutions tended to decline quite precipitously, thirty-three out of forty-nine testaments (67%) included a bequest to a hospital.[23] A similar incidence of testamentary bequests to hospitals has been found elsewhere, such as in the lower Rhône Valley. In Lausanne, 62 percent of testaments included at least one bequest to a hospital, at Viviers and Bourg-Saint-Andéol 68 percent of testators made bequests to hospitals, and just over a third of testaments from Avignon included hospital bequests.[24] A study of testaments from thirteenth- and fourteenth-century Saint-Quentin found that testators virtually always made charitable bequests, with one-third of all testaments including a bequest to the city's largest hospital, one-third including bequests to one or more of the city's other hospitals, and one-third including a bequest to the leprosary.[25]

A comparative study of testaments from early Renaissance cities in central Italy has established that there was a good bit of variation between different cities and across time in terms of where pious bequests were directed. In thirteenth-century Pisa, a higher proportion of testamentary bequests went to hospitals than to parishes, confraternities, nunneries, or mendicants. In Florence, in contrast, nunneries, parishes, and mendicants each received more than twice as many bequests as hospitals.[26] Still, it is clear that bequests

---

21. P. Godding, "La pratique testamentaire," *Revue d'histoire du droit* 58 (1990): 289–90 and note 46.

22. Brodman, *Charity and Religion*, 40. Michel Mollat, "L'hôpital dans la ville au moyen âge en France," *Société francaise d'histoire des hôpitaux* 47 (1983): 10.

23. De Spiegeler, *Les hôpitaux et l'assistance à Liège*, 176–83.

24. Le Blévec, *La part du pauvre*, 204–5.

25. Desportes, ed., *Testaments Saint-Quentinois*, xxxiii, xxxvi–xxxvii.

26. Samuel K. Cohn Jr., *The Cult of Remembrance and the Black Death: Six Renaissance Cities in Central Italy* (Baltimore: Johns Hopkins University Press, 1992), 36–37.

to hospitals had become a standard feature of Italian testamentary practice, with some communes, such as Siena and Assisi, even requiring citizens to make small testamentary bequests to particular institutions, such as the hospital of Santa Maria della Scala, in the case of Siena.[27] There were no such imposed charities in Champagne, and relatively few testaments from Champagne survive. Those that do are mostly from the second half of the thirteenth century. Yet, as was increasingly true in various parts of Europe, many of the testators in Champagne clearly felt a social and religious "charitable imperative" to leave legacies for the poor and sick. Even when someone like the Reims cleric Remy, known as "Chevalier," made a bequest to a family member, in this case his niece, who was married, the donor was also thinking about the city's poor and the hospital that cared for them. While bequeathing his house in Reims (upon his death) to his niece, Remy stipulated that if his niece should ever sell his house, half of the proceeds should go to the city's hospital and the other house to the cathedral chapter, to be distributed to the poor.[28]

The Social Class of Hospital Donors

The thirteenth century represented a turning point in terms of the class makeup of donors to charitable and religious institutions. Members of Europe's aristocratic class had long had a special relationship with religious communities and church leaders (most of whom came from this class), serving as their financial patrons in exchange for their prayers. By the thirteenth century, however, townspeople, that is the urban bourgeoisie, had also emerged as significant patrons of religious institutions, thus signaling a rise in lay piety and the democratization of charitable giving. Like their aristocratic neighbors, the shoemakers, launderers, lawyers, carpenters, goldsmiths, roofers, pastry chefs ("talemetarii"), and bourgeois married couples who frequently appear as donors to Champagne's hospitals were associating with a greater number and variety of religious communities. Even while at times patronizing a lengthy list of religious orders and institutions, donors also showed a particular attachment to one institution or type of institution, bestowing it with their most significant gifts, appointing the head of the

---

27. Cohn, *Cult of Remembrance*, 12. As Cohn shows, in some cases these mandatory charities seem to have elicited additional voluntary gifts to the same institution, such as the communal hospital, beyond what was mandated. In other cases, however, the mandatory charities appear to have discouraged additional, voluntary giving.

28. AMC (Reims): FH-HD B62, no. 19 (October 1300).

institution as the executor of their will, and even requesting burial in its cemetery. As we shall see, such expressions of a special attachment to a hospital were common. The largesse of these donors represented an attempt at forging and cementing strong social bonds with an individual hospital that had been or could potentially be useful to them, whether by paving the way for one day joining (or having a family member join) the hospital community, securing a life rent, or facilitating future property transactions or negotiations about rights and privileges.

The democratization of charity is particularly evident among the donors to Saint-Nicolas in Troyes. Although this hospital, which was connected to the cathedral chapter, was not a lay foundation, as many of Champagne's hospitals were, it nonetheless received strong lay support. Of sixty-six donations made prior to 1285 whose records are extant, 70 percent came from lay men and women and 30 percent from clerics. Unlike the hôtel-Dieu-le-Comte in Troyes, however, which was a comital foundation and continued to receive significant financial support from Champagne's counts, the hospital of St-Nicolas flourished without any comital support. Since St-Nicolas could not rely on this kind of support from Champagne's counts, it was even more dependent on bequests from others. While it received some support from aristocrats, it was unusual in having a higher proportion of bourgeois donors, who made up more than one-third of all its donors. This was also true of the hôtel-Dieu of Reims, which was also a dependent of the cathedral chapter. Many of the same families that patronized the cathedral chapter also supported the hospital, and during the thirteenth century the bourgeois Rémois were increasingly prominent benefactors of these institutions, while aristocrats became less so.[29] Of the lay donations that the hospital of Saint-Nicolas in Troyes received, 15 percent came from single women, principally widows, and 22 percent were made in the name of a married couple. The hospital's donors included a launderer and his wife, a lawyer from the court of Troyes (Bernier de Pont Sainte-Marie), a crusader from the prominent d'Arcis family, and a former comital officer and notary at Champagne's fairs. Certain noble families, such as the Saint-Sépulchres, who donated their seigneurial lands at Froiderive and Chauchigny, also appear frequently as donors. In addition to lands and vineyards, the hospital received donations in the form of rents (both money and in kind), forgiven rents that the hospital owed, amortizations, granges, crops, granaries, liturgical books, and rights (such as the use of a forest). Although the majority of donors to Saint-Nicolas came

---

29. Desportes, *Reims et les Rémois*, 149–54.

from Troyes, some donors lived quite some distance away, indicating that the hospital's social network extended far beyond the city.[30]

Of the over one hundred extant late twelfth- and thirteenth-century donation charters to the hôtel-Dieu-le-Comte, over half came from either the count or countess of Champagne or a member of the noble or knightly class. Roughly one-quarter of the donors were ecclesiastics, including a large number of curates, a curious fact since in general, parish priests were known to compete with hospitals for parishioners and burial rights. Among the donors to the hôtel-Dieu-le-Comte was Feliset de Paiens "dictus Judeus," possibly a Jewish convert, whose sister, Emelina Judea, approved the donation.[31] Comparing the names of donors to Saint-Nicolas de Troyes (thirty-nine unique donors before 1300) and the hôtel-Dieu-le-Comte (seventy-five donors), one finds virtually no overlap. In fact, apart from some testaments that included bequests to both hospitals, the only non-testamentary donor common to both hospitals was Lady Aude, wife of Thibaut de Rosières, the lady of Countess Blanche. The aristocrat, Jean de Saint-Sépulchre, who was lord of Villacerf and who made at least five separate donations to Saint-Nicolas, never seems to have given to the hôtel-Dieu-le-Comte. The rivalry between the hôtel-Dieu-le-Comte and the hospital of Saint-Nicolas may have extended to the donors who patronized the two hospitals. Unlike with Saint-Nicolas, relatively few of the donors to the hôtel-Dieu-le-Comte are identified as bourgeois townsmen. However, a significant number of women made bequests to the hospital on their own, and quite a few of them were widows.[32] The wealthy beguine Sebille de Donchery, who lived in Reims, bequeathed in her will of 1322 the sizeable sum of 220 l. par. to the city's largest hospital for the foundation of masses to be celebrated for her soul, "considering the works of mercy and charity which are done daily in our hospital of Reims for the members of Jesus Christ, eager as well to participate in the spiritual goods of the poor and the sisters of the same hospital."[33] Women

---

30. The priest, Odon de Froiderive, for example, who made a donation in 1264, lived in Saint Martin de Bossenay, some forty kilometers to the northwest of Troyes.

31. AD: Aube 40H1, no. 51 (April 1247). It is also possible that Feliset and Emelina's cognomen reflected the fact that an ancestor had been a convert and the epithet of "Judeus" was retained as a surname.

32. In some cases, women needed the consent of male family members (a son or a brother), but male donors also frequently required the consent of a wife. See Evergates, *Aristocracy*, 91–93. Touati has also found a significant percentage of women donors (24% overall), including a large number of widows, among donors to leprosaria in the province of Sens. See Touati, *Maladie et société*, 504–5.

33. Robert, "Les beguines de Reims," 271–72.

also made bequests with their brothers (who quite often were ecclesiastics), and it was also common for married couples to make bequests.[34]

Of the several hundred different donors to the hospital of Provins during the twelfth and thirteenth centuries, many of whom made multiple donations, the social class of some 125 individual donors is indicated in the cartularies: roughly half of all donors came from the noble and knightly class (comparable to the hôtel-Dieu-le-Comte in Troyes), 31 percent were ecclesiastics, and 19 percent were bourgeois. Just as the principal benefactors of Cistercian monasteries were knights, so too did they play a preponderant role in the patronage of the Provinois hospital.[35] The cartulary for the hôtel-Dieu of Provins contains twenty-eight copies (or confirmations) of testaments that included bequests to the hospital.[36] Of the testators, 57 percent were men, 32 percent were women (two of them widows), and 11 percent were couples (spouses or in one case, siblings). The social class is indicated for over 70 percent of the testators, and roughly one-third came from the urban bourgeoisie, one-third from the clergy, and one-third from the noble and knightly classes. Whereas the clergy preferred rural property, bourgeois donors tended to give urban property both in their testaments and in "inter vivos" donations, that is, gifts that took effect while both giver and recipient were still alive. The counts and nobles frequently bequeathed rents to the hospital, with the counts showing a preference for money rents over rents in kind. The martyrological obituary for the hospital of Provins is less explicit about the social class of the 510 donors it lists, particularly bourgeois donors. However, the manuscript consistently labels donors who were priests and religious as such, and 105 of the donors (21%) can be classified as ecclesiastics, including 46 members of the hospital personnel. Only 80 of the donors (16%) are identified as having been a knight, squire, count or countess, noble person, or lady. A sizeable proportion of the hospital donors in the obituary, 126 (25%), are women who acted alone, because they were single, widowed, or married but making their gift in their own name.

Jochen Schenk has found significant overlap between the landed families in Champagne and Burgundy who patronized traditional Benedictine

---

34. On some of the possible gendered differences in the nature of what was being given as pious bequests, see Francine Michaud, "Le pauvre transformé: les hommes, les femmes et la charité à Marseille du XIIIe siècle jusqu'à la peste noire," *Revue historique* 311, no. 2 (2009): 243–90. Michaud has found that 52% of known testators in Marseille (1248–1350) were women.

35. Constance Brittain Bouchard, *Sword, Miter, and Cloister: Nobility and the Church in Burgundy, 980–1198* (Ithaca: Cornell University Press, 1987), 102–49.

36. Most of these testaments were drawn up by the local rural dean, called the dean of Christianity. See Dupraz, nos. 50, 105, 163, 165, 168, 169, 176, 178, 182, 184, 187, 197, 204, 212, 213, 243, 323, 325, 347, 423, 424, 426, 429, 446, 461, 467, 468, B16.

monasteries, Cistercian houses, and houses of Templars.[37] As it turns out, many of the same families that supported the local Templars—Guy de Chappes, lord of Jully; Guy de Dampierre (whose brother-in-law, Guillaume de Baudement, was a Templar); and Clarembaud de Chappes—were also patrons of the hôtel-Dieu-le-Comte, perhaps because the Templars were considered a charitable religious order.[38] But there were also families that directed most, if not all, of their largesse to hospitals, in some cases to one particular hospital. The hospital of Saint-Nicolas of Troyes, for example, tended to be supported more by local townspeople, whereas the hôtel-Dieu-le-Comte and the hospital of Provins, which were probably regarded as more prestigious, were patronized by important aristocratic families and lords, such as the Villehardouin, the Chappes, the Plancy, and the Putemonoie for the hôtel-Dieu-le-Comte in Troyes and the Garlande, the Plessis-aux-Tournelles, and the Montmirail for the hospital of Provins.[39]

In examining the social class of hospital donors, what is striking is just how broad-based the medieval charitable revolution was, with men and women, lay and clerical, married, widowed, and single, from widely diverging social classes, from both the countryside as well as urban areas, all participating. There was certainly a tendency for people to give to institutions that were nearby or to which they felt some connection, with people in the countryside, for example, tending to give to country institutions and townspeople tending to give to urban institutions. The notable diversity of hospital benefactors reflected the diversity of individuals who worked in and were cared for by hospitals, and this distinguished hospitals from most monastic houses. In addition to wanting to support the caritative mission of hospitals, donors from a wide range of backgrounds experienced the power of these institutions, whether in a hospital's providing intercessory prayers, serving as a landlord, or caring for people with widely divergent needs. It was the mixed nature of these institutions, which brought disparate peoples together under one roof, as well as their multi-functionality that attracted such varied benefactors.

Admittedly, not everyone was equally eager to make charitable contributions, and sources occasionally reveal intra-family conflicts over what was perceived as excessive charity or avarice, depending on one's perspective. On the more theoretical level, several theologians addressed the question of whether a wife could give alms against her husband's will, suggesting

---

37. Schenk, *Templar Families*, 25, 77–79, 115.

38. Schenk, *Templar Families*, 148, 192.

39. On the Champenois aristocracy more generally, see Evergates, *Aristocracy*; on the Provinois aristocracy, see Verdier, *L'aristocratie de Provins*.

that perhaps the quandary was more than merely hypothetical. Raymond of Peñafort, Thomas of Chobham, and Godfrey of Fontaines all explored whether the virtue of almsgiving trumped a husband's usual financial control over his wife.[40] In responding in the affirmative, Raymond suggested that husbands did not always mean what they said in forbidding their wives to give alms. Even if a husband were to get angry with his wife for giving alms, the wife was nonetheless justified in giving moderate alms.[41] Thomas of Chobham went further, arguing that the wife of an avaricious husband who failed to pay alms was still obligated to give alms herself.[42] Other theologians, in contrast, argued that a wife must always obey her husband, even if it meant repressing her desire to give alms. In the eyes of these theologians, women's charity had the potential to disrupt the hierarchies of power within households.

In the *Chronique rimée*, a thirteenth-century rhymed chronicle about the kings of France, Philippe Mouskes (who was to become bishop of Tournai) suggested that Countess Jeanne of Flanders and Hainaut embodied the dangers of a woman's excessive charity. According to Mouskes, during the twelve-year period that Jeanne's husband was incarcerated, she was so reckless in her charitable donations that she brought the county to the brink of bankruptcy. When Jeanne's husband was finally released from prison, he had to rescind many of the donations that she had made. Although many of Mouskes's allegations are not borne out by charter evidence, as Erin Jordan has shown, his criticisms of the countess reflected a common male fear of excessive female charity.[43]

An example from Champagne of intra-family conflict over largesse, albeit one in which the husband was the more generous one, can be found in Jean of Montmirail, a wealthy castle lord who had been raised in the French royal court and who accompanied the king on crusade. As Jean turned away from knightly pursuits, such as tournaments, and became increasingly pious, seeking out lepers in need of assistance, and founding a hospital for the poor, a leper house, and a convent for his eldest daughter (who adopted the religious habit there), his wife, Helvide of Dampierre, became alarmed that

---

40. Dyan Elliott, *Spiritual Marriage: Sexual Abstinence in Medieval Wedlock* (Princeton: Princeton University Press, 1993), 189–90; Langholm, *Economics in the Medieval Schools*, 289–90.

41. Elliott, *Spiritual Marriage*, 189–90.

42. Young, *Scholarly*, 137; Sharon Farmer, "Persuasive Voices," *Speculum* 61 (1986), 517, 536–38.

43. Erin Jordan, "Exploring the Limits of Female Largesse: The Power of Female Patrons in Thirteenth-Century Flanders and Hainaut," in *Women and Wealth in Late Medieval Europe*, ed. Theresa Earenfight (New York: Palgrave, 2010), 149–70.

her husband's generosity was jeopardizing her future dower, and she made efforts to block his charitable bequests.[44] Following the death of their eldest son, Jean of Montmirail left his wife and young children to take the Cistercian habit at the abbey of Longpont.

Why Did People Give to Medieval Hospitals?

A hospital's relationship with those living outside the hospital walls was crucial as it competed for bequests. To fully understand hospitals' relationships with their patrons, there is a need to learn more about the diverse services these institutions provided the larger community, including the social networks that they were part of and the ways they functioned as power brokers. An investigation into the nature of donors' relationships with hospitals helps illuminate the complex motivations behind bequests and underscores the power of these religious and charitable institutions, both real and imagined.

It was common for twelfth- and thirteenth-century testaments to indiscriminately include bequests to all of the religious and charitable institutions of a city, regardless of whether the testator had any experience with this or that institution. In his famous will of 1248, the royal cook, Adam, made bequests to some one hundred different religious houses and seventeen leprosaries in the Paris region.[45] In 1219, Countess Blanche's sergeant, Jacques de Hongrie, made bequests in his testament directed to monastic houses, the hôtel-Dieu of Provins, the brothers of the hospital of Saint John of Jerusalem, and a *domus Dei* in Provins for students, which he acknowledged might never be built.[46]

Some testators, however, exhibited a particular proclivity to giving to hospitals and leprosaries, including those that were some distance away. Étienne Haudri and his wife Jeanne Barbou, a wealthy Parisian bourgeois couple who were draper merchants, not only founded a hospital for poor widows but also left testamentary bequests to lepers, the blind, orphans, prisoners, students who were without support, those suffering from ergotism, the poor who had fallen on hard times, hospices for the sick, and poor girls who wished to marry. The size of Étienne's charitable bequests was approximately ten times his bequests to churches and religious houses and about the same size as his bequests to family members, household servants, and individual

44. Evergates, *Aristocracy*, 93–94, 163, 236–37; Lester, *Creating Cistercian Nuns*, 159.
45. Touati, "Les groupes des laïcs," 146 and note 27.
46. Dupraz, no. 446; AD: Seine-et-Marne 11Hdt A12, fol. 129v–130.

clerics. But 80 percent of Jeanne's testamentary bequests were directed at hospitals and other charitable causes.[47] The curate of Sceaux-du-Gâtinais's testament included donations to hospitals and leprosaria in Provins (85 kilometers away), Sourdun (90 kilometers away), and Sens (65 kilometers away), as well as hospitals that were closer, such as in Boiscommun, Châtenoy, Pontfranc-les-Château-Landon, and Chenou.[48] The Dominican cardinal Hugues de Billom (d. ca.1297), who came from the powerful Aycelin family, left the staggering sum of 2,200 *l. t.* as well as other gifts to the hospital in his hometown of Billom, in central France.[49] The 1255 testament from Peter from Bar-sur-Aube, who was a convert from Judaism, shows that he had learned the conventions of the time in terms of Christian charitable giving, and among the many relatives and religious and charitable institutions that received bequests from him were the four principal hospitals in Troyes and the hospital and leper house of Bar-Sur-Aube. The executors of his testament, meanwhile, were tasked with distributing pennies to the poor on the first, third, and seventh day following his death.[50]

Some testators had a special relationship with a particular hospital, as evidenced by the donors making their most generous (or only) bequests to one hospital. Testators increasingly became "ardent materialists," in Martha Howell's words, because the material things that they bequeathed served as expressions of their social and religious values and helped them forge relationships. Donation charters and testamentary bequests to hospitals, for example, reflected a growing desire to quantify social and religious bonds by noting that the item being donated, such as a bed with linens or a liturgical book like a breviary was the donor's "best" one. In this way, the donor's attachment to the item being bequeathed expressed the donor's love for the particular hospital to which it was given.[51] Beds were clearly one of the most important possessions of hospitals, and so it was significant when a donor like Brice de Gouaix, the chaplain of Saint-Quiriace in Provins, chose to give his "better" bed to the poor of the hospital of Provins.[52]

47. Boris Bove, "Vie et mort d'un couple de marchands-drapiers parisiens d'après les testaments de Jeanne et Étienne Haudri (1309, 1313)," *Paris et Ile-de-France* 52 (2001): 19–81.

48. Dupraz, no. 243; AD: Seine-et-Marne 11Hdt A12, fol. 73v.

49. Pierre-François Fournier, "Les statuts de l'hôpital de Billom (Puy-de-Dôme)," in *Assistance et assistés jusqu'à 1610. Actes du 97ᵉ Congrès National des Sociétés Savantes, Nantes, 1972* (Paris: Bibliothèque Nationale, 1979), 129–46.

50. AD: Aube 3H336 (December 1255).

51. Howell, *Commerce before Capitalism*, 168–71. Francine Michaud has noted that it was only during the early thirteenth century that testators in Provence began showing a concern with the quality of items being given. See Michaud, "Le pauvre transformé," 282–83.

52. Dupraz, no. 213; AD: Seine-et-Marne 11Hdt A12, fol. 64 (1271).

The special attachment some donors felt to a particular hospital can also be seen in their requests that anniversary masses be said after their death, that a hospital's *magister* serve as the executor of their will, or, in a few cases, that they be buried in a hospital's cemetery. At times bequests were accompanied by expressions of gratitude for a service the hospital had provided (or that a donor hoped it might provide in the future), so there is a need to study these gifts in the larger context of the relationship between the donor and the hospital. What were hospitals doing to "earn" a donor's gratitude in the form of a gift? How common were bequests made as "entry gifts," that is, so that the donor would be received as a member of the hospital community? Are the gifts of some donors explained by a family's preexisting connection to a hospital or even a possible personal connection to poverty, illness, or disability? In analyzing the motivations of hospital donors and the social networks of Champagne's hospitals and patrons, we first need to consider the role that donors' concern with salvation played in their gift-giving.

Redemptive Almsgiving

Studies of gift-giving to monasteries have observed that the formulas used in charters recording pious donations changed during the later twelfth and thirteenth centuries, and these changes in the words used to describe gifts have been interpreted as signaling a larger shift in the meaning of pious gifts. The *pro anima* formula, indicative of a belief in the redemptive power of pious donations, which was pervasive during the twelfth century, was gradually supplanted during the thirteenth century by the phrase "in elemosinam" ("in alms"), although the two phrases at times appeared together. In his study of the wealthy Benedictine house Montier-la-Celle near Troyes, for example, Richard Keyser noted this shift, finding that by the latter half of the twelfth century, only 25 percent of gifts to the monastery included the phrase "pro anima." During the thirteenth century, the *pro anima* formula became even rarer.[53]

At the hospital of Provins, in contrast, donation charters continued to employ the "pro anima" phrase right through the thirteenth century, with one-third of donation charters continuing to use the phrase as late as the 1280s (down only from 46 percent in the 1210s). While the "in elemosinam" formula began to be employed more frequently than the *pro anima* formula in hospital bequests during the late thirteenth century (the phrase

---

53. Keyser, "Gift, Dispute, and Contract," 189–90.

"in elemosinam" is found in 86 percent of donation charters from the 1280s), the two phrases often appeared together. The central point is that unlike in the monastic context, late thirteenth-century hospital donors did not have a diminished sense of the inherent redemptive power of their donations. Perhaps pious gifts to the sick poor had come to be viewed as more powerfully redemptive in and of themselves, as opposed to gifts to monasteries, which were increasingly viewed as spiritually redemptive only in so far as the monks prayed for the souls of their donors. Moreover, some hospital donors conceived of their gifts as gifts to God as much as to a hospital and its sick poor, and this was made explicit in the language of charters. Thus, the furrier Hervé Pelletier of Lévêque and his wife Marie indicated in their charter of 1277 that they were giving a rent of wine "to God and the hospital" ("Deo et hospitali") of Saint-Nicolas of Troyes, a formulation that, while relatively rare in thirteenth-century charters, reflects the common association between pious gift and divine reward.[54] In their donation charter to the hospital of Saint-Nicolas, the squire Jean de Clérey, his brother, and their cousin made clear that they wished to support "the pious alms and works of mercy which are conferred upon the sick poor of Christ there."[55] Egidiul, the cantor of Langres and dean of Saint-Maclou in Bar-sur-Aube, made a donation in 1230 to the hospital of Saint-Nicolas in Bar-sur-Aube and "the brothers serving God there."[56] The testament of Thésie la Chiesoie was even more explicit about what inspired her to leave her house, her bedding, and some land to the hospital of Provins (as well as a money gift to Adam, the hospital chaplain): "considering God as the judge, and with the eyes of her heart fearing Him on account of the measure of her sins, hoping very much nevertheless for His mercy, knowing that mercy above others exalts judgment."[57] Thésie believed that her best chance of winning God's mercy was by supporting an institution that was dedicated to performing the works of mercy and thus that was seen (or saw itself) as embodying the *imitatio Dei*. These were not mere formulas. While a gift given for the donor's soul ("pro anima") was not an explicit request for a hospital's prayers in the way that a request for an anniversary Mass was, the use of the "pro anima" phrase nonetheless distinguished a gift intended to help a donor's soul from more commercial transactions. There had been a long history of material gifts being given in

---

54. AD: Aube 43H12, lay31, cote A, no. 38 (September 1277).
55. AD: 43H12, lay 31, cote A, no. 30 (May 1270): "pias elemosinas et opera misericordie qui sunt ibidem infirmos Christi pauperes visitando."
56. AD: Aube HD 33 / 50 (July 1230): "fratribus ibidem deo servientibus."
57. Dupraz, no. 165; AD: Seine-et-Marne 11Hdt A12, fol. 48v–49.

exchange for spiritual intercession (in the form of psalmody and Masses). Indeed, this was the cornerstone of the Cluniac system of exchange between monks and benefactors.[58] Addressing these clauses in the monastic context, Constance Bouchard has written, "From the point of the monks recording the transactions, a soul's salvation was just as real and solid as any other return."[59] What was different in the context of hospitals was that the spiritual counter-gift that donors found so appealing need not have been the result of intercessory prayer but could instead simply be from the works of mercy performed by a hospital. It was believed that the social and religious action of charity could reap the same (or even greater) spiritual benefits as intercessory prayer. Donations, in other words, whether to monasteries or hospitals, were understood as reciprocal and dynamic exchanges, whereby the donor reaped valuable and calculable assets in the form of spiritual benefits.

Some scholars of thirteenth-century monasticism have linked the decline of the *pro anima* formula in monastic bequests to the concomitant rise in bequests that were given on the condition that anniversary masses would be celebrated for the donor and his or her relatives and friends. It was no longer enough to merely state that a pious donation was being made for the salvation of certain souls; it was increasingly expected that pious donations would be rewarded with anniversary masses, which were regarded as the vital way to be remembered and have one's soul saved. At Montier-la-Celle, for instance, Richard Keyser found that whereas only 20 percent of gifts made between 1217 and 1280 were rewarded with anniversary masses, in the period from 1280 to 1349 that percentage had risen to 75 percent.[60]

The promise of anniversary masses was less common at Champagne's hospitals. At the hôtel-Dieu-le-Comte in Troyes only 18 percent of all late twelfth- and thirteenth-century donors were promised anniversary masses, and at the hospital of Saint-Nicolas in Troyes, 26 percent of donors were promised an anniversary. Nor was there a trend of anniversaries being promised more frequently in the late thirteenth century. At the hospital of Provins, the number of anniversary masses promised to donors did increase during the second half of the thirteenth century. However, the promise of anniversary masses for donations still occurred far less frequently than it did at many monasteries. During the 1250s, for instance, only 11 percent of donors

58. Arnold Angenendt, "Donationes Pro Anima: Gift and Countergift in the Early Medieval Liturgy," in the *Long Morning of Medieval Europe: New Directions in Early Medieval Studies*, ed. Jennifer R. Davis and Michael McCormick (London: Routledge, 2017), 131–54.

59. Bouchard, *Sword, Miter, and Cloister*, 241.

60. Keyser, "Gift, Dispute, and Contract," 334.

to the hospital were promised an anniversary mass. Even in the 1270s, when the largest number of hospital donations were rewarded with an anniversary mass, this still only represented 44 percent of all donations. Of all the bequests found in the cartulary for the hospital of Provins, only 22 percent were rewarded with an anniversary mass.[61] The percentage is even smaller for donations listed in the hospital's martyrological obituary, where only 45 of 506, or 9 percent, mention that the donor was promised an anniversary mass. It may be that the obituary was less systematic in recording anniversary masses, since much less information was recorded about gifts than in the cartulary, and the focus of the obituary was on inventorying all donors according to the date of their death (although generally not the year). Why were anniversary masses promised less frequently to hospital donors than to monastic donors, particularly during the late thirteenth century? It appears that even in the late thirteenth century, many gifts to hospitals had fewer strings attached, compared with gifts made to monasteries, which were increasingly conditional, contractual, and commercial in nature. This is not to suggest, however, that thirteenth-century donors to hospitals did not hope to reap spiritual or even material rewards from their gifts or that their gifts were not expressions of gratitude for services they had already received from a hospital.

Although not as many donors to Champagne's hospitals made the prayers of the hospital brethren a condition for their gifts, the language of the charters that record these gifts are replete with references to "pro remedio anime et salute," suggesting that the donors made their gifts with the belief that their souls (and the souls of their families and ancestors) might be saved partly as a consequence. Furthermore, even if a smaller percentage of donors were promised anniversary masses, the hospital brethren were nonetheless regarded as valuable spiritual intercessors. For example, Hagalon, a knight from Evry who made a very significant gift of 300 *l.* to the hôtel-Dieu-le-Comte, planned to visit the hospital's chapel each year on the day after Saint Bartholomew's Day for the celebration of the Mass of the Holy Spirit that had been promised to him and other benefactors, and he was also promised an annual Mass for the dead following his death.[62]

---

61. A significant percentage of the hospital donors at the hospital of Provins who were promised anniversaries—39%—were clerics, almost double the overall proportion of the donors who were of clerical status (22%). Likewise, at Saint-Nicolas in Troyes, 46% of donors who were promised anniversaries were ecclesiastics, even though ecclesiastics made up only 28% of all donors to this hospital. At the hôtel-Dieu-le-Comte, a somewhat smaller percentage of promised anniversaries, 27%, were made to clerics, roughly corresponding to their representation among the hospital's benefactors.

62. AD: Aube 40H1, no. 10 (August 1213); Aube 40H189, fol. 36.

Underlying some testators' bequests to hospitals was a profound sense of anxiety about the fate of their souls, particularly when they had engaged in what were considered immoral economic practices. This is reflected in the testament of Adam de Vervins, the notary for the officialty of the archdeaconry of Reims. As he lay on his deathbed ("jacens in lecto egridudinis") in 1303, still of a healthy mind, able to speak well and in a good cognitive state, he bequeathed his large house at Jard-aux-Drapiers in Reims to the city's principal hospital. Virtually all of his other testamentary bequests were directed at individuals, including, in many cases, the heirs to individuals, and it is possible that these were the heirs to people with whom he had had business dealings.[63] What is especially striking is how many of his bequests were given "in the name of restitution." The beginning of the testament not only included the common formula about the testamentary executors paying off Adam's debts but also called on his executors to restore to individuals and places those things of his that had been wickedly extorted or acquired illicitly.[64] This same anxious spirit also underlay the testamentary bequests of another Rémois, the wealthy bourgeois financier Perrecart de Villedommage, whose fortune may have approached 8,000 *l. parisis*.[65] Perrecart's father, Drouard de Villedommage, and his father-in-law from his first marriage, Estène le Boeuf, were business partners and usurers.[66] The late husband of Perrecart's first wife Isabeau le Boeuf, named Jacques Manjupoi, committed so much usury that after he died, Isabeau spent 700 *l. p.* to reimburse the victims of his ill-acquired gains; she spent an additional 300 *l.* in pious distributions for the salvation of her late husband's soul.[67] Perrecart's own testament, dated November 2, 1275, just days before his death, included significant bequests to his heirs, including his younger, second wife, their four children, the children Perrecart had had with his first wife, his sister, his nephews and nieces, and his servants. But with an eye to the salvation of his soul, Perrecart directed his executors to his account books and to the folios where he listed the victims of his usury, asking that restitutions be made to them. He further made bequests to pious and charitable causes totaling 1,200 *l. parisis,* including parish churches, abbeys, chapters, hospitals, and leprosaries, and 400 *l. p.* for parish poor relief societies ("chartriers") to provide assistance to the city's poor.[68]

---

63. Adam de Vervins also made bequests to his servants.

64. AMC (Reims): FH-HD B50, l. 3, no. 22 (October 1303): "et male extorta seu illicite acquisita restituantur personis et locis quibus sunt faciendum per manis executorum suorum."

65. Desportes, *Reims et les Rémois*, 144.

66. For the connections between these families, see Desportes, *Reims et les Rémois*, 137–45.

67. Desportes, *Reims et les Rémois*, 143.

68. Desportes, *Reims et les Rémois*, 144.

The belief in the redemptive power of giving alms to hospitals is also in plain view in the bequests made to hospitals by those about to leave on crusade. The seventeenth-century historian of Provins, Eustache Grillon, noted that among Count Henri the Liberal's crusading entourage that hailed from Provins, virtually all had made gifts to the Provinois hospital before departing.[69] This group included Guillaume le Roi, marshal of the count, who, before departing on crusade, made gifts to a number of religious institutions, including the hospital of Provins.[70] Milon de Provins, who was the son of the count's marshal and chamberlain, emulated his father in 1190/91 by giving a number of properties to the hospital of Provins before departing for the Near East. Milon ended up being captured by Muslims, and François Verdier has raised the intriguing question of whether a donation to the hospital in 1194/95 by Milon's brother, Fromond "le Borgne," was perhaps made with the hope that it would lead to Milon's liberation from captivity.[71] Before departing on crusade in 1202, the knight Geoffroy Chalot, who was a merchant-investor and had been sergeant of the archbishop of Sens, Guillaume aux Blanches Mains (the brother of Count Henri the Liberal), bequeathed his grange and lands in Sourdun to the hospital of Provins.[72] The central point is that a popular way for one to prepare one's soul before embarking on a crusade, which itself was regarded as a spiritually redemptive act, was to make bequests to a hospital's poor. In anticipation of the mercy they knew they might soon need, crusaders were eager to support the works of mercy being performed in local hospitals.

From charter evidence, it would appear that was it rare for hospital donors to make burial in a hospital's chapel or cemetery a condition of a bequest.[73] Among the records of 165 donations to the hospital of Provins found in the hospital's cartulary, there are only four cases of donors requesting to be buried in the hospital's cemetery. Out of the 510 donors listed in the obituary for the hospital, only two are mentioned as having been buried in the hospital's cemetery. For the hospital of Saint-Nicolas in Troyes, there is only one extant thirteenth-century donation charter that includes a request

---

69. Verdier, *L'aristocratie*, 150, 159.

70. Verdier, *L'aristocratie*, 151, 160. While in Marseille about to depart for the crusade, Geoffroy Éventé d'Egligny bequeathed his forest in Sourdun to the hospital.

71. Verdier, *L'aristocratie*, 160.

72. Dupraz, no. 440; AD: Seine-et-Marne 11Hdt A12, fol. 129; Verdier, *L'aristocratie*, 146–47.

73. It was also relatively rare for twelfth-century lay donors to be buried in monasteries in Champagne and Burgundy. See Keyser, "Gift, Dispute, and Contract," 198–99; Constance Brittain Bouchard, *Holy Entrepreneurs: Cistercians, Knights, and Economic Exchange in Twelfth-Century Burgundy* (Ithaca: Cornell University Press, 1991), 23, 66, 73–74.

for burial.[74] Some caution, however, needs to be taken in assuming that more donors were not buried in hospital chapels or cemeteries, since burial requests usually appear in testaments as opposed to donation charters, and relatively few testaments from this period survive for Champagne. Donors were almost certainly being buried in hospital chapels and cemeteries more often than charters' silence about the matter suggests. In the case of Pisa, Italy, where a large number of testaments do survive, Elizabeth Rothrauff has found that out of 280 testaments from the second half of the thirteenth century, fifty-nine testators (21%) requested burial at a hospital cemetery, reflecting a desire on the part of testators to be associated with the holy, caritative mission of hospitals.[75] Far from wanting to avoid any contact with the poor and the sick—groups we generally think of as social marginals during this period—these testators chose the cemeteries that were filled with the poor and sick as their eternal resting places.[76]

When donors to hospitals did request to be buried at a hospital or its cemetery, there was the potential for a conflict to arise with the donor's parish, which relied on burial fees for income. In late medieval London, where it has been calculated that 62 to 86 percent of testators chose to be buried in their parish cemetery, hospitals at times paid a rector when burying a parishioner from that rector's parish to compensate him for what would otherwise be a loss of revenue.[77] When Pope Celestine III accorded the hospital of Provins the right to have a cemetery in 1195, he made clear that the hospital needed to obtain the consent of the bishop and parish churches before it could bury not only the hospital brothers and sisters but the sick poor and hospital donors as well.[78] Still, it was not uncommon for hospitals to become embroiled in conflicts over burying parishioners in their cemeteries. The curate of Saint-Nizier accused the hospital of Saint-Nicolas in Troyes of stealing his parishioners and made the hospital promise to stop burying his parishioners in its cemetery.[79] A statute promulgated at Liège in 1288 sought

---

74. AD: Aube 43H12, layette 31, cote A, no. 35 (1274).

75. Elizabeth Rothrauf, "Charity in Medieval Community: Politics, Piety, and Poor Relief in Pisa, 1257–1312" (PhD dissertation, University of California, Berkeley, 2012), 102–3.

76. Admittedly, some wealthier donors were buried in hospital chapels as opposed to cemeteries. See Craig Cessford, "The St. John's Hospital Cemetery and Environs, Cambridge: Contextualizing the Medieval Urban Dead," *Archaeological Journal* 172, no. 1 (2015): 62.

77. Vanessa Harding, "Burial Choice and Burial Location in Later Medieval London," in *Death in Towns: Urban Responses to the Dying and the Dead, 100–1600,* ed. Steven Bassett (London: Leicester University Press, 1992), 122, 124; Imbert, *Les hôpitaux en droit canonique,* 90–95.

78. Dupraz, no. 1; AD: Seine-et-Marne 11Hdt A12, fol. 16.

79. AD: Aube 43H8 (August 1276).

to protect the rights of parish priests by insisting that they be present when a parishioner was drawing up his or her testament. If, despite the presence (and prodding) of the curate, the testator chose to be interred in a cemetery other than the parish's, a funeral mass would nonetheless first have to be celebrated in the parish church before the burial was performed elsewhere, thus ensuring that the parish's prerogatives (and income) were protected.[80]

The reality was that laymen and -women had a range of burial options besides the parish cemetery, including cemeteries at monasteries, friaries, and hospitals. The choice of where to be buried was a personal one that often reflected a donor's particular allegiances, sense of identity, and membership in a community. That Thomas, the chaplain of the church of Saint-Pierre in Provins, indicated in his testament his intention to be buried at the hospital of Provins, was not a surprise.[81] His late uncle, Adam, had been the *magister* of the hospital and was himself buried there. It was only natural that this priest, who had no spouse, should choose the hospital that his uncle had overseen as his final resting place. The rationale for the burial choices of other donors is a bit less clear. In 1252 Pierre de Montreant and his wife, Eramburge, drew up a testament in which they bequeathed their house and two *arpents* of land and abandoned a money and grain rent that the hospital owed them. They also appointed the *magister* of the hospital of Provins as their testamentary executor (along with the prior of the leprosary of Close-barbe). Separately, Eramburge bequeathed a feather bed and indicated her wish to be buried in the hospital cemetery.[82] Eleven years later, Pierre's new wife, Hodeborge, drew up her final testament, and she, too, requested burial in the hospital cemetery, and bequeathed two *arpents* of land, a small farm and dwelling place, pittances for bread for the hospital poor on the day of her death, an annual rent for the purchase of shoes and woolen cloth to be distributed to the poor of Provins, money for the chaplain and clerics of the hospital, a furnished bed, and three *sous* to install a statue of Our Lady in front of the hospital's door.[83] Although there is no mention in Pierre's testament of where he intended to be buried, that both of his wives indicated a desire to be buried in the hospital cemetery may suggest that he planned to be buried there as well. In the 1252 testament of Emanjarde, the widow

---

80. De Spiegeler, *Les hôpitaux et l'assistance à Liège*, 173–74.

81. Dupraz, no. 426; AD: Seine-et-Marne 11Hdt A12, fol. 124–124v.

82. Dupraz, no. 424; AD: Seine-et-Marne 11Hdt A12, fol. 123v–124. Although burial was considered a "free" sacrament, the monastic burial of lay men and women almost always involved a fee under the guise of alms for the deceased's soul. See Bouchard, *Sword, Miter, and Cloister*, 192.

83. Dupraz, no. 423; AD: Seine-et-Marne 11Hdt A12, fol. 123v.

of Herbert de Mointoingnon, she too, indicated her choice to be buried in the hospital of Provins's cemetery.[84] One wonders whether Emanjarde's husband was also buried at the hospital cemetery, or whether he chose to be buried in a different cemetery.[85]

Although relatively few donors to Champagne's hospitals seem to have made burial in the hospital's cemetery or chapel, or the celebration of anniversary masses a condition for their bequests, donors continued to display a strong belief in the spiritual power of redemptive almsgiving. That the *pro anima* clause was gradually disappearing from donation charters to monastic houses during the thirteenth century while still frequently being included in the records of bequests to hospitals suggests that alms given to hospitals for the "poor of Christ" were intrinsically understood as having the potential to produce spiritual and soteriological benefits.

Helping the Sick Poor

Some donors were thinking quite pragmatically about the ways their gifts might impact the sick poor, and this casts doubt on the frequently repeated argument that medieval charity was indiscriminate, with donors showing little to no regard for materially improving the lives of the recipients of their charity. Donors often made clear their desire to be associated with a hospital and its particular mission of caring for the poor and the sick. Donation charters for the hospital of Saint-Nicolas in Troyes, for example, were explicit in directing gifts to "the house of the poor," or "for the use of the poor," or "to sustain the poor," or simply for "the poor who lie down and rise up there."[86] When Marguerite "Gilbosa" gave some land at Froiderive to the hospital of Saint-Nicolas in 1265, the donation charter indicates that she conceived of her gift as supporting "the poor sick."[87] Likewise, in 1225, a certain Lord Nicholaus, who had formerly been the chaplain of a now-deceased lady, gave in perpetual alms for his soul, at his death, his house near the well of Varète and whatever other things he had "to the poor of the hospital of the domus Dei of Bar . . . with God having inspired him that it was worth spending a

---

84. Dupraz, no. B16; AD: Seine-et-Marne 11Hdt A13, fol. 47–47v.

85. Although spouses sometimes requested to be buried next to each other, many did not make such requests. See Christopher Daniell, *Death and Burial in Medieval England* (London: Routledge, 1997), 101–2.

86. AD Aube 43H12, lay 31, cote A, no. 3 (1216); no. 3 (1210); no. 4 (1208); no. 43 (1285).

87. AD: Aube 43H12, lay31, cote A, no. 26 (1265).

certain portion on his deathbed."[88] It was common for hospital donation charters to indicate that a gift was directed at the sick or the "sick poor," as opposed to the institution as a whole, or even the hospital's *magister*, brothers, and sisters. In the case of a leper house, such as Les Deux Eaux, outside Troyes, one donor, Hardouin des Eschèges, had a sister who was a leper resident of the hospital.[89]

Even beyond the wording of where a gift was directed, however, donors were giving thought to the hospital's needs and the work being done there. Guy de Chappes, lord of Jully, gave the hôtel-Dieu-le-Comte an annual rent of 20 *sous* to buy little pots and trays ("ollulas et scutellas") for the sick, and in addition, each year he gave three measures of red wine from his vineyards for the celebration of the Mass in the hospital's chapel, "considering how the domus Dei was generously open to the indigent and devotedly dedicated itself to the works of mercy."[90] In 1217 Erard de Villehardouin made a donation to the same hospital, "considering the works of mercy which are zealously and devotedly done in the *domus Dei* of Saint-Étienne, and wanting that I and my [relatives] be participants of those [works of mercy]."[91] Other charters refer to the "pious alms and works of mercy which are visited upon the sick poor of Christ in the same place."[92] For the knight Jean de Chappes, the decision to freely amortize some property from his fief that had been sold to the hospital of Saint-Nicolas stemmed from his recognition "of the poverty of the said house of Saint Nicolas de Troyes, the masses, alms, intercessory prayers that they do for the poor that are lying and standing there, and the many other kindnesses that they do not cease from doing day and night."[93] The knight Pierre des Barres confirmed a donation of a rent that his mother, Heloise des Barres, "made for the sustenance of the poor of the *domus Dei* of Provins, with love of God and in a spirit of piety."[94]

The types of gifts that donors made to hospitals at times reflected their desire to address the specific material and spiritual needs of the hospital. In recording the death of Lord Artaud, the knight from Nogent, who served as chamberlain and adviser to Count Henri "the Liberal" for over forty years,

---

88. AD: Aube HD 33/50 (1225): "pauperibus hospitalis domus Dei Barri . . . ubi deus sibi inspiravit in extremis aliquam portionem erogare valebit."

89. Harmand, *Notice historique*, 33.

90. AD: Aube 40H1, no. 28 (June 1218).

91. AD: Aube 40H1, no. 27 (June 1217).

92. AD Aube 43H12, layette 31, cote A, no. 30.

93. Arbois de Jubainville, "Etude sur les documents," 102–3.

94. Dupraz, no. B11; AD: Seine-et-Marne 11Hdt A13, fol. 21v.

the obituary for the hospital of Provins noted that it was Artaud who was responsible for building the refectory and dormitory for the hospital sisters.[95] In 1254, Mathieu, the lord of Montmirail and Oisy, bequeathed to the hospital of Provins an annual rent of 30 *sous* so that the hospital could buy incense for the chapel infirmary.[96] Was it Mathieu's idea to fund the purchase of incense for the chapel? Or did someone at the hospital suggest that he earmark his rent for this purpose, much as a development officer in a modern university, foundation, or charitable organization might do with a prospective donor? It is unclear, but a hospital's material and spiritual needs were surely well known. A potentially valuable source in this regard would be the recruiting messages of the *quaestors* who collected alms on behalf of hospitals. We know from a Parisian woman's testament from 1330, for instance, that alms seekers from thirty-nine leprosaria and seventeen hospitals converged each Monday on the "Grand Pont" in Paris.[97] The recruiting messages that they delivered from this bridge might reveal what hospitals believed would resonate with potential donors.

One way that hospitals sought to appeal to prospective donors and inform them about the charitable and spiritual work being performed there was by granting indulgences to those who gave alms, particularly while visiting the hospital. In that sense, as Nicholas Vincent has suggested, "indulgences were intended both to encourage alms and to serve as an early form of rent-a-crowd."[98] Indulgences, which were increasingly being granted over the course of the late twelfth and thirteenth centuries, did not offer the remission of sin, as Vincent has pointed out, but rather the remission "of a certain period of 'enjoined penance.'"[99] The granting of indulgences was used as a means of soliciting alms for various groups of needy people, religious and charitable institutions, and building projects, including bridges, roads, and fortifications.[100] Indulgences were frequently offered to those giving alms at the dedication of a church, monastery, or hospital, or on the anniversary of the dedication. The granting of these indulgences usually came about as a result of an institution's petitioning a bishop or pope. In 1191, the archbishop

95. AD Seine-et-Marne, 11Hdt/C5, fol. 11v; *Obituaires de la province de Sens*, 1:925. For more on Artaud, see Theodore Evergates, "Nobles and Knights in Twelfth-Century France," in *Cultures of Power: Lordship, Status, and Process in Twelfth-Century Europe*, ed. Thomas Bisson (Philadelphia: University of Pennsylvania Press, 1995), 31–33.

96. Dupraz, no. 87; AD Seine-et-Marne, 11HdtA12, fol. 29v–30 (1254).

97. Farmer, *Surviving Poverty*, 87.

98. Vincent, "Some Pardoners' Tales," 38.

99. Vincent, "Some Pardoners' Tales," 27.

100. Shaffern, *Penitents' Treasury*, 58–62.

of Sens granted an indulgence of ten days to anyone who gave alms while visiting the hôtel-Dieu of Provins during the seven days following the anniversary of its consecration.[101] In his letters granting an indulgence to a different hospital, Pope Boniface VIII stressed that by helping the sick poor, one was nourishing Christ.[102] Bringing people in to visit the hospital provided an opportunity not only to collect alms but also to showcase its most pressing needs and the valuable services it provided.

Clerics, mendicants, and personal confessors may also have played a role in shaping where testators and donors directed their bequests. It is difficult to know how much of an influence pastors had in spurring lay charitable giving, and in reminding laymen and -women of the Christian obligation to assist the *miserabiles*. Even apart from the question of whether and to what extent the laity internalized the moral lessons about charity from the kinds of sermon *exempla* that we examined in chapter 1, what role did clerics and confessors, many of whom were friars, play in the drawing up of last wills? In her study of late thirteenth- and early fourteenth-century testaments in Provence, Francine Michaud noted that 35 percent of testators cited clerics, and even more donors did so (59%) in their *inter vivos* bequests.[103] Confessors, for example, were frequently mentioned by merchant drapers and artisans in their testaments. Clerics and friars frequently served as executors of wills, and they were also appointed to oversee the distribution of alms to the poor.[104] Although clerics and friars may have had some influence on lay charitable practices, there is a danger in overstating their influence on the decisions and choices of the laity, particularly with something as consequential as naming the beneficiaries of their assets. In that sense, it is difficult to imagine that lay testaments and bequests did not, on the whole, reflect the personal preferences of testators and donors.[105]

---

101. In 1250, the archbishop increased this indulgence to twenty days. See Dupraz, nos. 22, 23; AD: Seine-et-Marne 11Hdt A12, fol. 19–19v.

102. Shaffern, *Penitents' Treasury*, 62.

103. Michaud, "Le pauvre transformé," 260.

104. Michaud, "Le pauvre transformé," 259–67.

105. This issue has long been the subject of debate among scholars, particularly over the extent to which wills reflected the voice of the notary (or were merely formulaic) or that of the testator. See Steven Epstein, *Wills and Wealth in Medieval Genoa, 1150–1250* (Cambridge: Harvard University Press, 1984), 34; Joëlle Rollo-Koster, "Item Lego . . . Item Volo . . . Is There Really an 'I' in Medieval Provençales' Wills?" in *"For the Salvation of My Soul": Women and Wills in Medieval and Early Modern France*, ed. Joëlle Rollo-Koster and Kathryn L. Reyerson (St. Andrews, Scotland: St. Andrews Studies in French History and Culture, 2012), 3–24; Clive Burgess, "Late Medieval Wills and Pious Conventions: Testamentary Evidence Reconsidered," in Michael Hicks, ed., *Profit, Piety, and the Professions in Later Medieval England* (Gloucester, 1990), 14–33; Chiffoleau, *La comptabilité*, 84–85.

Money rents that were donated to hospitals were at times earmarked for specific purposes. Philippe, lord of Plancy, adding to the gift that his mother, Odéard, had made a few years earlier to fund pittances for the poor in the hôtel-Dieu-le-Comte's infirmary, designated a rent to be collected from a fair for the brothers of the hospital to buy shrouds for burying the dead.[106] André de Nanteuil stipulated that his annual rent of 15 *sous* was "for the use of one lamp for the domus Dei to provide hospitality."[107] The knight Guillaume Putemonoie gave an annual rent of 20 *sous* for the purchase of three tunics and six pairs of shoes "for the poor of Christ."[108] In 1205 Countess Blanche made a donation of some land (that she had earlier purchased for 26 *l.*) in order to support the priest who served the altar of Saint Margaret the Virgin in the hospital's chapel.[109] In 1260, Count Thibaut donated two of his bakers to work in the hospital's mills and ovens, and earlier counts, going back to Henri the Liberal, had exempted the hospital's bakers from various seigneurial obligations.[110] In 1190 Geoffroi l'Eventi gave one-quarter of his woods at Maiel to the Provinois hospital so that the wood could be burned to keep the poor warm.[111] In addition to giving the hospital two houses (one near a garden belonging to the hospital), land, and part of a vineyard, Lucas de Laceon and his wife Emelina also endowed a chaplaincy so that the offices could be celebrated for their souls in the lower crypt of the hospital.[112] In June of 1270 the knight Renaud de Bar-le-Duc made a major bequest to the hospital of an annual rent of 200 *l.* on the entrance of wines. In addition, Renaud gave the hospital his house (located just behind the hospital), where he wanted both a chapel to be founded, dedicated to the Virgin Mary, and a small hospital to house six healthy, pregnant women, presumably to be cared for by the sisters of the hospital.[113] It is interesting that this knight wanted to create an annex or extension to the hospital specifically for pregnant women, perhaps because the statutes for the hôtel-Dieu-le-Comte, drafted seven years earlier, had specifically forbidden the reception of pregnant women due to their being a potential disturbance

---

106. AD: Aube 40H1, no. 23 (July 1218). Thomas l'Apothicaire (d. 1312) bequeathed property to the hôtel-Dieu of Reims so that it could buy cloth shrouds for the poor. See Desportes, *Reims et les Rémois*, 327 and note 35.

107. AD: Aube 40H1, no. 24 (February 1216).

108. AD: Aube 40H1, no. 39 (February 1232).

109. AD: Aube 40H1, no. 13 (August 1205).

110. AD: Aube 40H25 (1260); Boutiot, *Histoire de la ville de Troyes*, 1:348.

111. AD: Seine-et-Marne, 11Hdt/B1.

112. AD: Seine-et-Marne, 11Hdt/B1.

113. AD: Aube 40H1 (June, 1270); Arbois de Jubainville, *Histoire des ducs*, nos. 3660 and 3662 (for Thibaut's approval, since Renaud held this rent in fief from the count).

to the sick poor. But one also wonders whether Renaud had had some family experience that made him identify with the needs of pregnant women. It was certainly no coincidence that the chapel and hospital for these pregnant women was dedicated to the Virgin Mary, who was so closely associated with pregnancy, childbirth, and the healing of women.

This desire to materially improve the lives of the sick and poor in hospitals can be seen in some donors' bequests of pittances, usually on the anniversary of the donor's death. Out of the 165 donations to the hospital of Provins included in the cartulary, twenty (12%) include a gift earmarked for pittances, many of these in the context of a testament. Gauthier Bochard, a canon of Saint-Étienne in Troyes, wanted eight hens distributed as food in the hospital each year on All Soul's (or the next suitable day) to "the weaker and more sick ones."[114] A financial account for the hospital of Saint-Jean-en-l'Estrée in Arras for 1312/13 indicates that the distribution of pittances took place weekly, on various saints' days, and on the anniversaries of donors' deaths.[115] On All Saints' Day, for instance, the hospital distributed 8 *d.* to each sick person, spending over 36 *sous* for 59 sick individuals. At the hôtel-Dieu of Laon, it was the *magistra* who chose the foods for pittances and the lay brothers who actually distributed the food to the sick poor.[116] A testator in Reims requested that the pittances, which his donation to the hospital supported, be distributed by the hospital's female *conversae* to the poor in the form of eggs and cheese ("in ovis et caseis"), unless the hospital should choose some other thing to distribute.[117] Like with the celebration of anniversary masses, the distribution of pittances, usually in the form of either food or coin, was a way for donors' lives to be commemorated in the hospital. Indeed, the establishment of a fund for the annual distribution of a pittance was often associated with the hospital's celebration of an anniversary mass, and the distribution of the pittance usually took place either on the day of the donor's death or each year on the anniversary of his or her death. Unlike with an anniversary mass, however, this form of commemoration was meant to materially improve the lives of the sick poor, even if only momentarily. As hospital donation charters make clear, many of those making bequests showed an appreciation for the kindness and generosity with which a hospital's personnel cared for the sick poor, and these donors were eager to earmark even the

---

114. AD: Aube 40H1, no. 19 (1212): "debiliores et magis infirmi."

115. Jules-Marie Richard, ed., *Cartulaire de l'hôpital Saint-Jean-en-l'Estrée d'Arras* (Paris: H. Champion, 1888), 108.

116. Saint-Denis, *L'hôtel-Dieu de Laon*, 84–85, 97.

117. Varin, ed., *Archives administratives*, 999–1000.

most modest gift for a specific purpose that would help sustain that care and enhance the lives of the sick poor.

Entry Gifts

Prominent among Champagne's hospital donors were the brothers and sisters who worked in the hospitals, about whom more will be said in chapter 5. Of the 510 donors from the twelfth and thirteenth centuries listed in the martyrological obituary for the hospital of Provins, forty-six (9%) were members of the hospital personnel. Their gifts included landed property (arable, vineyard, meadow, forest), houses, rents, and money (in some cases to buy specific items, such as a liturgical book). The hospital brothers and sisters not only made gifts of their own but were sometimes joined by other family members. Jacob de Luserna gave a rent for the soul of his wife, Emanjarde, who was a hospital sister.[118] The hospital sister Ricent gave some land and woods at Boischevron along with her husband ("cum viro suo").[119] The mother of the hospital sister, Gile de Materello, Lady Emelina, gave the hospital a gift of 10 l. and a measure of wheat.[120] Roger and Emelina, who were the parents of Guillermus, a certain priest and brother of the hospital, made a gift of land and 45 l.[121] Robert de la Renouillère made a donation to the leprosary of Les Deux Eaux, outside Troyes, where his daughter was a *conversa*.[122] Gifts could also be tied to a hospital's promise to employ a donor's relative. A widow at Laon offered to found a chaplaincy at the hospital on the condition that her nephew be made the chaplain.[123] Clearly, the hospital personnel and their families could be an important source of revenue.

As was true at hospitals in other regions, there was an expectation that in order to take the religious habit, one first had to make an "entry gift."[124] In some cases, these gifts were specifically directed at the hospital *conversi*, who seem to have had their own funds or treasuries. In 1211, for example, Agnès Falconaria, who was in the process of taking the religious habit, most likely at the hospital of Bar-sur-Aube, and whose late husband, while approaching death, had given the hospital a half-measure of wine to be collected each year,

---

118. AD Seine-et-Marne, 11Hdt/C5, fol. 55; *Obituaires de la province de Sens*, 1:947.

119. AD Seine-et-Marne, 11Hdt/C5, fol. 61v; *Obituaires de la province de Sens*, 1:950.

120. AD Seine-et-Marne, 11Hdt/C5, fol. 92; *Obituaires de la province de Sens*, 1:964.

121. AD Seine-et-Marne, 11Hdt/C5, fol. 12v; *Obituaires de la province de Sens*, 1:926.

122. Harmand, *Notice historique*, 33–34.

123. Saint-Denis, *L'hôtel-Dieu de Laon*, 92.

124. Saint-Denis, *L'hôtel-Dieu de Laon*, 91–92.

gave the vineyard where this wine came from (at the "Valle de Tors") to the "convent of conversae of the domus Dei of Bar."[125] It is noteworthy that this gift was not made to the hospital as a whole but to the *conversae*, the female converts to the religious life. Likewise, in 1222 Hugues de Lignol made a donation to the hospital of Bar-sur-Aube for his salvation and that of his wife, Ermengarde. The donation, which consisted of the use of his forest at Lignol, with up to one cart full of deadwood (whatever was able to be pulled by one horse) each day, was also specifically given to the *conversae* sisters of the hospital at Bar-sur-Aube, and as part of his donation, Hugues requested that the sisters celebrate his wife's anniversary after her death.[126] It is interesting that Hugues did not request that his own anniversary be celebrated and that he chose the hospital sisters and not the brothers to celebrate her anniversary. In 1198 the *magister* and convent of the brothers of the hospital of Bar-sur-Aube conceded to the congregation of female *conversae* the use and fruits of a certain vineyard; the *conversae* gave 10 *l.* to the hospital from a gift that they had earlier received from a certain Magister Odo li Boceus in exchange for his anniversary being celebrated.[127] Most donation charters made no mention of the possibility that the donor might one day take religious vows and join the hospital community. However, some donors expressed an interest in the possibility of one day assuming the religious habit and wished for some kind of promise that, should they make this decision, the hospital would receive them. When Jean Fiz Samere and his wife Elizabeth bequeathed their house and property to the hospital of Bar-sur-Aube, the *magister* and the brothers not only promised the couple that they could take the religious habit whenever they desired but also conceded which of the properties Jean and Elizabeth could retain after having taken the religious habit.[128] When Gilles de Châlons and his wife, Sibille, made a donation "in pure and perpetual alms" of some pieces of arable to the hospital of Jonchery, near Reims, they promised not to make any claim on the donated land in the future provided that the cathedral chapter of Reims, which had jurisdiction over the hospital, not seek to deprive them unjustly or without reasonable cause of their role as the administrators of the hospital.[129] This married couple, in other words, explicitly tied their donation to their status as the overseers of this hospital.

---

125. AD: Aube HD 33/78 (1211).
126. AD: Aube HD 33/168 (September 1222): "proprie et specialiter pro sororibus conversis;" Arbois de Jubainville, *Histoire des ducs*, no. 1444 (September 1222).
127. AD: Aube HD33/87 (Feast of St. André, 1198).
128. AD: Aube HD 33/50 (November 1232).
129. AD: Marne (Reims), 2G454, layette 35, liasse 87, no. 3 (July 1256).

Hospital statutes often were explicit in forbidding the simoniacal entry of hospital brethren, but it was not difficult for hospitals to claim that donations made by entrants were not a quid pro quo requirement for joining the hospital community but rather separate gifts that they would have made anyway. A bourgeois woman from Troyes named Pasque, for example, made a gift in 1235 to the leprosary of Les Deux Eaux, which may have helped pave the way for her one day entering the hospital as a sister. While her donation charter suggests that she had not yet decided to take that step, it is clear that one of the central conditions of her gift was the promise that she would be received as a sister in the event that one day she decided to take the habit there.[130] According to a charter from 1182, another donor to the leprosary, Gauthier de Vanne, had given some land so that his daughter would be received as a *conversa*.[131] Furthermore, since hospital brethren at least in theory were expected to live religious lives without any personal property, it was only natural that they would need to divest themselves of their property before entering a hospital, and the hospital was the most obvious place for them to direct this gift. The gifts of hospital brethren represented an important source of revenue, so much so that church reformers worried that hospitals would be tempted to take on too many personnel so as to augment their revenues, when in the long term, an excess of personnel could divert resources away from the sick and poor and place a financial strain on the institution. This same argument was made with respect to the *donati* (or corrodians), who also were given a place in the community in return for a donation (which could sometimes be quite significant), although their status was somewhat distinct from the brethren and they ordinarily took no religious vows.[132] The main point is that a hospital's benefactors often included members of its personnel or their families. Whether financially, spiritually, or through their labor, the personnel of a hospital supported the very institution that provided them both with the opportunity for spiritual redemption and with the security that came from being part of a caritative religious community.

---

130. Harmand, *Notice historique*, 43–44. Pasque's donation charter stipulated several other conditions for her gift. While giving the leprosary one-half of a house in Troyes near the gate of Comporté, she insisted not only that she retain the use of this portion of the house during her lifetime but also that she be given the use of the other half of the house, which already belonged to the leprosary, for an annual rental fee of 10 *sous*.

131. Harmand, *Notice historique*, 30.

132. Charles de Miramon, *Les "donnés" au moyen âge: Une forme de vie religieuse laïque (v. 1180–v.1500)* (Paris: Cerf, 1999).

Family Connections and Special Relationships

Although Champagne did not have the kind of dynastic hospitals that Sethina Watson has found examples of in England—hospitals that served as familial sites of remembrance and even as family mausoleums—one does find many examples in Champagne of multiple generations of a family patronizing the same hospital, a common pattern in the benefaction of medieval monasteries as well.[133] For example, Agnès, the wife of the knight Eudes de Fontenay, gave the hospital of Provins a donation of half a *muid* of grain on a tithe, a donation that was confirmed in 1247, after she had already died, by her son, Guyard de Fontenay, a squire.[134] Guyard's sister, Margaret, it turns out, was a sister at the hospital. Another example comes from the hospital's obituary, which recorded the death of a certain Milesant, who was called "Donna soror," and who, according to the obituary, was very generous to the hospital. At her death, she left the hospital lands, meadows, vineyards, houses, and a good deal of moveable property.[135] In a charter from 1232, found in the hospital's cartulary, Milesant's son, Mathieu, gave the hospital a room and his rights on a grange, and he approved all past and future donations made by his mother to the hospital.[136]

Some donors (and families) made multiple donations to the same hospital, year after year. Jean de Saint-Sépulchre, the lord of Villacerf, who came from a prominent aristocratic family in Troyes, made as many as five separate gifts to Saint-Nicolas of Troyes. In his gift of 1264, he thanked the hospital for "all the goods and courtesies which he and his ancestors received and had from the same domus Dei."[137] When Colete, who was called "Naalete," who also came from the powerful Saint-Sépulchre family, made a donation in 1292, she thanked the hospital of Saint-Nicolas for "the welcome services and courtesies extended to her, as it is said, for a long time up to today."[138] As it turned out, however, Naalete had a very personal connection to the

---

133. Sethina Watson, "A Mother's Past and Her Children's Futures: Female Inheritance, Family, and Dynastic Hospitals in the Thirteenth Century," in *Motherhood, Religion, and Society in Medieval Europe, 400–1400: Essays Presented to Henrietta Leyser*, ed. Conrad Leyser and Lesley Smith (Farnham, U.K.: Ashgate, 2011), 213–50.

134. Dupraz, no. 102; AD: Seine-et-Marne 11Hdt A12, fol. 32.

135. Dupraz, no. 125; AD: Seine-et-Marne 11Hdt A12, fol. 36; AD: Seine-et-Marne, 11Hdt/C5, fol. 25v; *Obituaires de la province de Sens*, 1:934.

136. Dupraz, no. 125; AD: Seine-et-Marne 11Hdt A12, fol. 36.

137. AD: Aube 43H12, lay31, cote A, no. 19 (June 1264).

138. AD: Aube 43H12, layette 31, cote A, no. 46 (1292): "attendens et considerans grata servitia et curialites que et quas magister, fratres, et sorores dicte domus eidem Naalota impenderunt et dicitur diu in diem impendunt."

hospital, since her own brother, Jehan de Saint-Sépulchre, was the *magister* at the time. In thinking about the hospital's connection to the larger society, especially potential benefactors, it is significant that the administrative head of the hospital came from a powerful aristocratic family (with lordship over Villacerf) that had long been a benefactor of the hospital. Charter evidence suggests that the *magister* of St-Nicolas was a prominent political actor in Troyes, often being called upon to settle disputes (most of which had nothing to do with the hospital) and serving as the executor of the wills of Troyens. It is unclear whether the Saint-Sépulchre family's ties to the hospital predated Jehan's becoming *magister*. If so, he might have been inspired to join the hospital community because of his family's historical connection to the house. Still, one wonders what exactly the services and courtesies were that had been extended to Jehan's sister, Naalete.[139] It is quite possible that Naalete was living as a *donata* in St-Nicolas or in a property owned by the hospital. Fifteen years after her first recorded donation to the hospital, she made another substantial gift. Some bequests to hospitals were made as a result of the services these institutions provided and the relationships they developed with individuals and families, including ties between donors and particular members of a hospital community.

Among hospital donors were those who were members of a hospital community or in some way dependent upon the institution. The testament of Isabelle Papelarde "du Puits" from 1268, for example, makes clear that she was living in the hospital of Notre-Dame de Reims at the time as a dependent ("prebendaria").[140] "Seeing and paying attention to the fact that the life of man on earth is short, and wanting and desiring to provide well for the health of her soul during her full life," Isabelle bequeathed to the hospital, upon her death, her house, which was located behind the convent belonging to the Order of Preachers. She also bequeathed, in perpetuity, a small annual rent to support the lighting of the hospital's chapel of Saint-Loup. All of her moveable and immoveable property, present and future, was to go to the hospital for the needs of the poor, "in recompense for the comforts of

---

139. For this period, it is rare to find a reference like the one in a donation charter from 1439 to Saint-Nicolas, in which the donor thanked the hospital for its kindnesses over a thirty-year period, including nourishing and feeding her in the hospital. AD: Aube 43H12, layette 32, cote B, no. 7 (1439): "en recompensacion et remuneration de plusieurs biensfais, curalitez, confors et courtoisies que on lui a faiz oudit hostel depuis trente ans en ca et plus qu'elle a esté nourie et alimentee en icellui hostel Dieu."

140. AMC (Reims): FH-HD B54, liasse 6, no. 19: "manens in hospitali beate marie Remensis et prebendaria hospitalis eiusdem."

the hospital received by the same Isabelle over a long time in the same hospital."[141] Specifically, she requested that all the furnishings and utensils in her house—beds, covers, linen cloth, serge, pillows, cloth, spoons, pots, lamps, cauldrons—be sold and the money converted into pittances for the poor. Finally, she gave 100 *s. par.* to Maresonne, the niece of Hugues, a brother and chaplain in the hospital, for the salvation of his soul and in recompense for the services and labors that the same Maresonne had extended toward her.[142]

It is no surprise that Thomas, who was chaplain of the parish church of Saint-Pierre in Provins, made generous bequests to the main hospital of the city in his testament of 1267, including leaving the enormous sum of 225 *l. t.* for the celebration of the anniversary of his death as well as all of his books (including two breviaries and the fourth book of the *Summa*, probably Lombard's *Sentences*, which dealt with the sacraments), his bedding, and a chalice of two marks silver. Thomas's late uncle, Adam, who died in 1263, had served as *magister* of the hospital for twenty-two years. Although Thomas does not seem to have had any formal role in the hospital, his affection for its community is evident in the bequests he made to individual members of the community as well as in his decision to be buried not in Saint-Pierre, where he served as chaplain, but in the city's hospital, where his uncle was buried.[143]

Donations sometimes were intended to assist relatives or friends living and working in the hospital, a point that has also been observed with respect to donations made to local Templar houses.[144] In 1261 Pétronille de Vieux-Maisons bequeathed an annual rent of 20 *sous* to Emanjarde, a sister of the hospital of Provins.[145] Likewise, Jacques de Saint-Martin de Hupeello bequeathed a lifetime rent of oats and wheat to his sister, Alice, who was a sister of the hospital of Provins.[146] In 1270, the knight Henri de Saint-Benoît bequeathed a life rent of barley to his daughter Johanna, a sister of the hôtel-Dieu-le-Comte in Troyes; if his other daughter, Aalidis, a sister of Saint-Ouen, outlived Johanna, she would receive the life rent, and after both

141. AMC (Reims): FH-HD B54, liasse 6, no. 19: "in recompensationem bonorum ipsius hospitalis ab eadem Ysabella per longum tempus in eodem hospitali perceptorum."

142. AMC (Reims): FH-HD B54, liasse 6, no. 19: "Item legavit dicta Ysabella Maresonne nepti quondam domini Hugonis fratris et capellani dicti hospitalis tam pro remedio anime sue quam in recompensationem servicis et laboris ipsius Maresonne erga ipsam Ysabellam impensi et facti ut dicebat centum solidos parisenses super jamdictis bonis suis et rebus capiendos."

143. Dupraz, no. 426; AD: Seine-et-Marne 11Hdt A12, fol. 124–124v.

144. Schenk, *Templar Families*, 32.

145. Dupraz, no. 192; AD: Seine-et-Marne 11Hdt A12, fol. 57v.

146. Dupraz, no. 220; AD: Seine-et-Marne 11Hdt A12, fol. 66.

daughters had died, the rent would devolve to the hospital.[147] Members of a hospital community could and surely did encourage family members to direct their charitable giving to their community.

Even among donors who had no family connection to the hospital, however, there were some who had a special relationship with the hospital, and signs of this can be found in the hospital's own records. We do not know much about Alice de Jouy's relationship with the hospital of Provins. In 1250 she bequeathed all that she had in rents and customs in the parish of Gouaix, and in 1254 she is referred to as the widow of Evrard de Jouy, a bourgeois from Provins.[148] Yet as the obituary for the hospital made clear, she was not just one of the hospital's hundreds of donors: she was "the faithful friend of our house" ("fidelis amica domus nostre").[149] Underlying bequests to hospitals were often longstanding relationships, some due to a familial connection, with a bequest growing out of a family's multi-generational patronage of a particular hospital or a family member's being part of the hospital's personnel. Such bequests were still viewed as spiritually redemptive for the donor's soul, but they were simultaneously intended to further strengthen social and familial bonds.

Expressions of Gratitude

Some donations to hospitals were accompanied by expressions of gratitude for services the hospital had provided to the donor. What the hospital had done to help these donors is almost never specified, but these cases illustrate that the hospital's role in the larger society, outside of caring for those within its walls, could be directly tied to the bequests it received. In 12 percent of all donations made to the hospital of Saint-Nicolas in Troyes, the donors thanked the hospital for the kindness and courtesies it had shown to them. Interestingly, all of the statements of gratitude by donors appear in charters dated in the second half of the thirteenth century, when it was becoming increasingly common for donors to thank hospitals for their services, thus showing that there was a preexisting relationship between donor and hospital. Although, as we have seen, there was no surge of hospital donors being promised anniversary masses during the late thirteenth century, donors' expressions of gratitude at the time of making their gifts suggests that the

---

147. AD: Aube 40H1, no. 63 (April 1270).
148. Dupraz, no. 321; AD: Seine-et-Marne 11Hdt A12, fol. 96v.
149. AD: Seine-et-Marne, 11Hdt/C5, fol. 32v; *Obituaires de la province de Sens*, 1:938.

relationship between a donor and a hospital often did not begin at the time of a donation. In that sense, what we think of as being a donation (which, as we shall see, at times elicited a counter-gift from the hospital) sometimes was itself a kind of counter-gift for what the hospital had already given the donor. When Guillaume, the curate of Vailly, made a bequest to the hospital, he referred to "the welcome favors shown to him by the master and brothers of the domus Dei."[150] The absence of any reference to the sisters, who appear in other charters of the time, probably indicates that Guillaume's dealings with the hospital involved religious or business matters, as opposed to physical care. This was also the case with the donation of an annual rent in money and hens made by Jehan de Dosche, who lived in Bouilly, thirteen kilometers from Troyes, who was "not unmindful of the services, assistance, and courtesies which the master and brothers of the domus Dei Saint-Nicolas did and conferred, which were followed by no recompense."[151] Jehan regarded his donation as the long overdue recompense. In 1264 Jean de Saint-Sépulchre conceded to the hospital of Saint-Nicolas the right to build granaries and other buildings as recompense for the "goods and services" that he and his predecessors had received from the hospital.[152] In his testament of 1333, the dean of the cathedral chapter of Saint-Pierre made a bequest to the hospital of Saint-Nicolas and made clear that it was in recompense for the house that he had held from the master and brothers of the hospital.[153] These expressions of gratitude toward Saint-Nicolas are probably related to its lordship, extensive landholding, and market activities, including at times providing credit to those in need.

When the cleric, Jacques Bernier, a cleric in the diocese of Sens who had grown up in Provins, gave the hospital the use of houses, a pasture, two gardens, and fifty-two *arpents* of land (he had previously reserved the usufruct during his lifetime), he was rather explicit in thanking the *magister* and the brothers and sisters (and their predecessors) for their kindnesses, services, assistance, and many other favors they had continuously paid to him.[154] Eleven years earlier, Jacques donated a rent to the hospital, and then, too, he acknowledged "his devotion that he had had and continued to have

---

150. AD Aube 43H12, layette 31, cote A, no. 28 (1270).

151. AD Aube 43H12, layette 31, cote A, no. 43 (March 1283).

152. AD Aube 43H12, layette 31, cote A, no. 19 (March 1263).

153. AD Aube G2669, no. 6 (1333): "in recompensacione cujusdem domus quam ipse tenet a magistro et fratribus dicte domus Dei."

154. AD: Seine-et-Marne, 11HdtA12, fol. 149–50 (1296); Dupraz, no. 504; AD: Seine-et-Marne 11Hdt A12, fol. 149–50.

for the poor of the domus Dei and toward the house and the miserable poverty there."[155] Jacques evidently had some experience with the hospital and wished to express his gratitude to the community. Likewise, Pierre de Marolles, a priest living in Provins, bequeathed his grange near Mortery and some land, noting "the affection and love he has for the master and brothers of the larger domus Dei and their house."[156] The bourgeoise Jacqueline la Coypelle donated land out of a sense of "affection and devotion for the domus Dei and the sick poor."[157] The knight Jean de Lunay gave the hospital an annual rent of 12 d. "for the service that was done annually for him and his late wife in the domus Dei."[158] It is likely that the hospital brethren said prayers each year for this knight and his wife. Thibaut de Champfleury and his wife, Marie, donated their *cens* of 1 d. on a vineyard to thank the *magister* and the *ministri* for the assistance, courtesies, and services conferred on them from the property of the hospital.[159] Given the direct reference to the *magister* and *ministri*, as well as the use of the term *boni*, it seems most likely that the couple had been granted use of hospital property or had perhaps even been provided by the hospital with a loan of some kind. Jacques de Payns, who was the chaplain of the royal chapel, made a bequest to the hôtel-Dieu-le-Comte of Troyes "not unmindful of the favors, assistance, advice and even the gifts of honor that the master and brothers and sisters . . . had frequently done for and expended on him."[160] Magister André "de Porta," a canon at the church of Saint-Maclou in Bar-sur-Aube, gave the hospital of the same city his house as recompense for the many properties and gratuities he had received from his "faithful" and "dear ones" there.[161] Leprosaria were also given donations as an expression of gratitude for services they had provided or might provide in the future. In 1301, Jean Piquart de Sancey and his wife, Heliette, made a donation of 45 l. t. and all their property, which would be transferred to the leper house of Les Deux Eaux at their death, and they did so to thank the leper house for the good care it had given them and that it might give to them in the future.[162]

---

155. Dupraz, no. 358; AD: Seine-et-Marne 11Hdt A12, fol. 107–107v.

156. Dupraz, no. 431; AD: Seine-et-Marne 11Hdt A12, fol.125–126.

157. Dupraz, no. 460; AD: Seine-et-Marne 11Hdt A12, fol. 133v–134.

158. Dupraz, no. 191; AD: Seine-et-Marne 11Hdt A12, fol. 57v.

159. Dupraz, no. 345; AD: Seine-et-Marne 11Hdt A12, fol. 104.

160. AD: Aube 40H1, no. 67 (1276): "non immemor beneficiorum, auxiliorum et consiliorum ac etiam curialitatum que et quas magister, fratres ac sorores domus Dei comititis Trecenses eidem domino Jacobo pluries fecerunt et impenderunt."

161. AD: Aube HD33/66 (1275).

162. Harmand, *Notice historique*, 182.

When a donor thanked a hospital for its kindness and assistance, we should not rule out the possibility that the donor had been cared for by the hospital during an illness. As we shall see in chapter 5, some of the guests in Champagne's hospitals were sick but not poor, and it is likely that some of the donors who expressed gratitude toward hospitals did so as a result of the care they had received there. Consider a charter found in the cartulary for the hospital of Pontoise, northwest of Paris, which records a donation made in 1291 by Jehan de Lieux.[163] In donating his house in alms to the hospital, Jehan referred to the long illness that had detained him there. Jehan went on to express the inadequacy of the gift to repay the hospital for its courtesies. A number of donors to Champagne's hospitals likewise expressed their gratitude to hospitals for extending care to them, suggesting that perhaps like Jehan, they had spent time convalescing there. Donors' expressions of gratitude and their descriptions of their pious bequests as recompense for a hospital's kindness or specific service once again illustrates that these gifts often were not random but reflective of preexisting relationships between these institutions and their benefactors. Hospitals provided a wide range of different kinds of services—spiritual and financial as well as physical—and the bequests that they received reflected just how enmeshed they were in webs of reciprocity.

Counter-Gifts

Of the donors who made pious gifts to twelfth-century Cistercian monasteries in Burgundy, about 10 percent were rewarded with material counter-gifts.[164] Similar patterns have been observed at the abbey of Montier-la-Celle, near Troyes, where one-seventh of pious gifts elicited a material counter-gift from the abbey during the second half of the twelfth century. During the thirteenth century, this abbey gave far fewer material counter-gifts, perhaps because it was giving counter-gifts in other forms, such as anniversary masses.[165] In contrast, there was no decline during the first half of the thirteenth century in the frequency with which Champagne's hospitals gave material counter-gifts to donors, although the majority of pious gifts to hospitals still did not get rewarded with a counter-gift.

---

163. Joseph Depoin, ed., *Cartulaire de l'hôtel-dieu de Pontoise* (Pontoise, 1886), 78.

164. Some Cistercian monasteries gave counter-gifts as much as 34% of the time. Bouchard, *Holy Entrepreneurs*, 89–92.

165. Keyser, "Gift, Dispute, and Contract," 278.

Counter-gifts have sometimes been interpreted as exchanges or even disguised sales. However, historians increasingly argue that such gifts were a way of expressing gratitude for a gift and building up additional good will with a donor. Stephen White has suggested that it was the symbolic character of a counter-gift and its confirmation of social relations that mattered most, not its material value.[166] Counter-gifts were technically not exchanges, since exchanges tended to involve the transfer of properties or rights of roughly equal value, whereas counter-gifts were by definition of lesser value.[167] Charters, however, tended to frame counter-gifts as spontaneous and gratuitous acts, not as quid pro quo transactions. Nonetheless, the prospect of a counter-gift might have served as a further inducement for someone to make a gift, somewhat mitigating the material loss incurred by the gift itself.[168] Moreover, a clause was sometimes added to the donation charter to indicate that the hospital pledged a counter-gift in the form of a rent or monetary sum "lest it be called by the reproach of ingratitude."[169]

As Constance Bouchard has argued, in discussing gifts to monasteries, gifts were different from sales in the way that they created a complex and permanent relationship between a donor (and even his or her heirs) and the recipient of a gift: "A gift, rather than being a one-time event, established a long-term relationship between the donor and his kin (both living and dead), on the one hand, and on the other a group that included not just the monks but God and the saints."[170] As we have seen, hospital donations were themselves often expressions of gratitude for the services a hospital had provided to the donor. Yet the "logic of reciprocity" underlying all gifts, as Marcel Mauss long ago showed, did not end with a donor's gift.[171] Hospitals recognized the need to maintain good relations with their networks of donors so that they would continue to make (perhaps even bigger) bequests and possibly encourage other family members and friends to develop ties to the hospital as well. Just as many monasteries did, hospitals used counter-gifts

166. Stephen White, *Custom, Kinship, and Gifts to Saints: The Laudatio Parentum in Western France, 1050–1150* (Chapel Hill: University of North Carolina Press, 1988).

167. Bouchard, *Holy Entrepreneurs*, 87–94.

168. Emily Tabuteau, *Transfers of Property in Eleventh-Century Norman Law* (Chapel Hill, University of North Carolina Press, 1988).

169. Dupraz, no. 444; AD: Seine-et-Marne 11Hdt A12, fol. 129v: "ne de oprobrio ingratitudinis vocaretur."

170. Bouchard, *Holy Entrepreneurs*, 64.

171. Marcel Mauss, *The Gift: The Form and Reason for Exchange in Archaic Societies*, trans. W. D. Halls, foreword by Mary Douglas (New York: Norton, 2000).

to solidify their relationships with donors and, in some cases, as we shall see, head off the possibility of disputes over property.

In addition to serving as an expression of gratitude for bequests, counter-gifts were also given to a relative for approving a gift or to a lord for amortizing a donation that was part of the lord's fief.[172] Moreover, amortizations were themselves regarded as a form of charity, especially when they were given freely, and charters recording amortizations invoked the same pious language as donation charters. When amortizing property given to a hospital, some lords, such as Jean de Saint-Sépulchre, made clear that the hospital should do whatever it needed to do with the land—build houses, granges, or other buildings—that would fulfill its charitable work.[173] Hospitals did not take these amortizations for granted, particularly during the late thirteenth century, when Champagne's counts and other lords were becoming increasingly restrictive in making such concessions to ecclesiastical institutions. Counter-gifts were an important way for hospitals to show gratitude for a lord's amortization or a family member's approval of a gift.

Counter-gifts could also acknowledge the particular services that someone provided a hospital. The cleric Gérard de Polisy gave the hôtel-Dieu-le-Comte in Troyes one-half of a vineyard in Polisy in perpetual alms, and he sold the other half of the vineyard to the hospital for 10 *l.*[174] Recognizing Gérard's "kindness and generosity," as well as his "devotion" toward the hospital, and "not wanting to appear ungrateful," the hospital not only promised to celebrate anniversary masses for his mother and father, as well as for him, each year following his death, but it also counter-gifted with an annual lifetime rent of 20 *s.* so long as he participated in all of the "good things" that "are done and will be done day and night" at the hospital. It is clear that this counter-gift was conditional upon the cleric's continued service to the hospital. In the account books for the hospital of Saint-Nicolas from the late fourteenth century, there are even scattered references to the hospital's distributing small sums of money to individuals to thank them for a "free" service they had provided, for their efforts or troubles ("pour sa poigne"), for their courtesy, or in the case of a notary, for his friendship.[175]

172. Dupraz, no. 444; AD: Seine-et-Marne 11Hdt A12, fol. 129v.

173. AD: Aube 43H12, layette 31A, cotte 19 (July 1264).

174. AD: Aube 40H1, no. 40 (October 1232).

175. Julie Gesret, "Un hôpital au moyen age: L'hôtel-Dieu Saint-Nicolas de Troyes du XIIIe au XVe siècle, 'soustenir les povres'" (PhD dissertation, École des Chartes, Paris, 2003), 398–99; AD: Aube G2525, fol. 64 (Account book for 1382–83); Aube G2524, fol. 47 (Account book for 1381–82); Aube G2531, fol. 52 (Account book for 1389–90).

Many of the hospital donors and members of their families retained the use of the donated property during their lifetimes, yet this generally did not represent a counter-gift but was rather a condition placed upon the gift. Indeed, the hospital of Provins appears to have been more of an afterthought for the cleric Pierre de Durtein than the primary object of his charity. Pierre bequeathed a meadow (part of the hospital's lordship) to his sister Heloise, who, like the more famous Heloise, was a nun at the Paraclete abbey. After her death, the meadow would be transferred to their two brothers, and after their deaths, it would revert back to Pierre. Only after all four siblings had died would the meadow be transferred to the hôtel-Dieu.[176] In another case, Gauthier, a doctor ("medicus") from Troyes, gave an annual rent of 6 s. in 1222 to the leprosary of Les Deux Eaux for the annual celebration of his anniversary, and the leper house granted him the lifetime use of his donated rent. Two years later, Gauthier added a rent of 4 s. to his gift, and the leprosary again granted him the lifetime use of this additional rent.[177]

In other cases, however, hospitals granted donors the lifetime use of some other property in addition to the property they had donated. In 1235, for example, Thierry de Torci and his wife Heluyde, townspersons ("cives"), gave their house in Troyes to the master, brothers, sisters, and poor of the hôtel-Dieu-le-Comte.[178] The hospital permitted the couple to continue to use their house during their lifetime, while paying an annual rent of 20 s. in recognition of the hospital's title to the property. But the couple was also given a second house (on a different street) that belonged to the hospital, which the couple could hold for the rest of their lives so long as they remained "in the secular habit," with both houses reverting to the hospital upon the couple's death. Did the couple make their bequest to the hospital in order to acquire the use of this second house? And what did they plan to do with this additional house? If they rented it out, they stood to actually profit from their charitable donation.

Hospitals at times gave counter-gifts in the context of purchases, sales, and exchanges, and this further complicates the task of identifying gifts and counter-gifts. An example of these ambiguities can be seen in the transactions between the hospital of Meaux and a certain knight, Eudes Lagrue de Monthyon. According to a later charter from 1269, in April of 1222 the archdeacon of Meaux certified that the knight, Eudes, gave and conceded in

---

176. Dupraz, no. 254; AD: Seine-et-Marne 11HdtA12, fol. 79v.
177. Harmand, *Notice historique*, 225.
178. AD: Aube 40H1, no. 41 (1235).

perpetual alms eight *arpents* of arable near the grange of Touches to the hospital for the salvation of his and his family members' souls. In recompense, the hospital gave the knight 52 *l*.[179] A separate charter, however, from just a few months earlier, in January of 1222, records that Eudes conceded in alms to the hospital of Meaux eight *arpents* of land near the grange of Touches, and that Técelin, the curate of the place, paid the knight 50 *l*. on behalf of the hospital. In turn, the hospital agreed to pay the priest an annual life rent of two *muids* of wheat as well as twenty eels ("anguillas"); following the priest's death, the hospital would celebrate his anniversary and spend 5 *s*. on food for the poor each year.[180] A number of other charters recording the sale of land at Touches during this same period indicate that the market price for land was usually around 12 *l*. per *arpent*, whereas the counter-gifts for land in these transactions was closer to 6 *l*. per *arpent*. If these transactions, with their invocation of the conventional language used for pious gifts, are understood as "hybrid donation-sales," the knight was ceding his land for roughly half the market price.[181]

Hospitals frequently provided lifetime annuities as counter-gifts. When Adam, an Augustinian canon, donated to the poor of the hôtel-Dieu-le-Comte in Troyes a rent that he had purchased, the hospital counter-gifted with an annual lifetime annuity of 32 *setiers* of rye that he could collect from its grange.[182] When Gilebert Jalon and his wife, Aremburge, gave their house and grange with arable to the same hospital in 1239 "for the sustenance of the poor," they were promised a life rent of 16 *setiers* of grain.[183] The Augustinian priest, Odon, donated various pieces of land and a mill to the hôtel-Dieu-le-Comte, and the hospital counter-gifted a lifetime rent of 20 *s*. and set the amounts of grain that he could collect.[184] On account of the canon, Gautier Bochard's devotion in making a gift, the hospital brothers promised him a lifetime rent of 40 *s*. on a house that the hospital owned. However, the hospital was careful to stipulate that if the house were consumed in a fire or otherwise destroyed, the hospital would no longer be held to pay Gautier's rent.[185] In any case, upon Gautier's death the rent would revert to

---

179. AD Seine-et-Marne 9Hdt/B103 (1269, a *vidimus* charter).

180. AD Seine-et-Marne 9Hdt/B103 (January 1222).

181. On donation-sales, in which a sale is made significantly below market price as a form of charity, see Saint-Denis, *L'hôtel-Dieu de Laon*, 150.

182. AD: Aube 40H189, fol. 28 (1200); 40H1, no. 7.

183. AD: Aube 40H1, no. 43 (1239).

184. AD: Aube 40H1, no. 44 (December 1239).

185. AD: Aube 40H1, no. 19 (1212).

the hospital and be used to feed the poor. When Guy d'Hery, a canon from Notre-Dame-du-Val, conceded a *cens* as well as several customary rents in kind to the hospital of Provins "out of devotion and affection which he said he had toward the domus Dei and the poor of the said house," the hospital granted him the significant life annuity of 10 *l.,* an annuity that would revert to his mother if he predeceased her.[186]

In some of these cases, counter-gifts can be seen more as quid pro quo exchanges than spontaneous and gratuitous gestures, as charters cast them. It is clear, for example, that when the cleric, Guerri, gave the hospital of Saint-Nicolas in Troyes all the land that he possessed at Creney, he did so on the condition that the hospital pay him an annual rent of four *setiers* of wheat, and he asked that this rent be paid to his mother, Agnès, who was a *conversa* at St-Martin-de-Troyes, for the duration of her lifetime, should she outlive him.[187] Lambert de Bar "Coquins" and his wife, Supplitia, who were citizens of Troyes, gave all of their lands at Tennelières and Beli, but with the understanding that the hospital would counter-give with an annual life rent of wheat, oats, and two carts full of straw, as well as celebrate their anniversaries and distribute bread to the hospital's poor.[188]

Counter-gifting was frequently a way that hospitals sought to avoid or resolve conflicts with donors and their heirs, and such conflicts were not uncommon. When Gilles Ribuede disputed that his parents had given a house on rue de Busançois to the hospital of Provins, he was presented with official letters from the dean of Christianity, who served as the local rural dean, attesting to the legitimacy of the donation. This appeared to be a case of *calumnia*, a false claim against the hospital's rightful property. Before the provost of Provins, Gilles formally gave up his claim to the house, casting his abandonment of his claim as itself a charitable donation "for the souls of his parents."[189] Of the more than two dozen records of property disputes between the hospital of Provins and lay men and women found in the hospital's cartulary, the hospital almost always ended up keeping the contested property, usually in a kind of binding arbitration mediated by an *amicus*. However, the hospital was surely more intent on retaining records of disputes that it won than those that it lost, and so the cartulary's record of

---

186. Dupraz, no. 364; AD: Seine-et-Marne 11Hdt A12, fol. 109v–110.

187. AD Aube 43H12, layette 31, cote A, no. 6 (1220).

188. AD: Aube 43H12, layette 31, cote A, no.15 (December 1246).

189. When noble donors abandoned their (at times, unjust) claims to monastic property, they, too, often portrayed themselves as charitable for giving up their claims. See Bouchard, *Sword, Miter, and Cloister,* 209–10.

disputes may not be an accurate sampling. Even the disputes that the hospital won could still end up being costly, however, since many times it offered a counter-gift to claimants in return for the retraction of their *calumniae*.[190] Alice, the wife of Étienne le Bigot, renounced her claim to a dowry based on the house of the late Robert le Bigot, which apparently had become the hospital's property, only after the hospital agreed in 1213 to give her 40 *s*. The hospital warned Alice's husband that if he made any further trouble about his wife's claim, it would retract the 40 *s*.[191] At times, charters that at first appear to record a donation "given in perpetual alms," in fact record the resolution of a dispute. In 1222 Margareta, the daughter of the late Normande, gave the brothers of the hôtel-Dieu-le-Comte in Troyes some land that was contiguous to land already belonging to the hospital. The hospital brothers, meanwhile, abandoned the 16 *l*. that Margareta and her mother owed to them. This transaction, however, took place within the context of a dispute over lands that Margareta's mother had donated to the hospital, and the dispute was resolved by Margareta giving to the hospital as a pious gift what her mother had already given, also promising to not bother the brothers of the hospital over this again; in return, the hospital released Margareta from an obligation to pay a debt of 16 *l*.[192]

The disputes in which Champagne's hospitals found themselves embroiled often involved property or rights that hospitals had been given, and rents and annuities that the hospitals were obligated to give to others, thus underlining the social and economic networks in which hospitals participated. In one dispute, the hospital of Provins complained that Jean Malfardez and his wife, Marguerite, who had been tenants for two years in a house owned by the hospital, had not paid their rent. The couple, however, claimed that the hospital had not paid them a rent they were owed. As part of the settlement, the hospital agreed to let the couple remain in the house, free of charge, for an additional ten months, after which time they would pay the 8 *l*. rent owed to the hospital each year. As for the rent the couple claimed they were owed, the hospital agreed to pay them 12 *l*. as well as an annual rent of 60 *s*., a *muid* of wheat, and a weekly rent of eight breads each year during Marguerite's

---

190. Bouchard, *Sword, Miter, and Cloister*, 217–18. In winning a dispute in 1178 over an annual rent of wheat, the leprosarium of Les Deux Eaux was forced to promise Clarembaud de Chappes, the son of Clarembaud the Younger, that it would celebrate the anniversary of his father. In short, a condition for resolving disputes was not always monetary, but could involve the celebration of a Mass. See Harmand, *Notice historique*, 29.

191. Dupraz, no. 113; AD: Seine-et-Marne 11Hdt A12, fol. 34v.

192. AD: Aube 40H1, no. 32 (January 1222).

lifetime.[193] As these examples illustrate, medieval hospitals were not just receiving pious gifts and voluntarily dispensing charitable assistance; charitable institutions were also entangled in a complex web of contractual obligations, and failure to deliver on these obligations led to legal conflicts.

Conclusion

As we saw in chapter 1, the lay women and men living in twelfth- and thirteenth-century Champagne and other parts of Latin Christendom were steeped in a culture that celebrated the works of mercy as an antidote to sin and a way to secure salvation. Pious giving to hospitals was understood by contemporaries as a spiritual and penitential activity and was thus connected to the growing preoccupation with Purgatory and the rise of a confessional society. Although some monastic orders were known to be engaged in the works of mercy, the hospital, more than any other institution, embodied the performance of these works and was thus the natural place to direct bequests. The hospitals that were founded in Champagne during the twelfth and thirteenth centuries participated in the traditional Christian "spiritual economy," embroiled as they were in a soteriological system of good works and spiritual intercession. The broad support that hospitals received during this period, support that cut across social classes and gender lines, was also connected in various ways to the thriving local commercial culture of the time. It was the markets and fairs that both generated the wealth that funded charitable activities and provided a sense of need for almsgiving as spiritual expiation for profit making. Throughout the thirteenth century, records of bequests to hospitals continued to employ the *pro anima* formula, unlike at many monasteries, where the clause disappeared. Nor did anniversary masses become a common condition for donors' bequests to hospitals in the way that they did for monasteries. Hospitals had less of a need to reward a donor with an intercessory liturgical service, since caring for the sick poor—who were understood as stand-ins for Christ—was itself regarded as a service that would reap spiritual rewards for donors and caregivers. Furthermore, hospital donation charters frequently described bequests as being given not to the institution as a whole or even to its brethren but rather "to the sick poor" or even to God.

Beyond the way that gift-giving to hospitals was shaped by the larger spiritual economy, however, we have also observed that gifts were given to

---

193. Dupraz, no. 127; AD: Seine-et-Marne 11Hdt A12, fol. 36–36v.

hospitals to create or maintain social bonds, and it was the social context for each gift that imbued it with particular meaning. The pragmatic motivations behind many bequests to hospitals were similar to bequests made to monastic houses: a family connection, such as a relative who was a member of the community; a history of one's family patronizing the hospital; a desire to join the hospital's religious community; an expression of gratitude for a service that had been received; or a desire for intercessory prayers. But the works of mercy performed in hospitals also rendered these institutions different from monastic houses in the eyes of their benefactors, and this is evident in the language of donation charters. The work carried out by hospitals evoked the universal sense of the fragility and vulnerability of human life, embodied by the truism with which so many charters began, "that nothing is more certain than death, and nothing more uncertain than the hour of one's death." Hospitals conjured up the most visible form of human dependency, to say nothing of the universal dependency on human and divine mercy. And yet, as we have seen, the mercy shown by hospitals and hospital benefactors was by no means one-sided. Like the bustling commercial world outside the hospital walls, its benefactors and personnel and those for whom it cared engaged in transactional relationships and exchanges based on their mutual needs, with the works of mercy representing a kind of spiritual investment that involved payment and repayment, debts and credits.

Champagne's hospitals were not remote, abstract institutions that entered the consciousness of people only when they were making bequests, although patronizing hospitals was an important way for especially aristocrats to display their paternalism and enhance their status. The central location of many hospitals meant that people passed by them all the time. They might have known someone who worked there or might have taken a family member or neighbor there to convalesce or pray for a healing miracle, as the miracles of Saint Louis depict people doing at the hôtel-Dieu in Paris.[194] An inhabitant of Troyes, Provins, or Bar-sur-Aube might have seen (or might have been the beneficiary of) hospital workers distributing food and clothing in the streets on a particular feast day or at someone's funeral. He or she might have attended mass at the hospital. Champagne's hospitals also served as a kind of retirement home for people looking for material security and spiritual community, and some donors wanted to know that they could one day join the hospital as a *donatus* or *conversus*. Still others engaged in economic transactions with the hospital, buying, selling, or exchanging property, even

---

194. Farmer, *Surviving Poverty*.

turning to the hospital as a source of credit. Hundreds of tenants owed the hospital rents and other obligations, and the hospital's title to property or right to collect rents was sometimes challenged. In short, each hospital had a particular meaning for the inhabitants of a town and the surrounding region, and this is reflected in the donations that the institution received, many of which were the direct result of the relationships that the hospital had developed and the caring and non-caring services it provided to the larger community. To be successful in receiving bequests, a hospital had to carefully negotiate its relations with the public and weigh its short- and long-term needs and interests. Counter-gifts were one mechanism it used to create good will and strengthen its bonds with everyone from donors to those with whom it ran into conflict. Ultimately, a medieval hospital was a business, and like any institution, its ability to carry out its mission depended on the careful management of its resources, which included its social networks.

✖ CHAPTER 4

Managing a Hospital's Property

According to twelfth- and thirteenth-century reformers, some religious orders were using their financial resources for non-religious purposes. Jacques de Vitry, for instance, scolded the Trinitarians, an order founded in the late twelfth century for ransoming captives, for investing in various kinds of property and rents so as to secure future revenues. Rather than "investing" alms, which he viewed as a form of hoarding, Jacques thought that alms should be immediately and directly distributed as the almsgivers had intended.[1] The institutionalization of charity, however, required developing resources that could help sustain these institutions and their missions. Of the twenty hospitals in the bailliage of Troyes for which we have an estimation of the hospital's net worth, quite a few (Coulommiers, Chemin, Payns, Saint-Florentin, Maligny, Nogent) had assets worth only 20 or 30 $l.$[2] Many folded or barely survived from year to year. Others, such as the hôtel-Dieu-le-Comte, the hospital of Provins, and the hospital of

---

1. Bird, "Medicine for Body and Soul," 106. By the thirteenth century, the Trinitarians' charitable activities had come to include performing other works of mercy, including caring for the sick and poor in hospitals founded by the order.

2. In 1300, King Philip the Fair requested, as part of a census, to learn the revenue of different institutions in the bailliage of Troyes, which became part of the royal domain in 1285. These revenue figures for hospitals come from that census. Longnon, ed., *Documents*, 3:124–33.

Saint-Nicolas in Troyes were quite wealthy, both due to the number and size of the gifts they received and the investments they made in landed property, rents, agricultural cultivation, and commerce associated with the trade fairs.[3] While a fair amount of scholarly attention has been paid to the economic power of medieval monasteries, there has been little recognition of hospitals as central players in the medieval urban economy. This chapter will demonstrate the surprising economic power of hospitals and their prominent role in the larger society, including their relationships and conflicts with other institutions.

Thirteenth- and early fourteenth-century sources rarely permit a sense of the financial management of these institutions. An unpublished financial account book for the hôtel-Dieu Saint-Nicolas in Troyes that begins in 1300 and ends in 1303, however, reveals in remarkable detail the hospital's annual receipts and expenditures.[4] This account book, heretofore unstudied, represents one of the earliest and most detailed financial inventories of a medieval hospital.[5] Studied alongside the hospital's copious extant charters as well as charters from other hospitals, this account book sheds valuable light on how hospitals managed their properties and how some of them became remarkably wealthy institutions. The hôtel-Dieu Saint-Nicolas in Troyes was actually quite a bit less wealthy than the nearby hôtel-Dieu-le-Comte (or the hospital of Provins), with its property and rents estimated to have been about 600 *l.* in 1300, compared with 2,000 *l.* for the hôtel-Dieu-le-Comte and 1,600 *l.* for the hospital of Provins.[6] Yet the annual audit of Saint-Nicolas reflects the degree to which it was keeping careful records of its properties, income, and spending under the watchful eye of the bishop, dean, and canons of the neighboring cathedral chapter. Hospitals that were not under the jurisdiction of a chapter of canons would probably have been less likely to keep such financial records. In point of fact, contemporary registers of episcopal visitation of hospitals and monastic houses included frequent admonitions of the need to

---

3. The hôtel-Dieu of Reims, which was a dependency of the cathedral chapter, was also quite wealthy, as was the city's leper hospital, Saint-Ladre. In 1328 the hôtel-Dieu owned 42 houses, 3 stalls, more than 100 *jours* of land, and collected around 34 *l.* each year in lordly rents. See Desportes, *Reims et les Rémois*, 299–300, 413, 478.

4. BnF ms lat. 9111, fol. 282–301.

5. Alain Derville has studied a contemporary hospital account roll that was recorded daily for the hospital of Saint-Sauveur in Lille, beginning in 1285 and continuing through the mid-fourteenth century. See Alain Derville, *L'agriculture du Nord au moyen âge: Artois, Cambrésis, Flandre Wallonne* (Paris: Presses Universitaires du Septentrion, 1999), 91–132. For a study of comparable, albeit somewhat later account books, see Richard, ed., *Cartulaire de l'hôpital Saint-Jean-en-l'Estrée d'Arras*; and Victor Leblond, "Les deux plus anciens comptes de l'hôtel-Dieu de Beauvais (1377–1380)," *Bulletin philologique et historique (jusqu'à 1715) du Comité des travaux historiques et scientifiques* (1914): 163–344.

6. Longnon, ed., *Documents*, 3:124–33.

keep annual written accounts of their receipts and expenditures, something many of them were not doing the way that Saint-Nicolas was.[7]

Income

One of the striking features of the account book for Saint-Nicolas is how much of it concerns the hospital's cultivation of agriculture. With its rural granges in Froiderive, Belley, and Creney, the hospital was producing a significant amount of wheat, meslin, rye, barley, and oats. The account book indicates that in 1300 the hospital cultivated 65 *setiers* of wheat, 36 *setiers* of meslin, 26 *setiers* of rye, 63 *setiers* of barley, and 69 *setiers* of oats.[8] There was also livestock on these granges, with as many as 300 ewes, rams, sheep, and lambs at the institution's property at Belley.[9] In 1300 Saint-Nicolas had a cellar ("celarium") to store agricultural produce, and by the late fourteenth century, the account books were referring to "greniers" to store cereals, a "chambre aux lars" to conserve meat, "cuves" for the storage of wine, and stables for the horses of visitors and the *magister*.[10] While much of this agricultural production was consumed by members of the hospital community, the account book begins each year with how much grain remained from the previous year. Moreover, there was a surplus of all five grains for each of the three years covered by the account book. In 1300, for example, 25 percent of the meslin produced in 1299 had still not been consumed at the time of the accounting, which took place each year on March 12, the feast of Saint Gregory.[11] The hospital made a regular practice of selling its wheat, making 61 *l.* in 1300, 55 *l.* in 1301, and 62 *l.* in 1302.[12] The cultivation of wheat represented an even more important source of revenue for the hospital of Saint-Sauveur in Lille. Between 1285 and 1355, its sale of wheat to merchants in Flanders, Ypres, Witjschate, Poperinge, and elsewhere represented 57 percent of its total revenue.[13] The sources of revenue for the hospital in Troyes, however,

7. Davis, *Holy Bureaucrat*, 79–82, 92–103.

8. BnF ms lat. 9111, fol. 287–289.

9. Likewise, a charter from 1223 indicates that on one of the pastures belonging to the hospital of Provins, the hospital had up to 30 cows, 100 sheep, 40 pigs, and 12 horses and donkeys. See Dupraz, no. 482; AD Seine-et-Marne 11HdtA12, fol. 141–141v.

10. Gesret, "Un hôpital," 142.

11. BnF ms lat. 9111, fol. 282, 288.

12. BnF ms lat. 9111, fol. 291, 297.

13. Derville, *L'agriculture*, 94. Derville believes that the hospital in Lille was practicing a subsistence economy. Although it sold quite a bit of wheat and bought various foodstuffs, the hospital mostly consumed what it produced and received, making little attempt to invest its capital so as to make a profit. Derville, *L'agriculture*, 96.

were far more varied. In addition to selling wheat, meslin, rye, barley, and oats, the Troyen hospital received significant income from the sale of wine, cultivated at its vineyards at Troyes, Belley, La Vacherie, Chaillouet, Froiderive, and Gyé-sur-Seine. In 1300 the hospital collected 43 *l.* from the sale of wine cultivated at its vineyards in Troyes, and in 1301 it received an additional 100 *l.* from the sale of wines from Gyé, southeast of Troyes.[14] A study of the hôtel-Dieu of Paris during the fifteenth century has demonstrated that it, too, was not only selling grains and wine but also playing a "subtle game" of selling its produce when prices were high and buying when prices were low.[15] In short, medieval hospitals' involvement in agriculture and commerce was not limited to Champagne or the thirteenth century.[16]

In addition to participating in the agricultural market, hospitals like Saint-Nicolas were active in the rental market. In 1300 Saint-Nicolas collected 38 *l.* from the rental of fifteen houses and rooms, an oven (which brought in 7 *l.* each year), and a grange located in front of the Jewish cemetery in Troyes.[17] The annual rental income from houses ranged from as little as 4 *s.* to as much as 6 *l.* As we have seen, Champagne's hospitals frequently received houses (or portions therein) as bequests, and hospitals also purchased houses. In some cases, hospitals owned the right to rental income without actually owning the house or room that produced the rent. In 1250 the hospital of Provins received a charitable bequest from a cleric and his siblings of one-eighth of a house near the old butcher stalls in the neighborhood of Saint-Ayoul; the hospital purchased an additional one-eighth of the same house from the donors.[18] What were hospitals doing with the rooms and houses that they purchased or received in alms? In most cases, hospitals leased these properties, thereby producing a steady stream of rental income. The charter from 1249 that recorded the Provins hospital's purchase of a house for 34 *l.*

---

14. BnF ms lat. 9111, fol. 283v, 291. On the importance of the wine market in Provins, see Verdier, *L'aristocratie*, 172–74.

15. Christine Jéhanno, "'Sustenter les povres malades': Alimentation et approvisionnement à la fin du moyen âge: L'exemple de l'hôtel-Dieu de Paris" (doctoral thesis, Paris, 2000), 332.

16. See, for example, Lies Vervaet's work on St. John's Hospital of Bruges, which was one of the largest landowners in late medieval Flanders and received a large percentage of its revenue from leasing land. Lies Vervaet, "Lease Holding in Late Medieval Flanders: Towards Concentration and Engrossment? The Estates of the St. John's Hospital of Bruges," in *Beyond Lords and Peasants: Rural Elites and Economic Differentiation in Premodern Europe*, ed. Frederic Aparisi and Vicent Royo (Valencia: Publicacions de la Universitat de València 2014): 111–38; Vervaet, "Goederenbeheer in een veranderende samenleving."

17. BnF ms lat. 9111, fol. 282v–283. Ovens could produce significant rental income. In 1276–78, the rental of ovens in Provins raised 463 *l.* of revenue for the count of Champagne, 6% of his total revenue from the city. See Terrasse, *Provins*, 88.

18. Dupraz, nos. 134, 135; AD Seine-et-Marne 11HdtA12, fol. 38.

(located within its own lordship) noted that at that time the house was renting for 60 *s.* per year.[19] After about eleven years of renting this house, the hospital would have begun to make a profit beyond the purchase price. The specificity with which the terms of these leases was spelled out in charters reflected the hospital's vigilance in safeguarding its interests. The *censiers*, or landbooks, for the hospital of Provins also listed a tax ("ostauz" or "ostés") it collected on many of the houses that it leased.[20]

In some cases, a hospital's rental income was tied to the trade fairs. In 1141, for example, Count Thibaut II authorized the hospital of Provins to build houses in its enclosure and lodge foreigners there during the May fairs.[21] In addition, Thibaut conceded another significant privilege to the hospital by granting it immunity from the comital exaction of one-half of all rental income on houses located in the area of the May fair while the fair was taking place. Clearly, by the mid-twelfth century the hospital already owned houses, which it was renting during the fairs, and the count was willing to share his profits from the fair, a privilege that Count Henri I renewed in 1164.[22] In 1211, Countess Blanche gave the hospital a rent of 30 *s.* on a house that was leased during the May fairs.[23] As we noted earlier, another charter from the countess makes clear that drapery and belts were being sold in houses owned by the hospital of Provins.[24] Lambert of Provins, a canon in Troyes and son of Arnoul le Laineron (likely connected to the wool industry), bequeathed his family home, located in the heart of the wool market, to the hospital of Provins.[25] As this hospital's *censiers* make clear, many of the houses that the hospital leased owed one-half of the "toloneum" or sales tax, suggesting that these houses were involved in commerce.[26] One of the landbooks also refers to some of the houses owned by the hospital as being held by the weavers ("li tisseranz"), the launderers ("la lavanderie"), and a butcher ("le bouchier").[27] In 1232 Count Thibaut IV approved a rent of 20 *s.* that had been donated to the hôtel-Dieu-le-Comte in Troyes; the rent came from a house in which merchandise was sold on the basis of its weight.[28]

19. Dupraz, no. B15; AD Seine-et-Marne 11HdtA13, fol. 42v.
20. Morlet and Mulon, eds., "Le censier," 5–89.
21. Arbois de Jubainville, *Histoire des ducs*, 2:338.
22. Bourquelot, *Histoire de Provins*, 2:386–89.
23. Arbois de Jubainville, *Histoire des ducs*, vol. 5, no. 782, p. 66.
24. Verdier, *L'aristocratie*, 232 and note 244.
25. Dupraz, no. 119; AD Seine-et-Marne 11HdtA12, fol. 35; Verdier, *L'aristocratie*, 67.
26. Morlet and Mulon, eds., "Le censier."
27. Morlet and Mulon, eds., "Le censier," 31–32.
28. Arbois de Jubainville, *Histoire des ducs*, vol. 5, no. 2187, p. 314.

The hôtel-Dieu-le-Comte in Troyes also seems to have housed traveling merchants doing business at the fairs at a kind of annex to the hospital. It was of course common for medieval hospitals to house travelers in addition to the poor and sick, although these travelers tended to be pilgrims or needy in some way. However, the hospital at Troyes seems to have taken advantage of the economic opportunity provided by the fairs by renting some of its rooms to traveling merchants, something other Champenois hospitals did as well. The same hospital received revenue from boarders who stayed in one of seven guest rooms.[29] The nobleman, Guy de Dampierre, had also donated his servant, Theloneus, who, as the charter specifically indicates, was intended to help the hospital serve its merchant guests.[30] The hospital brethren may not have regarded housing traveling merchants as any different than their housing the poor or sick, even if the latter did not have to pay for their lodging and were housed in a different space from the merchants. In both cases, the hospital provided lodging to those in need, and the income from housing merchants could be used to care for the poor and sick.

Although a hospital's income and assets came from a variety of different sources, charitable bequests were a vital lifeblood for the institution's ability to carry out its mission of caring for its poor and sick guests. The cartulary for the hospital of Provins and its martyrological obituary together contain records of at least several hundred donations to the hospital from the late twelfth and thirteenth centuries.[31] Various kinds of proactive attempts were made to increase the alms that hospitals collected, and these attempts also came under criticism by church reformers. Jacques de Vitry, for example, leveled a blistering attack on hospitals' use of "quaestores," who traveled around in search of alms for hospitals, accusing them of not only being money hungry but also corrupt by posing under the guise of religiosity and displaying fake relics while soliciting alms.[32] The account book for the hôtel-Dieu

29. AD Aube 40H1, no. 11 (September 1204).

30. AD Aube 40H1, no. 15, no. 21. Guy de Dampierre was also one of the earliest recorded benefactors of the Templars in Provins. His brother-in-law, William of Baudement, was himself a Templar. See Schenk, *Templar Families*, 182.

31. Michelin and Le Duc identified 947 donors to the Provinois hospital during the thirteenth century, drawing on the cartulary and the martyrological obituary (an enormous increase from the twenty-eight donors they identified for the previous century). See Jules Michelin and Claude Léouaon Le Duc, *État des bienfaiteurs de l'hôtel-Dieu de Provins* (Provins, France: A. Vernant, 1887), 8.

32. See Bird, "Medicine," 101, 107. The obituary for the hôtel-Dieu de la Madeleine of Rouen refers to a "questor pauperum." See Louis Rousseau, "Les ressources casuelles de l'hôtel-Dieu de la Madeleine de Rouen (XIIe–XVIe siècles)," in *Assistance et assistés jusqu'à 1610. Actes du 97ᵉ congrès des Sociétés savantes, Nantes 1972* (Paris: Bibliothèque Nationale, 1979), 157.

Saint-Nicolas provides a sense of the relative importance of bequests in the hospital's annual budget. In 1300, Saint-Nicolas received a total of 132 *l.* in money receipts that were out of the ordinary ("extravagans"), a substantial percentage when one considers that its total income that year was 331 *l.*[33] On average, the hospital seems to have received about seven new individual bequests each year, mostly testamentary, ranging from 10 *s.*, to the occasional larger bequest of 60 *l.* in 1301 from Lord Robert de Mailly-le-Château.[34] For a point of comparison, in a typical decade the hospital of Provins received somewhere between ten and thirty-one donations. The "extravagans" income was in some ways more variable than other income, since it partially depended on the unpredictability of bequests. But this category of income also included the hospital's receipt of 100 *l.* in 1301 from the sale of wines from Gyé, far more than the 15 *l.* it had received the previous year.[35] And this section of the account book also included the income from paying boarders to cover their expenses, although as the account book made clear, a person like Michel de Froiderive was actually costing the hospital twice as much (6 *l.*) as what he paid to cover those expenses (60 *s.*).[36]

As we have seen, hospitals that were closely associated with the counts of Champagne—such as the hôtel-Dieu-le-Comte and the hospital of Provins—received enormous economic benefits from the vibrant commercial activity of their fair towns, something that was also true of comital chapters such as Saint-Étienne in Troyes.[37] Like comital chapters, hospitals were frequently exempted from commercial taxes and were given rents from fair revenues, merchant halls, and money-changing tables. In 1179, for example, Count Henri I approved Pierre de Langres's donation of the sales tax on fustians (a textile made of a mixture of linen and cloth) at the fairs of Bar-sur-Aube to the hospital of Bar. In fact, Pierre had bought two one-third shares of this sales tax so as to give them (along with the one-third share he already owned) to the hospital.[38] In that same year, Count Henri also gave the hospital of Provins a rent on each of the moneychangers' tables at the May fairs and confirmed the gift made by his brother, the archbishop of Reims, of 10 *l.* annual

---

33. BnF ms lat. 9111, fol. 283v, 291.

34. Occasionally, of course, hospitals received an extraordinary bequest, such as in 1267 when the hospital of Provins received a testamentary bequest of 225 *l. t.* from the chaplain of Saint-Pierre de Provins. See Dupraz, no. 426; AD Seine-et-Marne 11HdtA12, fol. 124–124v.

35. BnF ms lat. 9111, fol. 283v, 291.

36. BnF ms lat. 9111, fol. 283v, 289v, 291, 297.

37. Evergates has shown that Saint-Étienne's enormous wealth was directly tied to the trade fairs in Troyes and the commercial economy more generally. Evergates, *Henry the Liberal*, 48, 130, 175.

38. Benton and Bur, eds., *Recueil*, no. 509, pp. 636–37.

revenue from the sales tax of Provins.[39] In 1200, Agnès of Baudemont, the countess of Braisne, gave the hospital of Provins a rent of 40 *s.* on the weight of the Provins ("de pondere pruvini"), essentially from seigniorage revenue.[40] In 1219, shortly before his (and his eldest son's) death while on crusade at Damietta, Milon IV of Le Puiset, who was count of Bar-sur-Seine, gave the hospital of Provins a rent of 60 *s.* on the market and toll ("pedagio") at Bar-sur-Seine "for the use of the poor."[41] In 1230, Count Thibaut IV encouraged the hospital of Provins to build a market hall where he owned two houses, and the count henceforth required all merchants selling cloth, woolen fabric, and silk to sell their goods in this hall when the Provinois fair was not taking place. The revenue from the feudal tax and rent paid by the merchants would be equally shared by the count and the brothers of the hospital.[42] Rents payable by the counts to the hospital at the May fair totaled 43 *l.* 10 *s.* and came from the entrance of wines from Auxerre and elsewhere as well as from table changers, fiefs, mills, ovens, and sales taxes.[43] The fair of Saint-Ayoul brought in an additional 36 *l.* 15 *s.*[44] In total, the hospital of Provins received 81 *l.* each year from fairs.[45] By the second half of the thirteenth century, financial pressures made the aristocracy far more cautious about sharing the profits from commerce; there are many examples of aristocrats reigning in some of the grants they had earlier given to monastic houses and hospitals.[46]

Hospitals also had their own stalls at fairs, where they sold goods. A charter from 1173 shows that the hôtel-Dieu-le-Comte in Troyes paid the count 40 *s.* each year for the right to have a bread stall at the market, and Count Henri I redirected this rent to the chapter of Saint-Étienne.[47] A charter from 1202 refers to the hôtel-Dieu having a stall at the fair of St. Rémi in Troyes, one stall over from the Templars' stall.[48] In 1206 this same hospital was involved

39. Benton and Bur, eds., *Recueil*, no. 524, pp. 652–53.

40. Dupraz, no. 46; AD Seine-et-Marne 11HdtA12, fol. 24.

41. Dupraz, no. 51; AD Seine-et-Marne 11HdtA12, fol. 24v. On Milon IV, see Evergates, *Aristocracy*, 169–70, 215. A number of the rents that this hospital collected came from tolls, including those at Coulommiers, Augers-en-Brie, Tournan-en-Brie, Ferté-Gaucher, and Bar-sur-Seine. See Morlet and Mulon, eds., "Le censier," 44–45.

42. Arbois de Jubainville, *Histoire des ducs*, vol. 5, no. 2096, p. 298. As the cartulary of Provins makes clear, in later years the city was paying an annual rent of as much as 10 *l.* for the use of a small building ("loge") owned by the hospital, and it is possible that this was the same market hall that the hospital had built at the count's urging. See Prou and d'Auriac, eds., *Actes et comptes*, 225, 229, 265.

43. Dupraz, Table 5; Morlet and Mulon, eds., "Le censier," 44.

44. Dupraz, Table 5.

45. Dupraz, Table 5.

46. Bur, "Les 'autres' foires," 512–13.

47. Benton and Bur, eds., *Recueil*, no. 354, p. 446.

48. AD Aube 40H189, fol. 81v. This is a donation charter from the priest Manassere and his sister Jaquete.

in longstanding litigation over its claim to two stalls at the fair in Troyes, and the hospital won its claim to these stalls.[49] Two years later, Guy de Dampierre gave the hospital a stall where the moneychangers were stationed.[50] Leper hospitals also owned market stalls, with the leprosary of Les Deux Eaux, outside Troyes, paying a bourgeois from Troyes 12 *l.* in 1210 for two stalls at the Troyen market. In 1255, this same leprosary bought the rights to a stall that was adjacent to one owned by the hôtel-Dieu-le-Comte, in the section of the market where bread was sold.[51] The lepers of Saint-Ladre in Reims had long been accustomed to receiving a charitable gift of some thirty-nine "daily breads" from the hôtel-Dieu of Reims and the abbeys of Saint-Rémi, Saint-Nicaise, and Saint-Pierre-aux-Nonnains. At some point, however, the lepers, perhaps not needing as much food and in greater need of cash, began reselling these gifts of daily bread to bourgeois Rémois as lifetime rents.[52] It is unclear if this was the reason that at some point the hôtel-Dieu of Reims refused to continue furnishing the leper house with daily loaves of bread, but the hospital's refusal to perpetuate this charitable custom led to a dispute that, records show, literally continued to fester even into the seventeenth century.[53] In selling daily portions of bread to bourgeois Rémois, the leper house was merely emulating the nuns of Saint-Pierre and the monks of Saint-Rémi, who were regularly selling their surplus bread to the bourgeois of Reims. In 1331, the nuns of Saint-Pierre, who were baking as many as 1,300 loaves each day, sold fifty loaves as lifetime rents to forty townspeople, with one lifetime annuity of daily bread selling for as much as 30 *l. parisis.*[54]

The account book for Saint-Nicolas in Troyes indicates that the hospital received a relatively small sum each year from its tenants as a *cens* or nominal rent in recognition of its role as landlord. In 1300, the hospital received a total of 12 *l.* as *cens*, 10 *l.* the following year, and 8 *l.* in 1302.[55] The hospital of Provins collected a similar amount of *cens* in 1301.[56] Some tenants also paid hospitals a *modiatio* or *moisson*, an additional rent that tended to be greater than the *cens* and could be paid in either money or in kind.[57] The account

49. AD Aube 40H189, fol. 82 (November 1206).

50. Boutiot, *Histoire de la ville de Troyes*, 1:349.

51. Harmand, *Notice*, 53, 153.

52. Desportes, *Reims et les Rémois*, 387–88 and note 89; AMC (Reims): FH-FG, A6.

53. AMC (Reims): FH-FG, A6.

54. Desportes, *Reims et les Rémois*, 388.

55. BnF ms lat. 9111, fol. 283v, 291, 196v.

56. Dupraz, Table 4. The hospital collected 12 *l.* 18 *s.* 2 *d.*

57. Morlet and Mulon, eds., "Le censier de l'hôtel-Dieu de Provins," 50. Originally, the *moisson* (or *moison*) could be paid in terms of a certain measure of cloth or quantity of grains, but this rent was gradually converted into a money fee. See Terrasse, *Provins*, 82.

book for Saint-Nicolas itemized the *cens* by the location in which it was collected rather than by the name of individual tenants or pieces of property. Some hospitals, however, kept extraordinarily detailed landbooks of all the tenants who paid an annual rent as well as the property on which it was paid. An extant *censier* for the hospital of Provins, covering the period from 1191 to 1300, is 289 folios long and lists tenants in alphabetical order with the *cens* they owed.[58] While the amounts tended to be small, often just two or three *deniers* (or a set amount of wheat), the number of people who owed this nominal rent is quite extraordinary. A *censier* for 1264 for this hospital lists 536 *censitaires* outside of Provins who owed the hospital the *cens* at Saint-Rémi, 140 *censitaires* who owed the rent at Gouaix, and 35 at Saint-Loup.[59] The hospital collected a total of 37 *l.* 19 *s.* in *cens* that year.[60] That there are *censiers* extant for other individual years (1250–80, 1268, 1284, 1294, 1301) and for specific locations, such as Gouaix, Vulaines-lès-Provins, and Saint-Loup-de-Naud, makes it possible to trace the hospital's rental income over time and witness the diverse social and economic classes of the hospital's tenants. One tenant who paid the annual *cens*, for example, was Joçons de Coulommiers, a Jew who in 1291 bought a place in Provins within the hospital's *censive* from the wife and children of the late Salomon Pastorelle, a convert from Judaism.[61] Many of the hospital's tenants were peasants with extremely limited resources, precisely the kinds of people most likely to end up turning to the hospital for assistance as true dependents.

The hospitals' *censiers* also show just how zealous some hospitals were in recording the rents that they collected, thereby guarding their lordly right to this income, however small it tended to be. If a hospital's tenants failed to pay their rents, the hospital was quick to expel them. Champagne's hospitals were aggressive not only in claiming any *cens* that was overdue but in defending

---

58. AD Seine-et-Marne, 11HdtB177.

59. The *censier* for Saint-Remi is in AD Seine-et-Marne 11HdtB178; for Saint-Loup-de-Naud, 11HdtB179; for Gouaix, 11HdtB195. See also Morlet and Mulon, eds., "Le censier de l'hôtel-Dieu de Provins"; Dupraz, Table II; Françoise Baron, "Les possessions hors les murs de l'Hôtel-Dieu de Provins au XIIIe siècle," *Bulletin de la Société d'Histoire et d'Archéologie de l'arrondissement de Provins* 130 (1976): 51.

60. Dupraz, Table 2. This *censier* for the year 1264 is in AD Seine-et-Marne 11HdtB178.

61. AD Seine-et-Marne 11Hdt/B180; Jean Mesqui, *Provins: La fortification d'une ville au moyen âge* (Geneva: Droze, 1979), 200. In 1251 the hospital resolved a dispute with a Jew named Judelot who claimed possession over several rooms in the castle of Provins. See Dupraz, no. 130; AD Seine-et-Marne 11HdtA12, fol. 37. Provins had a sizeable Jewish community in the thirteenth century, with synagogues, a school, a cemetery, an oven, and possibly even a Jewish leprosarium. See Félix Bourquelot, *Histoire de Provins* (Paris, 1839; repr. 2004), 264–65; Verdier, *L'aristocratie*, 49; Touati, "Domus judaeorum leprosorum."

their right to these rents through litigation. Hospitals were also eager to buy rents, since they provided a reliable source of additional income. In 1223, for example, the hospital of Provins bought a *cens* that the knight Philippe Poile-chien owned on thirty-seven *arpents* of land.[62] When donors ceded property to hospitals in perpetual alms, they frequently retained the *cens*, a symbolic sign of their continuing lordship. Someone donating property to a hospital might promise to free the hospital of the obligation to pay the *cens* at a later date, as a chaplain at the cathedral of Reims did in his donation of a house to the Rémois hospital in 1260, but there was no guarantee that this would ever happen.[63] Nonetheless, hospitals searched for ways to extricate themselves from paying these recurring rents.

Expenditures

The account book for the hôtel-Dieu Saint-Nicolas details the hospital's annual expenditures on everything from the 70 *s.* it spent in 1300 for almonds, pepper, and other "apothecis," suggestive of items that had healing properties; to the 72 *s.* it spent for oil; the 22 *s.* it paid for lard; the 25 *l.* spent on meat, fish, and other foods; the 12 *l.* for the sisters and their servants ("familiae") as well as pittances; the 26 *l.* for the salaries of the servants and their expenses on the granges at Belley, Creney, and Froiderive; the 3 *s.* to repair the latrines for the sick; the 50 *s.* to cover the priests' dormitory and the rooms of the hospital; and the 18 *s.* needed to buy one *setier* of beans.[64] The list of the hospital's expenditures reveals a great deal about social life inside hospitals and the nature of a hospital's annual budget. By comparing the annual expenditures over several years, one gets a sense of what the regular expenditures were as compared with special, non-recurring expenses. As the account book makes clear in its itemized description of the expenses it incurred on its granges, there were significant costs associated with cultivating wine, with 34 *l.* spent in 1300 on the vineyards of Troyes, Froiderive, and Gyé.[65] These costs included supporting the custodians who were charged with overseeing the vineyards.[66] Every year the hospital spent between 18 and 26 *l.* on mowing its pastures and making hay.[67] There were also recurring

62. BM Provins ms. 85, no. 52.
63. AMC (Reims): FH-HD B62, no. 17 (1260).
64. BnF ms lat. 9111, fol. 284–287.
65. BnF ms lat. 9111, fol. 284–284v.
66. BnF ms lat. 9111, fol. 284–284v.
67. BnF ms lat. 9111, fol. 285, 292, 299.

expenses of 21 to 24 *l.* for the smith responsible for a four-horse team and the horses' harnesses.[68] There were also irregular yet frequent expenditures for building repairs; or the purchase in 1301 of ten pigs and eight meat cows; or the cost of materials needed for tanning hides.[69] Whereas the hospital's ordinary expenses totaled 71 *l.* in 1300, a year later they had increased to 152 *l.*[70] The hospital's overall expenditures also jumped from 320 *l.* in 1300 to 442 *l.* in 1301, but even then, receipts exceeded expenses by almost 30 *l.*[71] This was in contrast to the hospital of Saint-Sauveur in Lille, which already in the 1280s and 1290s was facing indebtedness due to a slump in the price of wheat and the rising cost of salaries for servants ("maisnies"). These challenges only increased during the first decades of the fourteenth century—a period of war, disorder, and famine in the far north of France—with the hospital's account rolls showing the disappearance of foodstuffs (butter, eggs, wine, and fresh meat and fish), a drastic reduction in the hospital's annual purchase of clothing, and even a two-thirds reduction in agricultural cultivation.[72]

As Daniel Le Blévec has shown in his study of charity in the Lower Rhône, hospitals could be major landholders, and as such, they profited from the economic growth of the late twelfth and thirteenth centuries.[73] Since the greatest potential for wealth lay in landed property, religious and charitable institutions could not merely rely on the collection of alms. Rather, a hospital's long-term survival required that charitable revenues be reinvested in the acquisition of new fiefs and other income-producing investments. While there is not much evidence for Saint-Nicolas's purchasing properties, the hospital of Provins, in contrast, made substantial investments in landed property. In 1269, 1273, and 1304, the hospital made individual purchases of 130 *l. t.*, 80 *l. t.*, and 300 *l. t.*, the latter for eighty-six *arpents* of woods near Plessis-aux-Tournelles.[74] Both the scale and frequency of this hospital's purchases was significant. Over the course of the thirteenth century, the hospital acquired or received in donation some 62 houses, 28 rooms, 29 gardens, 1,524 *arpents* of arable, 858 *arpents* of woods, and 1,248 *l.* in money rents as well as numerous rents in kind.[75] The references in charters to the hospital's

---

68. BnF ms lat. 9111, fol. 284v, 292, 299v.

69. BnF ms lat. 9111, fol. 285v, 292v.

70. BnF ms lat. 9111, fol. 284v–186v, 292v.

71. BnF ms lat. 9111, fol. 287, 293v.

72. Derville, *L'agriculture*, 96, 126–30.

73. Le Blévec, *La part du pauvre*, 720.

74. Dupraz, nos. 158, 483, 516; AD Seine-et-Marne 11HdtA12, fol. 46–46v, 141, 154.

75. Michelin and Le Duc, *État des bienfaiteurs*, Table.

ownership of mills, presses, and serfs suggest that the hôtel-Dieu was pro-ducing grain, wine, and oil both for its own needs and for sale on the market.

Some of the fiefs that the Provinois hospital purchased were part of its own *censive*. In these cases, the hospital bought back a fief from its tenants, another indication of its ability to invest liquid capital.[76] The hospital broth-ers at Provins seem to have made a concerted effort to purchase properties adjacent to those the hospital already owned so that its assets were more consolidated, easier to manage, and thereby more profitable. The frequency with which Champagne's hospitals exchanged landed property with other religious houses and individuals suggests that they, too, were strategic in con-solidating their property.[77] From 1269 to 1280, the Provinois hospital spent 236 *l. t.* in a systematic effort to buy and consolidate the lands of Briotte, some ninety *arpents* of land split up among six different individuals.[78] There are records of the hospital making fifteen purchases during the 1270s, some of them quite substantial. In 1304 it paid the exorbitant sum of 300 *l. t.* for eighty-six *arpents* of woods at Buignon.[79] By 1331, however, it seems to have been selling those same woods, paying 294 *l. t.* for eighty-four *arpents* of the woods at Buignon, perhaps indicative of the economic recession that char-acterized this period before the Black Death.[80] The hospital must not have been too strapped, however, since by 1335 it was again making a significant purchase of land for 112 *l. t.*[81] Four years later, however, it sold fifty-two *arpents* of woods at Le Corbier for 208 *l. t.*[82]

Much of the landed property that the hospital purchased or received in alms was in the form of fiefs. In order for a fief to be alienated, the lord had to grant a license, or amortization, which was usually accompanied by a fee. As Theodore Evergates has shown, whereas counts and barons in the early to mid-twelfth century often showed their generosity to the church by consenting to the transfer of fiefs held by their knights free of charge, by the

76. As Evergates has shown, lordly repurchases of fiefs were common in Champagne. Indeed, Countess Blanche repurchased fiefs so that she could donate them to the hôtels-Dieu in Château-Thierry and Argensolles. See Evergates, *Aristocracy*, 75.

77. To give just one example, a record from 1257 shows that the hospital of Meaux ceded a gar-den to Baudin the Jew and the Jewish community of Meaux in exchange for several *arpents* of land. AD Seine-et-Marne 9Hdt/B19 (copy).

78. Dupraz, no. 483–89; AD Seine-et-Marne 11HdtA12, fol. 141–143v.

79. Dupraz, no. 516; AD Seine-et-Marne 11HdtA12, fol. 154. This is in contrast to the hospital of Saint-Sauveur in Lille, which made very few purchases of land and which received little income from the sale of wood. See Derville, *L'agriculture*, 93–94, 96–97, 124–25.

80. Dupraz, no. 517; AD Seine-et-Marne 11HdtA12, fol. 154.

81. Dupraz, no. 519; AD Seine-et-Marne 11HdtA12, fol. 155–155v.

82. Dupraz, no. 518; AD Seine-et-Marne 11HdtA12, fol. 154.

late twelfth century they increasingly sought to restrict and tax the transfers of their fiefs to religious houses.[83] In the case of fiefs alienated to hospitals, however, thirteenth-century counts generally continued to grant amortizations without charge, perhaps indicative that the counts regarded hospitals in a different light than most monastic houses.[84] These free amortizations were one way that counts displayed their generosity toward hospitals and saved them from an additional expense. In addition to granting free amortizations, counts sought to ensure that a hospital could have unencumbered access to the valuable resources in the comital *censive*. Thus, in 1190 Count Henri II forbade his foresters from impeding the hospital of Provins from taking wood from comital forests so long as the hospital had a license from the owner of the woods.[85] Count Thibaut V granted the hospital permission to grind grain twice a week at his mill without paying any fees.[86]

The majority of the free amortizations granted to hospitals for their newly acquired lands came from members of the knightly class.[87] Free amortizations certainly helped facilitate the growth of a hospital's property holdings, since fiefs that were alienated to the hospital essentially became allodial land, outside the former lord's jurisdiction. At times a hospital compensated a lord for his grant of amortization, and it is not clear whether such compensation was demanded by the lord for his grant or whether this was a freely given counter-gift. When Thomas de Mirvaux, for example, amortized 131 *arpents* of woods that had been given or sold to the hospital of Provins, thereby authorizing the future exchange of woods between the hospital and one of his tenants, the hospital compensated him with ten *arpents* of its own woods at Orbies, a palfrey given by the countess of Angoulême, and 60 *s.* that Thomas owed.[88] As we have seen, it was common for hospitals to express their gratitude toward donors by presenting them with counter-gifts, and while these represented another expenditure, particularly when they were in

---

83. Evergates, *Aristocracy*, 76–77.

84. Dupraz, p. 51. The cartulary for the hôtel-Dieu contains fifty-one records of amortizations, a number of them comital. Anne Lester points out that Champagne's counts also tended to grant free amortizations to Cistercian nunneries. See Lester, *Creating Cistercian Nuns*, 197–99.

85. AD Seine-et-Marne, 11Hdt/B1–5. On the management of woodlands in medieval Champagne, see Richard Keyser, "The Transformation of Traditional Woodland Management: Commercial Sylviculture in Medieval Champagne," *French Historical Studies* 32, no. 3 (2009): 353–84.

86. Dupraz, no. 56; AD Seine-et-Marne 11HdtA12, fol. 24v.

87. Abbeys, ecclesiastics, and occasionally bourgeois also provided hospitals with free amortizations on properties and privileges that they acquired. Lords granting free amortizations were often still eager to retain the *cens*.

88. Dupraz, no. B7; AD Seine-et-Marne 11HdtA13, fol. 73v.

the form of an annual rent, hospitals clearly believed they were worthwhile in sustaining good relationships. When the knight Jean de Montceaux-en-Brie gave an *arpent* of arable at Rupéreux and a *cens* of 1 *d.* on a meadow, the hospital of Provins thanked him with a counter-gift of 10 *s. t.*[89]

In its role as a lord, hospitals were also asked for permission to grant their vassals the right to alienate property, and whereas hospitals were often the beneficiary of free amortizations, they were not always as generous in granting amortizations to others. Granting amortizations presented hospitals with the opportunity to assert their lordship and collect additional income. In 1279, when a priest with a benefice at Saint-Quiriace complained that the hospital of Provins was preventing him from collecting a rent of 40 *s. t.* on a house in the hospital's *censive*, the hospital explained that it had not yet granted amortization on the house and therefore could collect the rent for itself. An accord was reached whereby the priest collected 35 *s. t.* and the hospital 5 *s. t.*[90] The abbey of Jouy, on the other hand, seemed eager to thank the hospital for a rent of 12 *s.* that the hospital had amortized; the abbey (over) compensated the hospital for abandoning a *cens* of 3 halfpennies by paying 50 *s. t.*[91] Instead of demanding an amortization fee, the hospital sometimes demanded an increase in the *cens* that was paid annually. In other words, rather than receiving a one-time amortization fee, the hospital could increase the rent that it was owed in perpetuity.[92]

What did hospitals do with the properties that they acquired? In some cases, they infeudated property so that it was held in tenure as a fief. In 1252, for example, the hospital of Provins farmed out a meadow that it owned outside the city walls (and that bordered a tannery and another meadow that the hospital had already farmed out) to a group of men for an annual rent of 182 *s.* and an annual *cens* of 46 *d.* The men were expected to build houses on the meadow within a period of two years, which presumably would increase

---

89. Dupraz, no. 469; AD Seine-et-Marne 11HdtA12, fol. 137. For another example of a counter-gift, see Dupraz, no. 217; AD Seine-et-Marne 11HdtA12, fol. 65. On the ways that monks used counter-gifts to strengthen their relationships with their secular neighbors (and donors) and prevent disputes, see Bouchard, *Sword, Miter, and Cloister,* 217–19.

90. Dupraz, no. 69; AD Seine-et-Marne 11HdtA12, fol. 27–27v.

91. Dupraz, no. 77; AD Seine-et-Marne, 11HdtA12, fol. 28v. The hospital also at times entered into agreement with religious houses so that they could freely acquire fiefs from one another's estates.

92. The abbey of Sainte Colombe de Sens did this in granting an amortization free of charge, but also increasing the *cens* from 2 *d.* to 8 *s.*, a forty-eight-fold increase. See Dupraz, no. 157; AD Seine-et-Marne 11HdtA12, fol. 45v–46.

the value of the fief.[93] The hospital also owned a significant number of houses that it had acquired either through charitable donation or purchase. In 1273, for instance, Ythier "Barberius" and his wife sold a house and grange to the hospital for 80 *l. t.*[94] By renting this property, the hospital could count on regular, dependable sources of revenue. Jehan Jeucard, a notary of the court of Sens, and his wife Pétronille, rented a house in Provins from the hôtel-Dieu for 12 *l.* per year.[95] Leprosaries also raised revenue by essentially renting out land that they owned. In 1198, the leprosary of Les Deux Eaux, near Troyes, ceded some land to two brothers for their lifetimes, and they paid the leprosary 25 *l.* and an annual *cens* of 20 *s.* After their deaths, the land would revert back to the leprosary.[96]

As Richard Keyser has shown, the value of wood spiked in Champagne as demand for fuel and lumber increased during the thirteenth century.[97] This increased demand stemmed from an increase in the population and the clearing of woodlands, which reduced the overall supply of wood. Lords placed greater restrictions on the use of their forests, including how much wood could be used, how often it could be taken, what kinds of wood could be taken, from which part of the forest, and for what purposes. The "gruaria" tax and license fee for collecting firewood could be steep, sometimes amounting to as much as half the sale price of the wood.[98] Just the sale of woods could generate significant revenue. Keyser has shown that 15 percent of the comital revenue for 1252, a whopping 7,600 *l.,* came from woods, primarily commercial wood harvesting.[99] Thus it is not surprising that hospitals often had to spend significant resources on the wood they needed for heating, cooking, and building. In 1304 the hospital of Provins paid 300 *l. t.* for eighty-six *arpents* of woods near Plessis-aux-Tournelles.[100] Donations to hospitals sometimes came in the form of woodlands or the right to collect wood from particular forests. In 1234 Gautier, the lord of Vignory, gave to God and the hospital brothers of Saint-Nicolas in Bar-sur-Aube (along with two other

---

93. Dupraz, no. 196; AD Seine-et-Marne 11HdtA12, fol. 59–59v.

94. Dupraz, no. 158; AD Seine-et-Marne, 11HdtA12, fol.46–46v.

95. AD Seine-et-Marne, H suppl. B83. Note that the hospital had agreed to rent this house to Jean for the duration of his lifetime. Since the amount of the rent was fixed, the hospital ran the risk that inflation could erode the value of the rent.

96. Harmand, *Notice historique*, 34.

97. Keyser, "Transformation," 353–84.

98. Keyser, "Transformation," 379.

99. Keyser, "Transformation," 378.

100. Dupraz, no. 516; AD Seine-et-Marne 11HdtA12, fol. 154.

houses) the daily use of three cartloads of deadwood, whether standing or fallen, from his forests. The brothers were also given three standing beech trees ("fagos vinas et stantes") each year for their necessities. Gautier made this donation for the salvation of his soul and that of his wife, father, and ancestors, and the hospital promised on its own volition ("spontanea") to celebrate an anniversary mass each year in its church for Gautier, his wife, and his father.[101] Twelve years earlier, Gautier had given the same hospital the right to collect deadwood from his forest in Lignol once a day, and this donation was directed at the hospital's *conversae*. A stipulation of the gift was that it could not be sold, as Gautier seems to have wanted to make sure that his gift was actually used to provide heat for the sisters.[102]

Hospitals wanted both to purchase more rents (*cens, moisson*) that were paid in recognition of a landlord's rights and to extricate themselves from the obligation to pay these rents. Moreover, it was not uncommon for hospitals to pay what was sometimes a significant sum either to own the right to these rents or to free themselves of such a monetary obligation. When Régnier de Bannost and his wife, Burgis, gave the hospital of Provins a small garden in the *censive* of two knights in 1231, the knights agreed to free the hospital from the *cens* of 5 *d*. if it agreed to pay them 4 *l*. 10 *s*., or the equivalent of 1,080 *d*.[103] Since it would have taken the hospital 216 annual payments of the *cens* before it recouped what it had paid to be free of the *cens*, it seems likely that the knights provided the hospital with an additional service or good not mentioned in the charter. There are plenty of other cases, however, where those managing the hospital's assets were evidently thinking about the house's long-term growth in their willingness for the hospital to wait many years before recovering what it paid for a rent. In 1217 the hospital of Provins paid 6 *s*. for a *cens* worth 2 *d*., so it would have taken the hospital thirty-six years before it recouped its purchase price.[104] In 1266 the hospital paid 6 *l. t*. for a *cens* worth 4 *s. t*., so in this case it would have taken thirty years to recover what it had paid.[105] In 1267 the hospital of Provins paid a cleric 20 *s*. for a *cens* of 12 *d*., so after twenty years the hospital would have recouped the

---

101. AD: Aube HD33/209.

102. AD: Aube HD33/168.

103. BM Provins ms. 85, no. 58.

104. The hospital purchased the *cens* from Gerard Halegrin. Dupraz, no. B8; AD Seine-et-Marne 11HdtA13, fol. 45 v.

105. The hospital purchased this *cens* at Vinneuf from Marguerite de Vallery, a *domicella*. Dupraz, no. 333; AD Seine-et-Marne 11HdtA12, fol. 99v–100.

purchase price.[106] The hospital's landbook shows that by the later thirteenth century, it mostly owed lordly rents to churches and monastic houses, and these only totaled 53 s. 5 d.[107]

Like other kinds of rents, tithes represented a potentially lucrative investment, and hospitals showed great interest in acquiring them. As the account book for Saint-Nicolas indicates, the hospital received a significant amount of wheat each year in the form of a tithe it possessed at Creney. A thirteenth-century censier for the hospital of Provins also shows that it regularly received various grains as tithes (and other rents that it was owed), and it also received hens, wine, and a certain number of loaves of bread as tithes and rents.[108] Tithes were sometimes given as charitable bequests, but hospitals also purchased them. In 1215 the hôtel-Dieu-le-Comte purchased one-fourth of a tithe at Clérey for 270 l. from Hugues, a knight from Fresnoy, but the hospital did not make this large purchase on its own. A certain priest from Bucey contributed to the purchase on the condition that he and his cleric could share part of the use of the tithe's revenues.[109] There were other instances of hospitals engaging in collaborative investments. In 1202 the hôtel-Dieu-le-Comte in Troyes pooled its resources with Warren l'Archer, building at their common expense a mill at Nuisement after agreeing to share equally what was produced at the mill and the resulting revenue.[110] Some hospital purchases, including of tithes, came about because of an individual's indebtedness or need to raise liquid capital. The hospital of Provins, for example, bought a tithe at Plessis from the lord Baudouin Bréban, who was just about to depart on crusade (sometime around 1248) and needed to raise a large amount of capital to finance his expedition. In addition to selling the tithe to the hospital, Baudouin sold Count Thibaut IV the lordship over some two hundred serfs, the tax on his men at Vanvillé, and 111 arpents of woods.[111]

Like monasteries, some hospitals fulfilled the role of bank lender, providing credit to those in need.[112] That some hospitals were able to provide loans

---

106. The cleric who ceded this rent to the hospital was Master Mathieu de Pigy. Dupraz, no. 189; AD Seine-et-Marne 11HdtA12, fol. 157.

107. Morlet and Mulon, eds., "Le censier," 62–63.

108. Morlet and Mulon, eds., "Le censier," 46–47.

109. Arbois de Jubainville, Histoire des ducs, nos. 923–924.

110. Arbois de Jubainville, Histoire des ducs, no. 564.

111. Verdier, L'aristocratie, 202–3.

112. Robert Génestal, Rôle des monastères comme établissements de credit étudié en Normandie du XIe à la fin du XIII siècle (Paris, 1901). During the thirteenth century the hospital of St. John the Evangelist in Cambridge supplied credit to Christians wishing to free themselves from their indebtedness to Jewish moneylenders. See Rubin, Charity and Community, 217–26.

demonstrates that they had liquid capital available and that creditors thought to turn to them for help. It is noteworthy that creditors often gave hospitals tithes as surety for their loans. While a hospital waited to collect its debt, it collected the income from the tithe or whatever property had been given in surety. The mortgage that the hospital advanced in return for the tithe or other property was usually less than if the hospital had been buying the property outright. While the borrower could buy back the property within a certain period of time, it was reasonable for the hospital to hope that the borrower would not be able to do so, with the result that the hospital would be able to keep it.[113] In one instance, the hospital of Provins was confronted with an angry borrower, who, conceding an inability to buy back the property (in this case, an annual tithe of 26 *setiers* of grain), demanded what amounted to an adjusted sale price for the mortgaged property.[114] Even if the borrower did buy the property back, the hospital was able in the meantime to collect the income on it. It was particularly common for hospitals to lend money to members of the noble and knightly class. In 1221, for example, the knight Robert Baucanz de la Grange mortgaged his tithe on a parish to the hospital of Provins for 53 *l*.[115] In 1223, the noblewoman Reine du Plessis-aux-Tournelles, whose father, Robert de Pentecôte, had earlier engaged in various transactions (and conflicts) with the hospital of Provins, found herself in debt. She and her husband, Pierre du Plessis, turned to the hospital for help, mortgaging a tithe in the parish of Cucharmoy that they had inherited from Reine's father to the hôtel-Dieu for 53 *l*. The following year they received an additional 10 *l*. of mortgage from the hospital, with the intention of buying it back before the upcoming harvest.[116] In 1228 they gave half of the tithe to the hospital and the other half to the chapter of Notre-Dame-du-Val for the salvation of their souls, and these two religious institutions counter-gifted an annual life rent of several measures of wheat and oats.[117] Likewise, the knight Jean d'Atilly and his wife Emeline mortgaged their tithe in the parish of

---

113. Bouchard, *Holy Entrepreneurs*, 33–43.

114. Dupraz, no. 219; AD Seine-et-Marne 11HdtA12, fol. 65v–66. Upon the borrower's abandonment of the tithe, the hospital renounced its original loan of 70 *l. t.* and instead agreed to pay 60 *l. prov.*

115. Dupraz, no. 214; AD Seine-et-Marne 11HdtA12, fol. 64. On the mortgaging of fiefs, see Evergates, *Aristocracy*, 72. As Bouchard has pointed out, the term *decimas* did not always refer to property rightfully belonging to the church; the term was also applied to income levied as a percentage of crops or yield. It was common, however, for members of the laity to own tithes (in the narrower sense of the term) and purchase them from churchmen. See Bouchard, *Sword, Miter, and Cloister*, 181–83.

116. Dupraz, no. 366; AD Seine-et-Marne 11HdtA12, fol. 111; Verdier, *L'aristocratie*, 155–56.

117. Dupraz, no. 217; AD Seine-et-Marne 11HdtA12, fol. 65.

Cucharmoy for 70 *l.*, and if Emeline's sister did not approve of this mortgage upon becoming an adult, the hospital would free her half of the tithe and the couple would repay the hospital for the loan they had taken out in Emeline's name.[118]

Not all loans that hospitals provided, however, had a profitable result, especially when the loan was provided to another charitable institution. The hospital of Saint-Abraham in Troyes, for example, provided a loan of 50 *l.* to the nearby leprosarium of Les Deux Eaux, with the archdeacon of Langres, Jacques de Troyes, acting as guarantor.[119] In 1244, the master of Saint-Abraham forgave the 50 *l.* that the lepers had borrowed. While loans could be profitable for hospitals, loans provided by medieval hospitals could also serve a charitable function, helping an individual or institution that was in need of short-term capital.

Granting lifetime annuities was another expenditure hospitals were frequently making that, as we observed in chapter 3, could serve a charitable function but also served the function of strengthening relationships with donors and those associated with a hospital. The 1301 account book for Saint-Nicolas indicates that the hospital was giving a rent of 30 *s.* to the nieces of the deceased archdeacon, Radulph.[120] The cleric Gérard de Polisi had given the hôtel-Dieu-le-Comte half of his vineyard in Polisi and sold the other half for 10 *l.* Noting Gérard's kindness, generosity, and devotion to the hospital, the hospital brothers conferred on him an annual rent of 50 *s.* at the feast of Saint Rémi.[121] After four years of paying this rent, the hospital's counter-gift would equal the value of Gérard's donation, and thereafter, the hospital would continue to pay this rent, thereby lessening the value of the original gift. In 1215, the hospital of Meaux received a donation of some land from a cleric named Élie du Clos, but a condition for the gift was that the hospital was required to pay a life rent of eight *setiers* of wheat each year (cultivated from the donated land) to Jeanne, a nun from Fontaines. The *cens* of 10 *s.* was also to be paid to Jeanne, and after her death, this *cens* was to be used to pay for a lamp in the hospital's infirmary.[122] When Guy d'Hery, a canon from Notre-Dame-du-Val, conceded a *cens* as well as several customary rents in kind, "out of devotion and affection which he said he had toward the domus Dei and the poor" of Provins, the hospital counter-gifted with a life annuity

118. Dupraz, no. 216; AD Seine-et-Marne 11HdtA12, fol. 64v–65.

119. Harmand, *Notice*, 48–49.

120. BnF ms lat. 9111, fol. 285.

121. AD Aube 40H189 (cartulary for the hôtel-Dieu-le-Comte), fol. 60–60v.

122. AD Seine-et-Marne 9Hdt/B75, no. 1.

of 10 *l. t.*, an annuity that would revert to his mother if he predeceased her.[123] Given that hospitals were in the practice of granting pensions, it is perhaps not surprising that the mendicant friars asked hospitals to serve as intermediaries, holding and distributing a rent-pension that someone had wanted to give to an individual friar, thereby freeing the friar from the appearance of owning a rent. Indeed, Paul Bertrand has termed the hospitals in Liège "annuity factories."[124]

Lifetime annuities were not necessarily given by hospitals to compensate someone for a gift or service, nor should we assume that they were simply another form of charity; hospitals also sometimes sold annuities to raise capital. During the second half of the thirteenth century, theologians at the University of Paris were debating whether such life rents and annuities were even licit. Henry of Ghent took the position that annuities constituted a form of usury for both the seller and the buyer. Most other theologians, however, argued otherwise, with Matthew of Aquasparta, for example, making the case that annuities were legitimate due to the uncertainty as to how long the buyer of such a rent would live. As he pointed out, it was rarely clear whether the buyer or seller of a life rent stood to gain more.[125] Like other religious institutions, though, hospitals viewed the sale of life rents as a way of raising capital, notwithstanding that such rents might financially burden the institution in the long run. Thus, the hospital of Saint-Nicolas in Troyes sold Master Guillaume de sur-Seine an annual rent of six *setiers* of wheat (worth about 5 *l.*) for 40 *l.*[126] If Guillaume ended up living longer than eight years, the hospital would likely have lost money on this annuity, and if he lived fewer than eight years, the hospital would have profited. On the other hand, by selling such an annuity, a hospital had immediate access to liquid capital. This was one way that some medieval city governments borrowed money from their citizens, who paid a lump sum to the city in return for an annual fixed life rent.[127] In some cases, charitable institutions were seeking not short-term capital but precisely the regular income stream that annuity rents could provide. Indeed, in fifteenth-century Bruges, the lay-run parochial "poor tables," which distributed meals to the "shame-faced,"

---

123. Dupraz, no. 364; AD Seine-et-Marne 11HdtA12, fol. 109v–110.

124. Bertrand, *Commerce*, 250. Bertrand also points out that hospitals served as the agents of friars in buying, selling, and redeeming rents and other properties.

125. Ian P. Wei, *Intellectual Culture in Medieval Paris: Theologians and the University of Paris, c. 1100–1330* (Cambridge: Cambridge University Press, 2012), 323–45; Ceccarelli, "'Whatever' Economics," 482–83, 499–504.

126. BnF ms lat. 9111, fol. 283v.

127. Nicholas, *The Growth of the Medieval City*, 242–43.

"respectable" poor, were largely dependent upon the regular income from annuity rents on real properties. These rents made up the bulk of the revenues of the seven poor tables of Bruges, since alms represented at most only 6 percent of their annual income.[128]

Conclusion

Champagne's largest and wealthiest hospitals received income from ovens and mills; the sale of grain and wine; various kinds of rents and tithes (some of which they purchased); the sale of arable land, vineyards, and forests; and the provision of interest loans. The diversity of these hospitals' holdings is remarkable, as is the degree to which these charitable and religious institutions were engaged in various kinds of markets, including at their own stalls at the trade fairs in Troyes, Provins, and Bar-sur-Aube. The account book for the hospital of Saint-Nicolas at Troyes indicates that this hospital was relatively self-sufficient, producing enough grain, cider, and wine to meet its needs. Relatively little of its annual budget was spent on ordinary foodstuffs such as meat, fish, and beans even though it had a fairly sizeable community to support, including clerics, lay brothers and sisters, and servants as well as its poor, sick, and traveling guests. Those managing the properties belonging to this and other hospitals were very much thinking about the long-term economic growth of their institutions. In the eyes of Jacques de Vitry and other church reformers, what these hospitals were doing with the alms they received was regarded as "hoarding," since they were not immediately dispensing alms to those most in need, but investing in income-producing fiefs, arable land, vineyards, forests, houses, mills, and various kinds of rents. There was also an apparent disconnect between the way these hospitals managed their properties and the messages relayed on behalf of the hospitals by alms collectors, who pleaded for alms that would help support the works of mercy. Alms collectors painted a dire picture of those suffering from abject poverty and illness. A donation to help "Christ's poor" was described as a literal loan to God, one that would be repaid a hundredfold in the world to come. And while it was certainly true that the alms given to hospitals were used for pittances of food and clothing for the sick poor or to pay a hospital chaplain who supplied what was thought to be life-saving sacramental medicine or the countless other needs these institutions had, the reality was that

---

128. Michael Galvin, "Credit and Parochial Charity in Fifteenth-Century Bruges," *Journal of Medieval History* 28, no. 2 (2002): 131–54.

unlike some of the weak and vulnerable guests they served, some hospitals were powerful landlords and major players in the urban economy.

As landlords with extensive assets and privileges, the hotels of Champagne's cities and towns were not just associated with the religious discipline of an Augustinian community or the works of mercy they performed for those in need of assistance. Hospitals also made their power felt for large numbers of people living outside their walls. Even those with no intention of one day joining the staff of a hospital or being a recipient of its care experienced the reach of its institutional power. After all, hundreds of people were its tenants and owed it various kinds of rents and obligations. Some tenants surely resented having to fulfill these obligations, and it was not uncommon for individuals or groups to challenge a hospital's title to property or right to collect rents. Others viewed hospitals as a source of credit, which may explain why a number of donors to hospitals expressed gratitude for the past kindness they had been shown. For others, a hospital was the source of a lifetime annuity, which in some cases represented a form of charity but could also serve to repay or thank a donor or someone who had worked for the hospital. Economics—a mixture of obligations, dependency (and interdependency), charitable assistance, and desire for gain—lay at the heart of a hospital's relationships with individuals living both inside and outside its walls.

While hospitals made their power felt in a variety of ways, they were also profoundly dependent on the social and economic landscape. Since much of their property was in the form of fiefs held from other lords, hospitals also owed their own share of rents. These institutions also depended upon good relations with the inhabitants of the region, since these inhabitants represented potential benefactors or parties from whom a hospital might one day buy, sell, or exchange property.

To be sure, a hospital's social and religious roles were inextricably tied to its economic power. While in some of their property dealings hospitals appear to have acted charitably, it is difficult to determine when hospitals were in fact primarily acting to safeguard their own interests. Ultimately, however, a hospital's careful management of its resources and its efforts to increase those resources were aimed at advancing the institution's spiritual and charitable mission. For hospital donors, for the religious community that lived and worked in hospitals, and for the sick and poor who sought refuge and care there, what was at stake was nothing short of salvation itself, whether that deliverance was bodily, financial, or otherworldly.

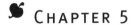

❧ Chapter 5

"In Service of the Poor"

Hospital Personnel in Pursuit of Security

In the main, the martyrological obituary for the hospital of Provins is a dry, administrative document, recording the dates of death for the hospital's donors and personnel.

There are scant words of affection, and those that are there are generally reserved for someone like Praxedis, "our sister and the prioress of our house, who for a long time, faithfully worked in the service of the poor."[1] But there are also some unusual entries that provide clues as to the wide range of people who provided services to the hospital. There is the entry for a certain Bernard, "who for a long time faithfully buried the bodies of the poor, and provided service around them to those in charge of them."[2] There is also mention of Master Jean Furnerius, a physician ("phisicus"), who also appears as a witness in 1281 and 1283 in the hospital's cartulary.[3] This is one of the rare mentions of a physician in a French hospital before the fourteenth century. Unlike the vast majority of hospitals, the hospital at Provins might have

---

1. *Obituaires de la province de Sens*, 1:934; AD: Seine-et-Marne: 11Hdt/C5, fol. 26.

2. *Obituaires de la province de Sens*, 1:940; AD: Seine-et-Marne: 11Hdt/C5, fol. 35v.

3. *Obituaires de la province de Sens*, 1:943; AD: Seine-et-Marne: 11Hdt/C5, fol. 43; Dupraz, nos. 431, 353. See Touati, *Maladie et société*, 457–58. See Danielle Jacquart, *Le milieu médical du XIIe au XVe siècle* (Geneva: Droz, 1981), 127–37, 73.

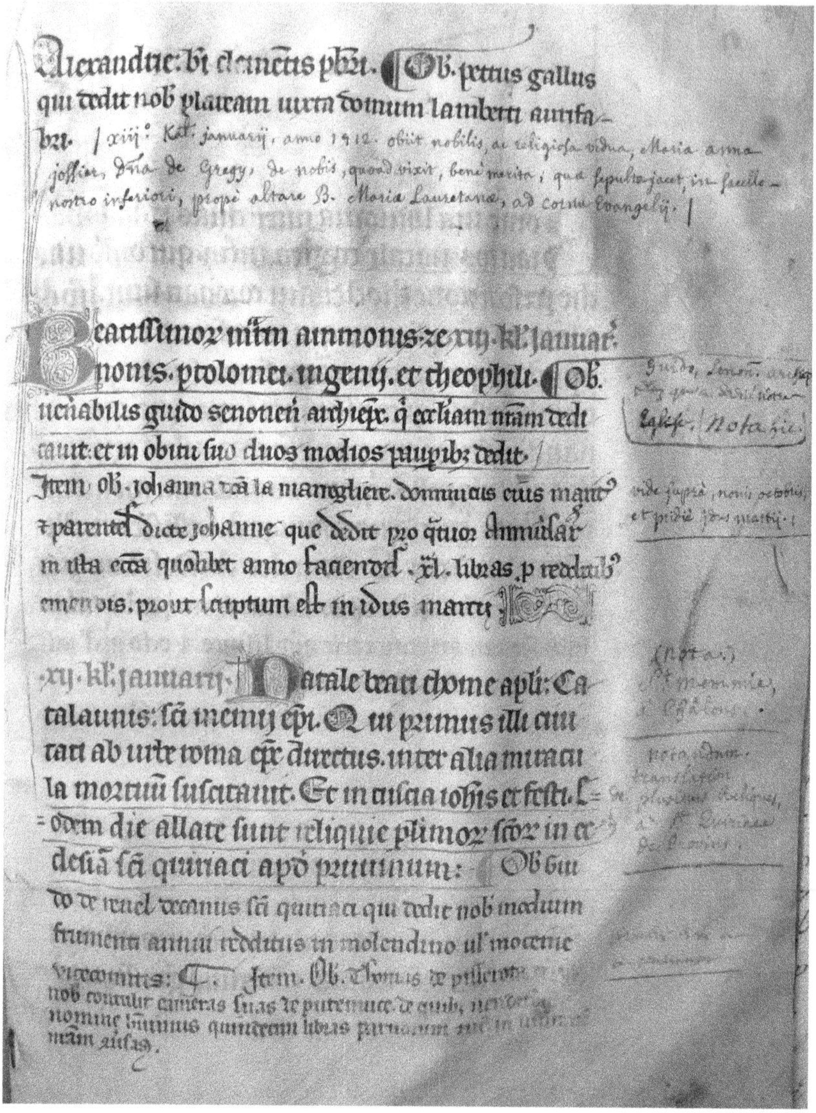

FIGURE 4. The martyrological obituary for the hôtel-Dieu of Provins (1250 with later additions). Archives départementales de Seine-et-Marne: 11Hdt/C5, fol. 97.

been able to provide at least some medical care from a trained physician. The hospitals, which by the late twelfth and thirteenth centuries dotted the European countryside and were regular features of most cities and towns, could not have functioned without a staff of devoted workers of various kinds, from the chaplains who celebrated Mass and heard confession, to the sisters and brothers who cared for the poor and sick, to the paid maidservants who laundered the bed linens and clothes, to the serfs who cultivated the hospital's land.[4] Medieval hospitals were unusual religious institutions in the degree to which they were mixed, often including chaplains, lay brothers and sisters, servants, serfs, and *donati* (or corrodians) who, as the name suggests, gave themselves and their property to a hospital so as to be associated with the works of mercy performed there.

As this chapter will show, there was a good deal of variety in the makeup of a hospital's personnel. Within the larger, wealthier, and better documented hospitals, such as those in Troyes, Provins, and Bar-sur-Aube, the personnel were strikingly diverse in terms of the social classes represented, the workers' place of origin, the kinds of tasks they were charged with doing, and the reasons to join a hospital in the first place. This chapter contends that it was piety and a pursuit of security that underlay the inspiration to serve in hospitals. Some workers were clearly attracted by the opportunity to perform the works of mercy and acquire the spiritual rewards associated with these works. As preachers sought to remind hospital communities, serving the sick poor was not any ordinary work, but a penitential expression of piety, rich in the possibilities it offered for spiritual rewards. Joining a hospital community represented an attractive religious alternative to taking holy orders (in the case of men) or taking formal monastic vows, although the brethren in hospitals that followed the Augustinian Rule did take vows. In the eyes of the laity, however, living a religious life in a hospital would have been less religiously stringent than what was expected in most monastic houses. And if, as medieval *exempla* frequently suggested, helping the poor and sick was understood as providing assistance to Christ, disguised as a poor or suffering hospital guest, then joining a hospital community held that additional lure. The examples of recent charitable saints, many of whom had worked in

---

4. The account books from the 1380s for Saint-Nicolas in Troyes include expenses for pastry chefs, cooks, bakers, chaplains, chambermaids, barbers, and the people who worked at the hospital's press. AD: Aube G2523 (account book for 1379–80); G2526 (account book for 1383–84). For an unpublished edition of the account book for 1379–80 (G2523), see Gesret, "Un hôpital au moyen âge," 414–569.

hospitals, and the growing sanctification of charitable service more generally would also have motivated some women and men to follow these saintly examples. In addition, however, this chapter reveals that joining a hospital community also represented a way to obtain greater social and material security. Hospitals housed, clothed, fed, prayed for, and in some cases even paid some of their workers. By being part of a fraternal, caritative community, one essentially lived with the guarantee of being cared for if one became too infirm or frail to continue working. Moreover, some who joined a hospital's community may already have had certain physical needs at the time of their joining. In short, as this chapter will illustrate, the boundaries between those giving and receiving assistance in medieval hospitals were remarkably permeable.

The hospitals in Champagne that are the focus of this book were mostly independent in the sense that they did not belong to a hospital or religious order, such as the Hospitallers, Antonines, or Trinitarians, although they were often located in towns and cities where there were hospitals affiliated with such orders. Unlike in England, where the religious and constitutional status of hospitals tended to be dictated by the founder's wishes, many northern French hospitals, such as the ones in Champagne, adhered to a more monastic-like model, drawing their inspiration (if not their observance) from the Augustinian Rule.[5] This monastic influence is evident in the statutes that were composed, including those for the hospital of Provins and the hôtel-Dieu-le-Comte in Troyes.[6] Moreover, during the thirteenth century, ecclesiastical reformers in northern France sought to regularize hospitals that were under episcopal jurisdiction, subjecting them to stricter religious discipline. Did the increasing institutionalization of charity, largely imposed from the outside by bishops, undermine the charitable ethos or provide the structure needed to have this ethos realized?

The Inspiration to Serve

It is difficult to reconstruct the roles that the medieval hospital personnel played, since there are no narrative accounts of life inside these institutions. In Guillaume de Saint-Pathus's account of the miracles associated with the tomb of Saint Louis, he relates that when Jehanne of Serris, who was

---

5. On the constitutional status of English hospitals, see Watson, "Fundatio."

6. Le Grand, ed., *Statuts d'hôtels-Dieu*; Le Grand, "Les maisons-Dieu: Leurs statuts au XIIIe siècle," *Revue des questions historiques* 60 (1896): 95–134.

paralyzed, spent time at the hôtel-Dieu of Paris, the sisters made crutches for her and helped her get out of bed and walk to the altar.[7] The late medieval statutes for the hospital of Saint-Nicolas du Bruille, in Tournai (1460), described the experience of hospital work in rather bleak terms:

> You will be called upon . . . to attend the sick day and night, often to assist them to rise, to tolerate their infirmities, their filth and their vermin, to endure harsh words and answer them gently; you will often have to fast, often confess that you are at fault and be harshly admonished, and you will have to bear this with grace and without rancour and suffer for the love of God. . . . You will have to get up when you want to sleep, rise when you are exhausted and want to rest, work when you long for recreation.[8]

The author of these statutes made no attempt to gloss over the self-sacrifice involved in working at a hospital. Rather, the statutes sought to communicate what was expected of the hospital personnel. Why would anyone have volunteered for this kind of burdensome work?

One explanation relates to hospitals' employment of women and men who themselves needed help. Guillaume de Saint-Pathus's account of the miracles associated with the tomb of Saint Louis includes the story of a certain swineherd named Moriset, who hailed from Poitiers. When Moriset developed a leg paralysis, he sought help from his stepmother, who, after the death of Moriset's father, had worked as a maidservant in the hospital at Saumur. When Moriset arrived at the hospital, he discovered that his stepmother had herself recently died, but finding his half-brother there, Moriset decided to stay at the hospital and remained there for about three months.[9] Hospitals, in short, could provide much-needed employment to a woman like Moriset's stepmother, who had suddenly become widowed. That Moriset and his half-brother would turn for assistance to a hospital where their mother (or stepmother) worked also illustrates that institutional and familial support were not mutually exclusive. Hospitals could bring together several members of a family in need of assistance or employment.

---

7. Farmer, *Surviving Poverty*, 120–21.

8. Carole Rawcliffe, "Hospital Nurses and Their Work," in *Daily Life in the Late Middle Ages*, ed. Richard Britnell (Stroud, U.K.: Sutton Publishing, 1998), 43.

9. Guillaume de Saint-Pathus, *Les miracles de Saint Louis*, ed. Percival B. Fay (Paris: H. Champion, 1931), 46–47.

Religious piety was another motivation for devoting one's life to working in a hospital, and this seems to have been particularly true for aristocratic and royal women, as illustrated by the examples of Elizabeth of Hungary and Marguerite of Burgundy. As Lynn Courtenay has written, "Following the Gospels and the spirit of the *imitatio Christi*, the true follower of Christ was morally obliged not only to give alms, but also actively to serve the poor. Given this mentality, the rich became (demonstratively, as in the public piety of St. Louis) the servants of the poor. Menial tasks done with love and tenderness toward the afflicted and infirm (such as feeding, cleansing, dressing wounds, washing feet, and so on) became valuable currency in the 'economy of salvation' and part of the ritual of piety associated with hospitals."[10] The documents associated with Saint Elizabeth of Hungary (daughter of King Andrew II of Hungary), who founded and worked in a hospital for the poor at Marburg in Thuringia, demonstrate that some understood hospital work through a devotional lens.[11] These concrete descriptions of Elizabeth's activities in the hospital give a sense of the day-to-day roles of the personnel who worked there. Admittedly, the descriptions of Elizabeth's hospital work in many ways embodied the hagiographical genre of the "servant-saint," particularly her selfless devotion to the sick and poor.[12] One can well imagine how the reputation of "servant-saints," especially those who were known to have personally worked with the sick and poor in hospitals, might have served as role models for hospital workers, particularly for hospital sisters, and may even have inspired some lay women to join a hospital's staff. In addition to Saint Elizabeth, there were female saints from more modest backgrounds, like Ubaldesca da Calcinaia (d. 1206), a lay associate who, at age fourteen, came to Pisa where she begged for alms, lived an ascetic life, consuming only bread and water, and provided assistance to sick nuns in the female hospital of San Giovanni, in Pisa, a hospital affiliated with the Hospitaller Order.[13]

---

10. Lynn T. Courtenay, "The Hospital of Notre Dame des Fontenilles at Tonnerre: Medicine as *Misericordia*," in *The Medieval Hospital and Medical Practice*, ed. Barbara S. Bowers (Aldershot, U.K.: Ashgate, 2007), 104–5.

11. In addition to hagiographical accounts of Elizabeth's life, another valuable source is the witness testimony that was part of canonization inquests that occurred just after her death in 1231. See Ancelet-Hustache, *Gold Tried by Fire; The Life and Afterlife of St. Elizabeth of Hungary: Testimony from Her Canonization Hearings*, trans. Kenneth Baxter Wolf (New York: Oxford University Press, 2010).

12. Michael Goodich, "Ancilla Dei: The Servant as Saint in the Late Middle Ages," in *Women of the Medieval World: Essays in Honor of John H. Mundy*, ed. Suzanne F. Wemple and Julius Kirshner (Oxford: Basil Blackwell, 1985), 119–36.

13. Vauchez, *Sainthood*, 200; Anthony Luttrell and Helen J. Nicholson, "Introduction: A Survey of Hospitaller Women in the Middle Ages," in *Hospitaller Women in the Middle Ages*, ed. Anthony Luttrell and Helen J. Nicholson (Aldershot, U.K.: Ashgate, 2006), 17–18.

The reputations of saints like these set a new standard for what constituted holiness, linking the works of mercy to the apostolic life. These saints not only helped popularize the Christian ideology of charity discussed in chapter 1 but demonstrated that an apostolic life devoted to charity could be well suited to lay women—even members of a royal family.

Indeed, the charitable example of Elizabeth of Hungary, along with the pious and charitable role models among the French nobility of the time, helped inspire Marguerite of Burgundy, who was also from a royal family (she was Queen of Sicily and Jerusalem and hereditary Countess of Tonnerre).[14] After becoming a widow (she had been the wife of Charles of Anjou, the brother of King Louis IX) at the age of thirty-six, Marguerite decided to remain single, and in 1293 she founded the hospital of Notre Dame des Fontenilles on her property in Tonnerre, where she lived out the rest of her life and where she was buried.[15] In the hospital's foundation charter, Marguerite made clear that her donation was motivated both by the biblical injunction to imitate God's mercy and by a desire to earn eternal life, the ultimate "recompense":

> We, Marguerite, by the grace of God, Queen of Jerusalem and of Sicily, countess of Tonnerre make it known . . . that we, considering the word of the Gospel where one reads: "Be merciful always, as your Father is merciful!" And considering the mercy of our Father . . . , in order not to be judged ungrateful or displeasing to God, having compassion for the poor of Jesus Christ, and wishing to obey the Gospel . . . not only because we ought but also because it is within our means and desire to extend corporeal mercy . . . with the aspiration of receiving the recompense promised in the Gospel to all those who are merciful [that is] to receive eternal life, and to avoid the pain of those who are punished and who were not merciful, namely, the eternal fire, found a hospital or "maison-Dieu," and we establish it at Tonnerre in the street of the said place called Fontenilles.[16]

---

14. Courtenay, "Hospital of Notre Dame des Fontenilles," 88.

15. Marguerite also founded both a leprosary and a hospital at Ligny-le-Châtel, twenty kilometers northwest of Tonnerre. See Lynn T. Courtenay, "Les chartes de Marguerite de Bourgogne: Une étude préliminaire," in *Les établissements hospitaliers en France du moyen âge au XIXe siècle: Espaces, objets et populations*, ed. Sylvie Le Clech-Charton (Dijon: Éditions Universitaires de Dijon, 2010), 41; Sylvie Le Clech-Charton, *L'hôtel-Dieu de Tonnerre: Métamorphose d'un patrimoine hospitalier, XIIIe–XXe siècle* (Langres, France: Éditions Dominique Guéniot, 2012), 21.

16. Courtenay, "Hospital of Notre Dame des Fontenilles," 84. For the full text of this foundation charter, see Ambroise Challe, *Histoire du comté de Tonnerre* (Auxerre, France: Imprimerie de Gustave Perriquet, 1875), 203–20.

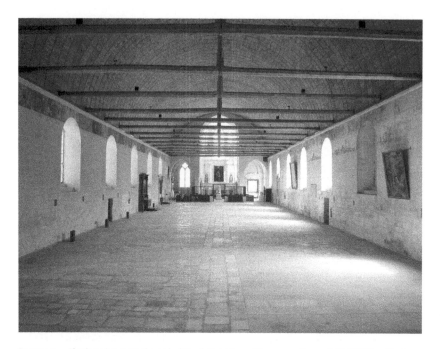

FIGURE 5. The interior central ward of the hôtel-Dieu of Tonnerre. NemesisIII / Wikimedia Commons / CC BY-SA 3.0.

As Lynn Courtenay has observed, what made Marguerite different from most other female patrons of religious houses was "her long-term physical participation in the works of mercy."[17] To ensure that she was involved in the day-to-day caring for the "poor of Christ" herself, Marguerite had the hospital ward connected by stairs and an outside corridor to the castle where she lived. She continued to live as a secular countess in a conventional aristocratic household even while assisting with the hospital's care of the poor and sick.[18] Overseeing the hospital were a master, four chaplains, four choirboys (who

---

17. Lynn T. Courtenay, "Seigneurie et charité: L'exercise du patronage de Marguerite de Bourgogne, comtesse de Tonnerre," in *Les établissements hospitaliers en France du moyen âge au XIXe siècle: Espaces, objets et populations*, ed. Sylvie Le Clech-Charton (Dijon: Éditions Universitaires de Dijon, 2010), 21.

18. Marguerite was not the only royal or aristocratic woman to establish a hospital within her own residence. She may have been emulating Countess Jeanne of Flanders, who in 1232 created a hospital within her residence in Lille, later known as the Hospice Comtesse. Jeanne's sister, Marguerite, who succeeded her as countess of Flanders, also went on to found a hospital, this one within the comital palace in Seclin. See Grant, "Royal and Aristocratic Hospital Patronage," 109.

were to receive instruction in grammar and music at the hospital), a *magistra*, and between twelve and twenty sisters.[19]

The hospital ward, which, with the adjoining chapel, was one hundred meters long, had forty alcoves for beds, and was able to hold up to eighty poor and sick guests, making it an unusually large hospital. Above the entrance portal to the hospital was a sculpted representation of Christ performing a blessing, welcoming those who entered the hospital. Inside the narthex porch stood a sculpted depiction of the Last Judgment, reminding those who worked in the hospital that performing the works of mercy might save them from eternal punishment. There were four altars in the hospital chapel, with the central one dedicated to the Virgin Mary and the other three dedicated to John the Baptist, Mary Magdalene, and Marguerite's near contemporary, Elizabeth of Hungary.[20] The hospital's decorated glazing and painted walls also contained secular imagery and symbols of aristocratic patronage, an indication of the way that Marguerite's vision of a hospital embodied both lordship and religious charity.[21]

Several model sermons from northern France that were directed at hospital audiences illustrate how preachers and reformers sought to reaffirm the importance of hospital work and inspire those working in hospitals to perform the works of mercy with piety and compassion. Preaching was a common occurrence in hospitals not only by members of a hospital's own religious community but also by outside visitors, and it represented an important opportunity for moral and religious edification. The sermons a hospital's personnel would have heard illustrate how preachers sought to exhort, commend, comfort, and correct these workers. Sermons thus provide a window into the particular moral and religious environment of these houses of mercy, showing the ways that the themes of a sermon both shaped and were shaped by the particular social context of the preaching.[22] Some of the northern French "ad status" sermon collections—containing sermons addressed to particular types of audiences—include sermons directed to hospital workers. These sermons may well have served as material (or "talking points") for sermons that were preached in Champagne's hospitals during the thirteenth century.

---

19. Courtenay, "Hospital of Notre Dame des Fontenilles," 88–89.

20. Courtenay, "Hospital of Notre Dame des Fontenilles," 84.

21. Courtenay, "Seigneurie et charité," 29.

22. See Adam J. Davis, "Preaching in Thirteenth-Century Hospitals," *Journal of Ecclesiastical History* 36, no. 1 (March, 2010): 72–89; Alexander Murray, "Piety and Impiety in Thirteenth-Century Italy," *Studies in Church History* 8 (1972): 83–106.

One of the central messages of these sermons was the penitential power of works of mercy, which may suggest both why some women and men devoted their lives to working in hospitals and why these institutions were such popular objects of benefaction. Surely one way for an outside preacher to win the favor of a community of hospital workers was to persuade them that he appreciated the difficulties of their daily lives. In an *ad status* sermon directed at those working in hospitals for the sick and poor, the French Dominican, Humbert of Romans, reassured his listeners that of all the works done in the service of the Creator, the works of mercy surpassed them all, and the greatest work of mercy was that of helping the sick poor in hospitals. In a passage that is noteworthy for its scholastic divisions—despite being intended for a popular audience—Humbert enumerated the heavy demands and sacrifices that nursing entailed:

> Nurses of poor patients do works of mercy through the sense of touch, when the patient is lifted, or put down, or taken out to the lavoratory, or brought what he needs, or has his bedclothes taken off, or put on, and when he is dressed and undressed, and so on. They do it through the sense of sight by comforting him with compassionate looks. Again, they show mercy through the sense of hearing by patiently putting up with their charges' impatient remarks, and the groans at night which stop people sleeping. And they show it through taste, too, when the nurse misses a meal, as happens sometimes, to look after a patient. . . . Thus nurses show mercy through all five senses.[23]

Humbert here was seeking to convey to the hospital brothers and sisters what was expected of them and that he fully grasped the burdens that were inherent in their job.

Preachers may have felt a need to reassure hospital workers of the value of their work so that they did not get discouraged by those who spoke ill of them. This seems to have been the case in a sermon that the secular master Gérard of Reims preached at the hôtel-Dieu in Paris.[24] In discussing the ways that "denigrators" seek to negate all that is good, Gérard cited the example of a denigrator who cynically interprets charitable activity (giving alms, feeding a poor person, lifting or putting him or her to bed) merely as an

---

23. The translation is from Alexander Murray, "Religion Among the Poor in Thirteenth-Century France: The Testimony of Humbert de Romans," *Traditio* 30 (1974): 297; Humbert, "De eruditione praedicatorum," 1.2.40, in *Maxima bibliotheca veterum patrum*, ed. de la Bigne (Lyons, 1677), 25:476.

24. See Bériou, *L'avènement*, 2:428–31.

attempt to win praise. By invoking this particular example, Gérard may have been trying to combat a kind of cynicism that some hospital workers had encountered or likely would encounter. At the Council of Paris in 1213 and the Council of Rouen in 1214, there had been criticism of the lay men and women, including married couples, who entered hospitals and leper houses under the pretext of religion so as to escape the power of secular lords and exploit the charitable resources of these institutions.[25] It was in the context of these kinds of criticisms that Gérard sought to bolster the spirits of his listeners.

In addition to linking works of mercy to God, preachers also used various analogies to equate God/Christ with both the charitable hospital worker and the poor or sick hospital resident. By representing the poor and sick in the image of Jesus, preachers sought to galvanize hospital workers to help the less fortunate. As we saw in chapter 1, by the thirteenth century it was increasingly common in devotional art, literature, and sermons to emphasize the humanity and suffering of Jesus and to associate him with the beggar and leper.[26] Preachers told hospital workers that they could help Jesus and draw spiritually closer to him by helping the *pauperes Christi*. As Guillaume de Chartres put it in a sermon in Paris, "We ought to receive Christ in our arms through good works, especially through works of mercy, by leading them [the poor] to our house and serving and warming them. Then may we dwell near the same Christ, when we support the poor with our arms."[27] Humbert of Romans sought to dramatize the reciprocal relationship linking God, those who worked in hospitals, and the sick and poor they served: "the Lord will restore those who restore His sick in His name."[28] As another thirteenth-century preacher put it, just as a king must pay his soldiers in order to win battles, so too must the ordinary Christian help the poor so as to be able to overcome the flesh, the world, and the devil. "The poor," he proclaimed, "are our soldiers."[29] Thus, a work of mercy might bestow as much benefit on the one performing the work as the recipient of the mercy. This notion was dramatized by the *vita* of Hugh of Lincoln, written by Adam of Eynsham, which contrasted Saint Martin, who had allegedly healed lepers by kissing them, with Hugh, who had reportedly been healed of his own sickness of

25. Mansi, ed., *Sacrorum conciliorum*, vol. 22, col. 835–36, 913.

26. On the notion of *Christus quasi leprosus*, see Rawcliffe, *Leprosy*; Farmer, "Leper in the Master Bedroom."

27. Bériou, *L'avènement*, 339n176.

28. Humbert, "De eruditione," 476.

29. Bériou, *L'avènement*, 339n178.

spirit by kissing lepers. A fundamental principle of the economy of salvation, in other words, was that the act of doing works of mercy could be spiritually curative and salvific for the person performing the charitable service.[30]

The Franciscan Guibert de Tournai, who drew heavily on the ideas of Jacques de Vitry, made mercy the central theme of his *ad status* sermons directed "to servants and hospitallers."[31] In the *thema* of his first sermon to hospital workers, Guibert quoted Micah 6:8 to assure his listeners that by doing works of mercy they were fulfilling God's expectations: "I will show you what is good and what the Lord requires from you, especially to do justice and to love mercy and to walk solicitous with your God."[32] In his discussion of mercy, Guibert seemed especially interested in exploring the theme of dependency and love, and he drew a parallel between the dependency of humans on God and the dependency of the sick poor on the brothers and sisters of a hospital. Guibert told the hospital workers that by helping their neighbor—the sick poor—they were helping God. But Guibert then went further, stressing the importance of motivation and intention in a charitable act. Above all, the Franciscan insisted that works of mercy be done out of love, and that this love of one's neighbor grow out of God's love for us: "Because works of mercy are worth little unless love of neighbor is established in the conscience, let him therefore take the form of Him who loves us, and from His love, the works will pay us mercy."[33] Guibert then drew on the metaphor from Proverbs 19:17 discussed in chapter 1 in which charity is described as a loan to God. Here, Guibert, specifically applied this metaphor to the works of mercy performed by hospital workers and quoted one of Saint Augustine's sermons in which Augustine had imagined Jesus speaking: "You had me as a lender; make me a debtor so that I may have you as a lender."[34] Performing works of mercy was one form of lending that a Franciscan like Guibert could unhesitatingly embrace, and he exhorted his

---

30. *Magna vita sancti Hugonis: The Life of St Hugh of Lincoln* [by Adam of Eynsham], ed. D. L. Douie and D. H. Farmer (2nd impression, 2 vols., Oxford, 1985). See also Catherine Peyroux, "The Leper's Kiss," in *Monks and Nuns, Saints and Outcasts: Religion in Medieval Society: Essays in Honor of Lester K. Little*, ed. Sharon Farmer and Barbara H. Rosenwein (Ithaca: Cornell University Press, 2000), 172–88; Rawcliffe, *Leprosy*, 144–45.

31. Paris, BnF MS lat. 15941, f. 273v–273r; 275r–277r; 277r–278v.

32. Paris, BnF MS lat. 15941, f. 273v.

33. Paris, BnF MS lat. 15941, f. 276r: "Quia parum valent opera misericordie nisi dilectio proximi solidetur in mente, conformetur igitur ei qui nos diligit et ex dilectione sua nobis misericordiam impendent."

34. Paris, BnF MS lat. 15941, f. 274v: "Augustinus in parabola domini, 'habuisti me largitorem, fac me debitorem ut habeam te feneratorem." See Augustine, Sermon 123.5.5, in *Patrologia Latina*, vol. 38, 686.

listeners to be lenders to God by caring for the *pauperes Christi*. By building up credit with God before their death, hospital workers, just like hospital donors, might hope to shorten the time they spent in Purgatory.

In one of his *ad status* sermons directed to the hospital personnel, perhaps based on the kinds of sermons that he had already preached in hospitals in various parts of Europe and the Near East, Jacques de Vitry praised the *hospitalarios* for being living examples of humility and charity, and he then told them that in helping the poor and sick, they were "refreshing Christ in his members every day, choosing to be abject in the house of the Lord [*domo domini*], that is, in a hospital."[35] "Spiritually," he told the hospital workers, "it is said that you are the mother of Christ for whom you feed and nourish Christ in his members."[36] Here Jacques was playing with the idea of hospital workers being maternal, like Jesus' mother, in nourishing the body of Christ through his "members," the sick poor. By "refreshing Christ in his members," it was believed that hospital workers nourished the fullness of Christ's body both in head (Christ) and members (Church). The *thema* for this sermon was from Psalms 41:1, "Blessed is the one who considers the destitute and the poor. On the day of trouble the Lord will deliver him."[37] Other biblical verses were cited, such as Matthew 25:40, a popular verse in sermons dealing with works of mercy: "Whenever you have done this for the least of my brethren, you have done it to me." The intended lesson was that in showing charity to a neighbor, one was in fact doing charity to God. If hospital workers were persuaded that those they cared for were literally stand-ins for Christ, they might be more likely to treat hospital guests like their lords, as some hospital statutes enjoined them to do.

If this was not enough of a motivation, though, Jacques de Vitry went on to suggest that the more the hospital workers suffered and sacrificed in their works of mercy, the more they would please God and earn salvation. As the lives of the saints demonstrated, the works of mercy represented a powerful form of self-mortification and were considered a central part of the penitential system. The most heroic works of mercy were those that were most revolting and involved the greatest sacrifice, such as the kissing of lepers. Moreover, by enduring the stench of hospitals, the brothers and sisters would obviate the need to experience the far worse stench of Hell: "Indeed, it is useful to sustain a moderate stench so that you will be strong enough to

---

35. Bird, "Texts on Hospitals," 115.
36. Bird, "Texts on Hospitals," 115.
37. Bird, "Texts on Hospitals," 113.

avoid the stench of hell."[38] In his *Historia occidentalis*, which Jacques de Vitry wrote only a few years after the Fourth Lateran Council of 1215, he sought to lay out his vision for the implementation of the new religious and moral reforms.[39] As part of this vision of reform, he singled out hospital work, when done well, as a "holy martyrdom":

> The more abject they are in the Lord's house [*domus Dei*] upon the way, the more exalted position they will attain in their [eternal] homeland. Because they frequently endure so many of the sick's filthinesses and the nearly intolerable assault of [various] stenches, inflicting injury upon themselves for Christ's sake, I believe that no other kind of penance is comparable to this holy martyrdom, precious in God's sight. The Lord will transform the odors of these squalors, which they use like manure to fertilize their minds for bearing fruit, into precious stones and instead of a stench there will be a sweet fragrance [in heaven].[40]

The correlation that Jacques drew between the misery of hospital work and the heavenly reward that would follow was a popular theme in hospital sermons. On the eve of Pentecost, 1273, in the hôtel-Dieu of Paris, the Franciscan Simon the Norman reassured his listeners that on Judgment Day, the ultimate reward would be bestowed on those who had endured many tribulations "and done works of mercy toward the indigent and the sick just as is done in this house" (*sicut sit in domo ista*).[41]

As we have seen, sermons and saints' lives articulated how the spiritual ideal of charitable service figured in the economy of salvation. Let us now move from this spiritual ideal to the specific realities of those who made up the medieval hospital's personnel. Sketching a taxonomy of the medieval hospital's diverse membership will help us better understand the different roles these hospital members played and why they joined a caritative religious community in the first place.

---

38. Bird, "Texts on Hospitals," 119.

39. On the relationship between Jacques's sermons and his *Historia*, see Jessalynn Bird, "The Religious's Role in a Post–Fourth Lateran World: Jacques de Vitry's *Sermones ad status* and *Historia occidentalis*," in *Medieval Monastic Preaching*, ed. Carolyn Muessig (Leiden: Brill, 1998): 209–29.

40. Bird, "Texts on Hospitals," 110: The translation here is Bird's.

41. Bériou, *L'avènement*, 249.

Hospital Personnel: Chaplains

The capitular reform movement, which sought to reform and regularize chapters of canons, injected the hospital movement with additional energy by providing hospitals with regular canons who were committed to pastoral and charitable service and a well-defined, yet relatively flexible, structure in the Augustinian Rule. Through the Councils of Reims and Paris in 1213 and Rouen in 1214, Robert of Courson sought to make the church more directly responsible for hospitals.[42] In the eyes of Robert and other French reformers, the laity could express their apostolic enthusiasm by joining a hospital's religious community and performing the works of mercy, but they had to do so under the aegis of the church and within the confines of the Augustinian Rule. The reformer Jacques de Vitry expressed concern about the foundation of new hospitals that were not connected to a chapter or abbey, and that were therefore without a predetermined conventual organization, controlling body, and statutes.[43] What really concerned these reformers were hospitals that were not actively under ecclesiastical control and that made no attempt to follow a religious rule. Despite the best efforts of these reformers, however, there was no clear or consistent principle in canon law that placed all hospitals under the jurisdictional authority of bishops. While the Fourth Lateran Council took up many of Robert of Courson's conciliar decrees from Paris and Rouen, it ignored the decrees dealing with hospitals. During the thirteenth century, charitable institutions in northern Italy, the Low Countries, and the German Empire were increasingly municipalized, such that, even within episcopal cities, hospitals were frequently under the

---

42. The discussion that follows is informed by Sethina Watson's astute analysis of Robert of Courson's legatine councils and a network of northern reformers who articulated a new vision for how hospitals should be regulated. Watson convincingly argues that one important influence for this vision of a new form of religious life inside hospitals was the early beguine movement. Courson's hospital decree in his legatine councils sought to impose a religious rule on hospitals, with residents required to take vows and live a common life. Yet as Watson demonstrates, these regional reforms failed to be adopted as canon law or church policy more broadly, although their reform efforts influenced the organization of some hospitals. See Watson, *On Hospitals*, 13–14, 18–19, 37–39, 261–94, 319–20 (for the text and translation of Courson's hospital decree).

43. De Spiegeler, *Les hôpitaux et l'assistance à Liège*, 147; Bonenfant-Feytmans, "Les organisations hospitalières," 17–45; Bird, "Medicine for Body and Soul." As we have observed, even when a hospital was "attached" to a chapter of some kind, the hospital often exercised significant autonomy. Some cathedral hospitals, such as those at Amiens, Beauvais, and Noyon, were even located in a different neighborhood from the cathedral. See Montaubin, "Le déménagement," 69–70.

jurisdiction of the cities, not the bishops.[44] In that sense, the episcopal and reformist context of northern France was different from much of Europe in placing limits on the laicization of charity.

A hospital's *magister* was often a priest in addition to being a brother, and he oversaw both the hospital's spiritual and temporal affairs, although in some hospitals, like at Amiens, it was not the *magister* but rather a "provisor" or "procurator exteriorum," who was charged with managing the hospital's finances and external relations.[45] In hospitals where the Augustinian Rule was observed, Augustinian canons often served as the arbiters of the Rule's precepts, ensuring that the lay brothers and sisters adhered to its prescriptions. In addition to serving as hospital administrators, clerics above all played a vital role in overseeing the liturgical life. As will be discussed in greater depth in the next chapter, sacramental medicine was at the heart of a hospital's caretaking mission, and there was therefore a fundamental need for priests to celebrate Mass, recite the canonical hours, hear confession, preach, anoint the sick, and perform other pastoral services for the sick poor and the hospital's other personnel. In this sense, clerics were understood as being just as much the caretakers of a hospital's sick poor as the lay sisters and brothers who tended to be more involved with providing for the physical needs of the sick and poor. The liturgical life inside hospitals was also critical to the institutions' donors, who expected that prayers and masses were regularly said for them and their ancestors. In addition, it is clear that some hospitals were offering parishioners outside their walls a range of pastoral services—as an example, the master of the hospital of Saint-Nicolas also performed the weddings of artisans in Troyes—and this kind of pastoral care could be perceived as threatening to local churches and their clergy.[46] From 1245 to 1276, for example, the hospital of Saint-Nicolas in Troyes found itself in a protracted conflict with the curate of Saint-Nizier, who accused the hospital of "stealing" his parishioners and usurping parish rights and revenues. Ultimately Saint-Nicolas had to agree to stop burying parishioners of Saint-Nizier in its cemetery.[47] From the time that a chapel was endowed by a knight in 1233 in the hospital of Jonchery-sur-Vesle, just west of Reims, it was agreed that all of the residents of this hospital would be subject to the curate of the town and that the hospital's chaplain, who was required to live outside the hospital, would not begin the celebration of the Mass before

---

44. De Spiegeler, *Les hôpitaux et l'assistance*, 124.
45. Montaubin, "Le déménagement," 57.
46. Gesret, "Un hôpital au moyen âge," 398.
47. AD: Aube, 43H4, layette 35, no.1.

the curate of the parish reached a certain section of the Mass.[48] In addition to the pastoral services being provided within hospitals, the clerics of these hospitals were also providing services to remote communities. According to a seventeenth-century source, the wealthy and powerful lord of Mortery ran into conflict with the curate of Grisy-sur-Seine when the lord appointed one of the clerics from the hospital of Provins to serve the new chapel of Notre-Dame de Grisy, which he had arranged to build.[49]

As we have seen, not all canons or clerics were considered brothers, nor were all hospital brothers clerics (the term *lay brother* marked a brother as non-clerical). Some clerics living in hospitals were carrying out roles that were not religious in nature. At the hospital of Saint-Nicolas in Troyes, a certain hospital brother who was also a priest was charged with overseeing the production of wine and the management of the hospital's lands that were under tenure.[50] While some hospital clerics resided within the hospital, others did not and might even be salaried. A chaplain for the hospital of Laon who lived outside the hospital bequeathed significant property to the hospital.[51] Account books for the hospital of Saint-Nicolas in Troyes list the total expenses for salaried chaplains. The account book for 1300–01 also indicates that there was a dormitory specifically for priests, who slept in a separate space from the brethren.[52] Visitation records from fourteenth-century hospitals in the diocese of Paris indicate that it was common for those who joined a hospital as a lower-level cleric to be promoted to the priesthood during their time at the hospital.[53] In this way, hospitals could serve as a training ground for priests.

Hospitals could also provide much-needed social security to clerics. Elderly, infirm, or disabled clerics were at times on the receiving end of care from hospitals, and yet they might still also provide the hospital with pastoral services. Take the example of Jehan, a priest from Payns, who in 1217 gave the hôtel-Dieu-le-Comte all of his property in houses, lands, and meadows, excluding his brother's house. In exchange, the hospital granted him a lifetime of sustenance ("victum") as well as an annual clothing stipend of 4 *l*. so

---

48. AD: Marne (Reims), 2G454, no. 1 (June, 1233).

49. Verdier, *L'aristocratie*, 112 and note 403.

50. The account books from 1382 and 1389 indicate that the hospital priests and a certain brother, Felix Boutet, carried out these administrative roles with the *magister*. Gesret, "Un hôpital au moyen âge," 181.

51. Saint-Denis, *L'hôtel-Dieu de Laon*, 88.

52. BnF ms lat. 9111, fol. 285v.

53. See, for example, the 1351 visitation record for Gonesse, in Le Grand, ed., "Les maisons-Dieu et les léproseries," 246.

long as he physically lived at the hospital and performed the office of chaplain suitably. If Jehan ended up taking the religious habit, he would receive a lesser clothing stipend of 60 *sous*, and if he were to go on pilgrimage to Jerusalem, the hospital would give him the value of his clothing stipend for three years up front. Most interesting for our purposes, however, is that the hospital made these arrangements, according to the charter, as recompense for an earlier donation of personal property that Jehan made to the hospital when he was sick and presumably being cared for by the hospital.[54] It appears that at some point before becoming a chaplain of this hospital, Jehan may have been one if its sick guests. He then made a donation of some personal property to thank the hospital for its care and made yet another donation of landed property upon becoming one of the hospital's chaplains (being promised room, board, and a clothing stipend), with the possibility that he might still take the religious habit.

Although some hospitals were specifically established to house poor and aged clergy, such as the one established in mid-thirteenth-century Amiens by Bishop Gérard de Concy, even general hospitals often cared for clerics who were in need of assistance, and the employment of such clerics could itself constitute a form of charity.[55] Among the skeletal remains excavated from the chapel of the English hospital of St. Giles by Brompton Bridge, in Brough, were those of a disabled priest who had been buried with a chalice and paten. An analysis of his bones revealed that as a young man he had had an untreated slipped proximal femoral epiphysis, which meant that he could not put weight on his right leg and would have used a crutch over a period of many years. It is unclear whether he served a pastoral and liturgical function at this hospital or was there purely as the recipient of care, but if he worked there, it might well have been because he could not find employment elsewhere due to his disability.[56]

The Magister and Prioress

The hospital's *magister* served as the administrative and spiritual head of the community. In some cases he also seems to have been regarded as a leader in

---

54. AD: Aube 40H1, no. 26; AD: Aube 40H189, No. 165, fol. 33v. The original charter is dated January 1217, while the cartulary copy is dated as January 1207: "Et hoc in recompensationem mobilium eius que ante in elemosinam predicte Domui Dei in infirmitate sua contulerat."

55. Montaubin, "Le déménagement," 76.

56. Roberta Gilchrist, *Medieval Life: Archaeology and the Life Course* (Woodbridge, U.K.: Boydell Press, 2012), 65–66.

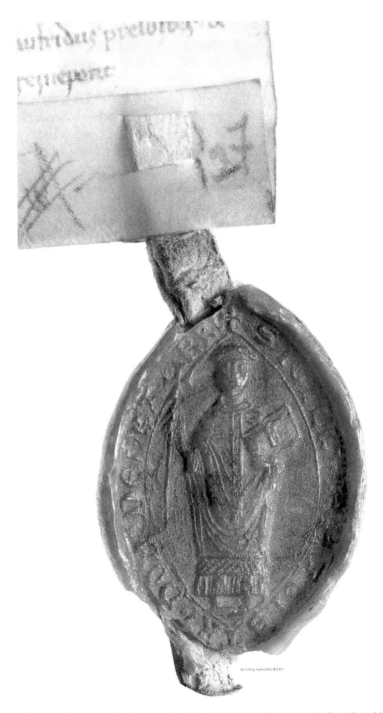

Figure 6. A seal representing Magister G. of the hôtel-Dieu of Bar-sur-Aube (1183). Archives départementales de l'Aube, 3H1183.

the urban religious and political community and was asked to serve as a mediator in various conflicts outside the hospital. *Magistri* also frequently served as the executors of wills. Some of the *magistri* in Champagne's hospitals served very long tenures, and this was in contrast to the *magistri* of the hôtel-Dieu of Laon, who were all cathedral canons and who generally returned to the cathedral chapter after serving as *magister* for only a couple years.[57] From 1185 to 1220, the hospital of Provins was run by a certain Eudes. From 1241 until 1263, the hospital was overseen by Magister Adam. Jean Gaultier served as *magister* for forty-one years, from 1263 until 1304.[58] According to a seventeenth-century source, when Pierre Britaud, the count's viscount, was ruling while the count was on crusade and was faced with the decision of whom to appoint as the *magister* of the hospital of Provins, he turned to Guibert, one of Henri the Liberal's chaplains.[59] At the hôtel-Dieu-le-Comte in Troyes, a certain Hébert is identified as the hospital's master or procurator in 1206, and in 1222, he was still in this position.[60] It is possible that this is the same "Magister Herbertus medicus" who held a prebend at the chapter of Saint-Étienne in 1199 and whose prebend Thibaut III gave to the poor of the hospital. If so, this might suggest that the *magister* was a physician.[61] It was common to spend many years serving as a hospital brother before being elected or appointed as *magister*. Henri Coci, for example, served as a brother at the hospital of Gonesse in 1328 and became *magister* twenty-three years later.[62] Some *magistri* served much shorter tenures. From 1220 to 1228, for example, the hospital at Provins had four different *magistri*, with each serving for only a year or two. Although the foundation charter for the hospital at Tonnerre gave the *magister* enormous responsibility over the temporal and spiritual administration of the hospital, he was actually only required to be in residence for a minimum of six months out of the year, a sign perhaps that the *magistri* were quite often absent.[63] This may have been why at Tonnerre and elsewhere, a female *magistra* was appointed to help oversee the hospital.

Having a prioress or *magistra* present also made it easier to oversee the hospital sisters and the sick poor who were women, given the desire to maintain

57. Saint-Denis, *L'hôtel-Dieu de Laon*, 79–80.
58. Dupraz, List.
59. Verdier, *L'aristocratie*, 150.
60. AD: Aube 40H189, fol. 75v, 82 (cartulary for hôtel-Dieu-le-Comte).
61. Guignard, ed., *Les anciens statuts*, xvii.
62. Le Grand, ed., "Les maisons-Dieu et les léproseries," 246.
63. Challe, *Histoire du comté de Tonnerre*, 219.

gender separation as much as possible.[64] The hospital at Provins had a sister who served as prioress, and the hospital's obituary singled out three prioresses, Sisters Emelina de Vernon, Praxedis, and Cecilia "for having worked for a long time in the service of the poor."[65] Sister Emelina is mentioned in the cartulary as having donated her sheets, towels, and murra stones to the hospital.[66] As was also true for Champagne's hospitals, the *magistra* of the hospital at Laon rarely appears in the sources. When someone endowed a pittance for the poor at the hospital of Laon, however, the prioress was often designated as the one to choose which foods were distributed, consistent with her regular contact with the hospital's poor.[67]

The Brethren

Hospitals varied a great deal in the size and makeup of their personnel. During Archbishop Eudes Rigaud's visitation of the hôtel-Dieu of Saint-Mary Magdalene in Rouen in 1266, for instance, he found eight canons living inside the hospital, eight additional canons living outside the hospital (presumably serving outside churches), twenty-two sisters, three brothers (and others living outside the hospital), and eleven maidservants.[68] The small hospital at Les Andelys, by contrast, had a staff of only three: a prior, a sister, and a maidservant.[69] Like other kinds of monastic houses, hospitals struggled to achieve the right number of workers relative to the hospital's size and financial resources. Hospital statutes limited not only the total number of hospital workers but also the number of priests, brothers, and sisters. Episcopal visitors sought to enforce these rules, since exceeding personnel limits could place a strain on a hospital's resources. The Council of Paris in 1213 had tried to limit the size of a hospital's personnel roster in order to ensure that the staff did not outnumber the sick poor or siphon off the resources intended to help them.[70] The statutes for both the hôtel-Dieu-le-Comte in Troyes and the hospital of Provins stipulated that there should be no more than eight

---

64. Saint-Denis, *L'hôtel-Dieu de Laon*, 84–85.

65. *Obituaires de la province de Sens*, 1:933, 934, 951.

66. Dupraz, no. 426; AD: Seine-et-Marne 11Hdt A12, fol. 124–124v (December 27, 1267).

67. Saint-Denis, *L'hôtel-Dieu de Laon*, 84–85.

68. *The Register of Eudes of Rouen*, trans. Sydney M. Brown, ed. Jeremiah O'Sullivan (New York: Columbia University Press, 1964), 645. On the hospitals of Normandy, see Neveux, "Naissance," 241–53.

69. *The Register of Eudes of Rouen*, 309.

70. Le Grand, "Les maisons-Dieu, leur régime intérieur," 99.

priests (including the *magister*), ten lay brothers, and ten sisters, but unlike in Provins, where these numbers were increased shortly after the statutes were drawn up, these numbers appear to have remained in force at the Troyen hospital during the later thirteenth century.[71] In 1261, at the hospital of Châlons-en-Champagne, the chapter of Saint-Étienne, which oversaw the hospital, sought to limit the number of *conversi* (that is, brothers and sisters who were converts from the laity) to twenty, and stipulated that they had to be at least twenty-five years old and no older than fifty.[72] A similar attempt was made at containing the size of a hospital's personnel at the hospital at Laon in 1294.[73] The statutes for the hospital at Angers, however, stipulated that the number of brothers or sisters could exceed the maximum of seventeen it had established if the new postulant could offer the hospital sufficient resources.[74] This provision seemed to embody the simony that most hospital statutes claimed to oppose. Bishops and church reformers were concerned that hospitals were losing sight of their core charitable mission of caring for the sick poor and instead turning into retirement homes for the hospital sisters and brothers.[75] Viewed another way, however, by fulfilling the needs of the sisters and brothers, these hospitals were fulfilling a different kind of charitable function, whereby the dispensers of charity were in fact also its beneficiaries, something that often seems to have been happening anyway.

The number of brethren at the hospital of Provins and the hôtel-Dieu-le-Comte in Troyes was quite similar to that of other hospitals in northern France, such as those at Laon, Noyon, and Rouen, although at some hospitals, the number of sisters greatly outnumbered the number of brothers.[76] To be admitted to the hospital community at Laon, men had to be at least twenty-five years old, and women had to be at least thirty, and both needed to be approved by the master, dean, and chapter. However, these age

---

71. In 1266, the master of the hospital of Provins received permission from Count Thibaut, the pope, and the archbishop of Sens for the maximum number of hospitallers to be raised to thirty-eight, with twenty-five sisters, eight lay brothers, four priests (one of whom was the *magister*), and one cleric-brother. AD: Seine-et-Marne 11Hdt/E6 (1266), a charter from the archbishop of Sens, Guillaume de Brosse.

72. Saint-Denis, *L'hôtel-Dieu de Laon*, 89n93.

73. Saint-Denis, *L'hôtel-Dieu de Laon*, 89.

74. Le Grand, ed., *Statuts d'hôtels-Dieu*, art. 17, p. 107.

75. Le Grand, "Les maisons-Dieu, leur régime intérieur," 102.

76. Saint-Denis, *L'hôtel-Dieu de Laon*, 90. The thirteenth-century *Register* of Archbishop Eudes Rigaud of Rouen also shows that the number of hospital personnel could fluctuate quite a bit over a short period of time, something that the archbishop did not like. When he visited the hospital of Pontoise in 1256, he found only five sisters. At his visitation in 1266, the number of sisters had tripled, with thirteen sisters and two more about to be veiled. See *The Register of Eudes*, 283, 654.

requirements were not always followed.[77] A statute for the hospital at Angers prohibited receiving as sisters any woman who was too young or too pretty out of fear that she would serve as a distraction.[78] At Troyes and Provins, all of the hospital brethren professed the three vows of poverty, chastity, and obedience. Indeed, the prologue to the statutes for the hôtel-Dieu-le-Comte at Troyes asserted that one could only be a true hospital brother or sister, living in a "state of religion," that is, "the perfection of the Holy Gospel," by observing all three vows.[79] According to the prologue, each vow was a metaphor for a part of "the house," that is the hospital—with obedience being the foundation, poverty being the walls, and chastity being the ceiling—and if any one of the three vows was not followed, the "meson de religion" would fall apart.[80] Shortly before the Fourth Lateran Council in 1215, church councils in Reims, Paris and Rouen sought to impose greater religious discipline on hospital communities, insisting that the brethren wear the religious habit, take the three vows, and follow the Augustinian Rule. This effort is reflected in the statutes that a number of hospitals, such as those at Troyes and Provins, promulgated in the thirteenth century. The prologue to the statutes for the hospital of Provins and the hôtel-Dieu-le-Comte at Troyes scorned "the many mesons Dieu" that had no religious rules or standards, where "just as people freely come there as they please, so too are they able to depart, believing that they are not obligated to take vows or oaths."[81] Imposing the rules of the religious life was likely much more difficult at tiny, rural hospitals, which might offer only a couple of beds. The existing sources for Champagne contain scattered references to many small, rural hospitals in places like le Chêne, Biesme, Rosnay, Mery, and Hans, but apart from knowing of their existence, we know virtually nothing about the people who lived and worked there. Many of these hospitals did not have statutes and the sisters and brothers might have carried the titles of sisters and brothers and even worn the habit, but they generally took no formal religious vows and were sometimes even married.[82] The most that episcopal authorities could demand of these lay hospital workers was that they practice charity and live in an honest and orderly way.

---

77. A document from 1282 makes reference to "fratres sorores et conversi existentes minori aetate." See Saint-Denis, *L'hôtel-Dieu de Laon*, 90–91.

78. Le Grand, ed., *Statuts d'hôtels-Dieu*, art. 38, p. 29.

79. Le Grand, ed., *Statuts d'hôtels-Dieu*, 103.

80. Le Grand, ed., *Statuts d'hôtels-Dieu*, 103–4.

81. Le Grand, ed., *Statuts d'hôtels-Dieu*, 103.

82. Le Grand, "Les maisons-Dieu, leur régime intérieur," 109.

Some of the brethren at Troyes and Provins were clerics, while others were referred to as "lay brothers" to distinguish them from clerical brothers. A brief note about the term *conversi*, a term whose meaning evolved over the course of the twelfth and thirteenth centuries and which could mean different things in different contexts. In earlier centuries, *conversi* denoted those who entered a monastery later in life. Similar to the later twelfth-century Cisterican context, where "conversi" sometimes referred to humble peasants considered second-class citizens compared to full-fledged monks and nuns, in some French and Italian hospitals *conversi* was another term for the *donati*, who generally did not take vows and in some cases even lived outside the hospital.[83] At the hôtel-Dieu of Laon, the term *conversus* was used to refer to those brothers who had not yet taken vows or adopted the religious habit, that is, those in the novitiate who were on their way to becoming fully professed brethren.[84] In many northern French hospitals, however, including at Provins, *conversi* seems to have simply been a synonym for the sisters and those brothers who were not clerics. In the Provins cartulary, the few times that the term appears, it is in the context of a relative making a donation to a *soror conversa*, perhaps because the donation was a reminder of the sister's blood ties and her relatively recent conversion to the religious life.[85] While many hospital records from northern France stressed the brothers' lay status, they did so not to suggest that the brothers did not lead religious lives, which they frequently did, but to differentiate them from those who had received holy orders (the "fratri sacerdotes" and "clerici" who were also considered brethren).[86]

Many statutes seem to have conceived of hospital sisters as the principal caretakers of the sick and poor, saying, as the statutes for the hôtel-Dieu-le-Comte put it, that the sisters ought to be "humble and suitable for filling the needs of the house and for serving the poor—God's messengers—with great diligence and in complete nobility."[87] According to the statutes, during the day the sick were to be visited devotedly by sisters, and at night two sisters

---

83. Constance H. Berman, "Distinguishing between the Humble Peasant Lay Brother and Sister, and the Converted Knight in Medieval Southern France," in *Religious and Laity in Western Europe, 1000–1400: Interaction, Negotiation, and Power* (Turnhout, Belgium: Brill, 2006), 263–86.

84. Saint-Denis, *L'hôtel-dieu de Laon, 1150–1300*, 89.

85. For examples of the term in the Provins cartulary, see Dupraz, nos. 104, 164, 290. The term *conversi* was used synonymously for lay brothers in the statutes for the hospital of Provins as well.

86. On the kinds of formulas used in the professing of vows to a hospital's *magister*, see the formula (in French) used at the hospitals of Pontoise and Lille, in Le Grand, ed., *Statuts d'hôtels-Dieu*, 142–43.

87. Le Grand, ed., *Statuts d'hôtels-Dieu*, 102.

or "girls" (presumably servants) were charged with keeping vigil over the poor and ministering to them.[88] According to the foundation charter for the hospital at Tonnerre, the sisters were expected to look after the sick and oversee the washing of the bedding, while the chaplains and choirboys said the canonical hours and Mass at least twice daily.[89] The statutes include no references to the brothers' involvement with the care of the sick poor. Likewise, when the bishop delegate of Paris visited the hospital at Gonesse, he found that the master and brothers oversaw the hospital's properties and its workers in the fields and vineyards, whereas the prioress and the sisters cared for the sick and housed travelers.[90] Interestingly, when the king of France, Louis IX, fed delicacies to the sick poor in the hospital of Vernon, he reportedly first asked the hospital sisters "what was wrong with" the sick poor, wondering "if they could eat meat and other things, and what was good and healthy for their meals."[91] The king clearly assumed that the sisters, not the brothers, would be most knowledgeable about the physical condition of each sick person and what would be an appropriate diet. The obituary for the hospital of Beauvais referred to one sister who had died, Ermentrudis, as "the mother of the poor," perhaps reflective of her special connection with the poor but also clearly tapping into notions of mothers as nurturing to those with needs.[92] In some cases, the hospital sisters' care of the sick required them to leave the hospital. The sisters of the hospital of Saint-Nicolas in Troyes, for example, at times attended to sick canons from the nearby cathedral chapter of Saint-Pierre. Since the hospital was under the jurisdiction of the cathedral, this is not all that surprising. However, it is interesting that sick canons did not move to the hospital but rather were cared for by the sisters in the canons' residences. In his study of the hôtel-Dieu at Laon, Alain Saint-Denis concluded that while the hospital brothers were initially charged with caring for the sick and distributing pittances, by the later thirteenth century they were increasingly occupied by the temporal administration of the hospital, including acting as the executors of wills, working with donors, and managing the hospital's agricultural cultivation.[93] Although the sisters at the hospital of Laon were not cloistered, they do not appear to have been involved in

88. Le Grand, ed., *Statuts d'hôtels-Dieu*, art. 94, 116.
89. Challe, *Histoire du comté de Tonnerre*, 207–8.
90. Le Grand, ed., "Les maisons-Dieu et les léproseries," 241.
91. Rawcliffe, "Hospital Nurses," 57.
92. Leblond, ed., "L'obituaire," 354.
93. Saint-Denis, *L'hôtel-Dieu de Laon*, 97.

the temporal administration of the hospital.[94] Many hospital charters from Champagne mention the *magister* and brothers but make no mention of the sisters even though we know that the hospital sisters outnumbered the brothers. For instance, Philippe Poil-de-Chien sold his *cens* on thirty-seven *arpents* of land to "the master and brothers of the domus Dei of Provins."[95] The absence of any mention of the sisters may reflect the fact that it was the *magister* and the brothers who were viewed as the managers of the hospital's properties.

On the other hand, a donation charter from 1219, from a certain widow, Belina, the wife of the late P. Godet, was clearly directed to the sisters of the hospital of Bar-sur-Aube, this even though there was a *magister* and brothers there as well.[96] While conceding a part of her vineyard and requesting that an anniversary mass be said every year after her death, this widow was thinking of the sisters, not the brothers. Although the masters at the hôtel-Dieu-le-Comte in Troyes and the hospital of Provins were expected to appoint a brother to solicit bequests and oversee the hospital's worldly business, there was also an expectation that the sisters would be involved in the administration of the hospital and its business affairs.[97] The statutes for both of these hospitals reference the sisters and brothers working by the labor of their own hands, with whatever they made becoming the property of the hospital community.[98] Some sisters from the hospital of Provins appear to have been involved in agricultural work. A papal bull from Celestine III, for example, mentions that both brothers and sisters were staying on a hospital grange, where they worked with the hospital's land, vineyards, and livestock.[99] The master was also expected to appoint a suitable sister as prioress to minister to the brothers, sisters, and the sick. The prioress could be sent to the hospital's granges, and in such a case, suitable brothers and sisters would fill in for her in dealing with the hospital's business matters.[100] Moreover, the statutes suggest that the sisters were involved in the administrative and business side of the hospital as well as caring for the sick poor.

---

94. Saint-Denis, *L'hôtel-Dieu de Laon*, 98–99.

95. BM Provins, ms. 85, no. 52.

96. AD Aube HD33/17 (1219). Arbois de Jubainville, *Histoire de Bar-sur-Aube*, 80.

97. Le Grand, ed., *Statuts d'hôtels-Dieu*, art. 97, p. 116.

98. Le Grand, ed., *Statuts d'hôtels-Dieu*, art. 96, p. 116.

99. Dupraz, no. 1; AD: Seine-et-Marne, 11HdtA12, fol. 16. The hospitallers who worked outside the hospital were still part of the hospital community and were expected to follow the rule. Moreover, in 1195 the pope granted the hospital the right to have a chapel built on the grange.

100. Le Grand, ed., *Statuts d'hôtels-Dieu*, art. 41, p. 110.

The hôtel-Dieu-le-Comte in Troyes had separate refectories and dormitories for the brothers and sisters.[101] For those who socialized with members of the opposite sex, the statutes threatened a penance of bread and water every Friday for seven years. Sexual relationships between a hospital brother and sister at Troyes could result in the brother's expulsion and the sister's being deprived of her habit and subject to a lifetime's penance of discipline and fasts.[102] A case from the hospital of Saint-Nicolas of Troyes in 1430, a bit beyond the period covered in this book, shows a hospital brother being found guilty of having a sexual relationship with a woman and placed in one of the hospital's prisons ("carceres dicti hospitalis").[103] An even more dramatic case unfolded in 1354/55 at the hôtel-Dieu in Paris where one of the hospital sisters gave birth to a baby that she reportedly conceived with one of the hospital brothers. The new parents were then accused of murdering their baby. While the fate of the father is not known, the mother spent the next fourteen years in the hospital's prison and was permanently stripped of her veil, although she appears to have stayed at the hospital after her release.[104] When the bishop delegate of Paris conducted hundreds of visitations of hospitals and leprosaries in the mid-fourteenth century, however, keeping a detailed inventory of what he found, he did not record a single instance of a sexual relationship among a hospital's personnel.[105] Even Archbishop Eudes Rigaud of Rouen, who was just as zealous a disciplinarian and meticulous recorder of visitations, found only one instance of fornication among the hospital personnel in Normandy.[106] In short, non-marital sexual relationships involving the personnel of medieval hospitals appear to have been quite rare.

Unlike at some hospitals, where the sisters and brothers held separate weekly chapter meetings, at the hôtel-Dieu-le-Comte and the hospital of Provins the brothers and sisters were permitted to hold their weekly chapter meetings for mutual correction together.[107] While guests were permitted in the hospital with the approval of the *magister*, male guests could only visit

---

101. Le Grand, ed., *Statuts d'hôtels-Dieu*, art. 42, p. 110. Charters differentiate between the refectory of the poor and the refectory of the brethren. A testament from November 1307 refers to a dormitory for the *conversae* ("dormitori conversarum") at Saint-Nicolas of Troyes: AD Aube 43H12, lay. 31, cote A, no. 49.

102. Le Grand, ed., *Statuts d'hôtels-Dieu*, art. 105, p. 117.

103. AD: Aube G1275, fol. 62 (June 30, 1430); Gesret, "Un hôpital au moyen âge," 144.

104. Jéhanno, "Entre le chapitre cathédral," 529.

105. Le Grand, ed., "Les maisons-Dieu et les léproseries."

106. Le Grand, "Les maisons-Dieu, leur régime intérieur," 109; *The Register of Eudes*, 645.

107. This was also the case at hospitals in Paris, Cambrai, and Le Mans. See Le Grand, ed., *Statuts d'hôtels-Dieu*, art. 112–13, p. 118; Le Grand, "Les maisons-Dieu, leur régime intérieur," 115.

with brothers and female guests with sisters. No man was allowed in the women's refectory, an injunction that even the prior could not overrule.[108] The statutes were generally quite lax, however, about visitors, even permitting male relatives and guests—potential donors, for instance—to stay with brothers in the dormitory and female guests to eat with sisters if the need to honor the guest required doing so.[109] And while the statutes sought to regulate outside expeditions by the brothers and sisters, such excursions were permitted if they involved the hôtel-Dieu's business affairs. Given the hospital's extensive properties and seigneurial rights, there would have been a frequent need for members of the community to travel, especially the *magister*. Hence, the statutes sought to regulate the conduct of members of the community when they ventured outside the hospital: they were expected to avoid visiting taverns that were of ill repute; they were not supposed to wander around the city without purpose; and any "open fornication" outside the hospital would result in warning and punishment. If these warnings went unheeded, the brother or sister would be ejected.

The statutes for both the hôtel-Dieu-le-Comte in Troyes and the hospital of Provins were adamant that no hospital brother or sister be permitted to retain any individual property. Even the poor and sick at the hospitals of Troyes and Provins were required to deposit any clothes or belongings upon entering the hospital; their belongings were returned to them when they left.[110] This was in marked contrast to the hospital of Laon, where sisters were permitted to keep property that helped them provide for their needs.[111] At the hospital of Reims, too, it appears that the hospital sisters retained some of their property. A charter from 1221 records a widowed *conversa* from the hospital giving a small annual rent of 2 *s.* to the nuns of Clairmarais.[112] Upon taking vows, the hospital sisters and brothers at the hôtel-Dieu-le-Comte and the hospital at Provins were required to renounce all claims to property, and if a brother or sister was found to have retained some property by placing it in the trust of someone outside the hospital, he or she would be punished; continued failure to renounce all right to property would lead to the brother or sister being stripped of their habit and thrown out of the hospital as an excommunicate. Any hospital brother or sister who died with

---

108. Le Grand, ed., *Statuts d'hôtels-Dieu*, art. 53, p. 111.
109. Le Grand, ed., *Statuts d'hôtels-Dieu*, 113.
110. Le Grand, ed., *Statuts d'hôtels-Dieu*, art. 74, p. 114.
111. Saint-Denis, *L'hôtel-Dieu de Laon*, 99 and note 153.
112. AD Aube 3H3784 (March 1221). The *conversa* was Agnès, widow of Eudes de Marhello.

property would be denied a funeral and burial in the hospital cemetery and, in the words of the statutes, be "thrown out into the countryside like dogs."[113]

Despite this warning, there are a number of cases, particularly at the hospital of Provins, of sisters who had presumably taken vows of voluntary poverty receiving a life annuity. I have only found one instance of this happening at the hôtel-Dieu-le-Comte in Troyes, where, in 1270, the knight Henri de Saint-Benoît made a donation to the hospital conditional upon his daughter, Johanna, a sister in the hospital, being promised a life rent of barley.[114] Yet it seems to have been fairly common for sisters in the hospital of Provins to receive life rents, in direct violation, it would seem, of the statutes' prohibition of the hospital brothers and sisters owning individual property. At Provins, Agnès de Courbouzon gave a lifetime rent of half a *muid* of wheat to her daughter, Marguerite, a *conversa* in the hôtel-Dieu. When Marguerite died, this rent would be transferred to the hospital in mortmain.[115] In 1261, Pétronille de Vieux-Maisons, who came from a well-connected family and was a frequent donor to the same hospital, gave Emanjarde, a sister in the hospital, the use of a life rent of 20 *s.* on some houses. Upon the sister's death, the hospital would be able to collect the rent and use it for a pittance for the poor.[116] It is likely that this is the same Emanjarde (or possibly her daughter) who was the widow of Eudes Poilechien and a neighbor of Pétronille's.[117] In the 1270 testament of Raoul Comtesse, the chamberlain of Count Thibaut, Raoul and his wife Marguerite bequeathed a house to the hospital of Provins so that their anniversaries would be celebrated and 20 *s.* given as pittances to the poor. In addition, they requested that a life annuity of 40 *s.* be given to their daughter, Edelina, a *conversa*, for her "necessities" in the hospital.[118] Although the statutes for the hospital of Provins, like those for Troyes, explicitly prohibited the sisters and brothers from having personal property, in fact the hospital and its charitable mission profited from donations to individual members of the hospital staff, and this may help explain why in 1283 Pope Martin IV authorized the hospital sisters and brethren to receive testamentary bequests.[119]

---

113. Le Grand, ed., *Statuts d'hôtels-Dieu*, art. 100, pp. 116–17.

114. AD: Aube 40H1, no. 63 (April 1270).

115. Dupraz, no. 104; AD: Seine-et-Marne, 11HdtA12, fol. 32–32v.

116. Dupraz, no. 192; AD: Seine-et-Marne, 11HdtA12, fol. 57v.

117. Verdier, *L'aristocratie*, 48–49. Both notable Provinois families, the Vieux-Maisons and the Poilechien, had residences in the Jewry and may well have been involved in money and exchange.

118. Jean Mesqui, *Provins: La fortification d'une ville au moyen âge* (Geneva: Droze, 1979), 199–200. On Raoul Comtesse and other members of the family, see Verdier, *L'aristocratie*, 64–65.

119. AD: Seine-et-Marne, 11HdtA4.

As Paul Bertrand has shown in his study of the economic structures of mendicant convents, even individual mendicant friars, who were among the strictest adherents of the vow of voluntary poverty, accepted life pensions as gifts, particularly when a legal loophole rendered the gift a licit transaction. For instance, a donor might confer the lifetime use of a rent (as opposed to ownership of the rent) on an individual friar (who often was a family member), with the ownership of the rent only being transferred from the donor to the friar's convent upon the friar's death (a *donatio post obitum*).[120] Those giving pensions to individual friars also used hospitals as intermediaries to hold the donated pension and then distribute it, almost as a form of charity, to the individual friar.[121] The central point is that just as friars found ways to justify the individual friar's receiving a pension, the brothers and sisters working inside Champagne's hospitals did much the same thing.

Champagne's hospitals received significant entry gifts from those wishing to join the hospital community as brethren. Hugues, the curate of Colombé-le-Sec, made a donation to the hôtel-Dieu of Bar-sur-Aube (which owned properties in his parish) in 1170 while he was becoming a brother at the hospital.[122] A charter from 1211 shows that during the period when Agnès Falconaria, a widow, was in the process of adopting the religious habit, she agreed, with her son's consent, to give a vineyard in the Val de Tors to "the convent of the conversae sisters" of the hospital of Bar-sur-Aube.[123] Agnès would not actually surrender the vineyard until her death or until she left the secular world by taking the religious habit, which she was in the process of doing, almost certainly at the hospital itself.[124] In other words, the vineyard was Agnès's "entry gift," and in that sense was very much part of an agreed-upon exchange. Charters from 1228 and 1232 that detail this same hospital's granting the lifetime use of several other vineyards reveal that one of the vineyards belonged to a certain "brother Bernard" and another to a certain "brother Berangerius" who had died.[125] A conflict in 1254 between the hôtel-Dieu-le-Comte and a priest, Guillaume de Hancourt, reveals that some disputed land in Dronay had been given to the hospital by Guibert, a

---

120. Bertrand, *Commerce*, 250–51, 336–37.

121. Bertrand, *Commerce*, 215–16, 472.

122. Arbois de Jubainville, *Histoire de Bar-sur-Aube*, 77.

123. Agnès's late husband, Ansericus, had assigned an annual wine rent (from the same vineyard) to the hospital while he was approaching death.

124. AD Aube HD 33/78, no. 16.

125. AD Aube HD 33/87 (two separate charters, dated 1228 and November 1232).

priest and brother of the hospital.[126] Hospitals were often tempted to take on additional personnel as a way of augmenting revenues from entry gifts. Anyone who wished to take the religious habit at the hospital at Laon, for example, was expected to make a donation in accordance with his or her means.[127] In contrast, the statutes for the hospital at Angers made clear that in recruiting personnel, no financial demands were to be made of postulants and no attention was to be paid to the extent of their wealth.[128]

The charters that record entry gifts at times provide a valuable glimpse into what motivated some people to join a hospital community. When the shoemaker Colet Neele made a donation to Saint-Nicolas of Troyes in 1346, he did so "in order that the master, brothers, and sisters would receive the same Colet in their community, and as a brother, and so that as long as he lived in the same place, they would minister to him and give him sustenance just as they did to their others."[129] The language of the charter makes it sound more as though Colet was being admitted as one of the sick or poor in need of care, rather than as a brother who would serve as a caregiver. While Colet may have decided to become a hospital brother in part out of a desire to lead a religious life and help the *pauperes Christi*, he was clearly also concerned about obtaining food and care during his later years of life. For Colet and many others, joining a hospital community offered a form of social security, just as it did for the sick and poor, but with a much greater sense of permanence. Moreover, the statutes for the hôtel-Dieu-le-Comte promised that if a brother became senile, infirm, or sick, he would be provided for in the infirmary specifically designed for the hospital personnel. The statutes even included a provision for any brother who contracted leprosy. Although the hospital did not admit lepers, it would still ensure that its own leprous member would be kindly ministered to at some location in Troyes, outside the hospital.[130]

---

126. AD Aube 40H1, no. 53.

127. Saint-Denis, *L'hôtel-Dieu de Laon*, 91. When Helwide d'Avin, who belonged to an important and wealthy bourgeois family in Laon, joined the hospital community, she made a donation to the hospital but also stipulated that at her death, part of her estate should go to the Cistercian abbey of Sauvoir-sous-Laon. The abbess, however, argued that Helwide's entry into the hospital was itself a kind of quasi-death and that the abbey could collect its portion of Helwide's bequest right away, a point that the hospital was quick to contest.

128. Le Grand, ed., *Statuts d'hôtels-Dieu*, art. 18, p. 26.

129. AD Aube 43H12, layette 31, cote A, no. 57 (1346): "ut ipsi magister, fratres et sorores, eundem Coletum in suum consocium recipiant, et in fratrem, et ut eidem, quamdiu vixerit, sicut uni eorum, victui tribuant et ministrent."

130. Le Grand, ed., *Statuts d'hôtels-Dieu*, art. 116, pp. 118–19.

Although it is difficult to learn much about the social background of the hospital brethren, one can occasionally acquire hints, and the picture that emerges is of hospital brothers and sisters made up of everyone from former serfs, to townspeople, to members of noble and aristocratic families. During the twelfth and thirteenth centuries, it was not uncommon for aristocrats to supply various kinds of religious houses with their daughters as well as with adult *conversi*.[131] Indeed, the majority of monks at the abbey of Clairvaux came from aristocratic backgrounds, and the prospect of recruiting monks or nuns from wealthy families along with the substantial gifts that they might bring led many monasteries to accept larger and larger numbers of professed religious, a frequent point of criticism by church authorities. In 1312 the bishop of Cambrai sent a letter to the sisters of the hôtel-Dieu Saint-Jean, who were apparently terrified to reject the entreaties by many nobles and powerful people that the hospital accept their "unsuited" and "useless" girls as sisters. According to the bishop, it was vital that the hospital have a strictly enforced limit on the number of sisters so that it could more easily turn away such requests even from those with power and influence.[132] We have seen that a number of the hospital sisters, in particular, had substantial landed properties that they bequeathed to hospitals. A charter for the hospital of Provins mentions that Marguerite, one of the hospital sisters, was the daughter of the noblewoman Agnès de Courbouzon.[133] Some hospital workers like Marguerite received gifts from family members while they were professed sisters. The sister of the Provinois squire Jacques de Saint-Martin de Huppello was a sister of the hospital of Provins and received a lifetime rent from her brother.[134] Maresonne, the daughter of the wealthy lawyer-clerk Guillaume de Clermont, became a *conversa* in the hôtel-Dieu of Reims. The wealth of this hospital sister's family is evident in the 600 *l.* inheritance that each of her brothers received, one of whom was a lawyer and professor of civil law and the other a canon at the chapter of Saint-Symphorien.[135]

As noted earlier, a number of thirteenth-century female saints and holy women who worked in hospitals, which in some cases they founded, came from aristocratic or even royal backgrounds. The royal ancestry of Elizabeth of Hungary (d. 1231), the daughter of the king of Hungary and the wife of the landgrave of Thuringia, made it all the more remarkable that she so

---

131. Evergates, "Nobles and Knights," 18–19.
132. Le Grand, "Les maisons-Dieu, leur régime," 102 and note 1.
133. Dupraz, no. 104; AD: Seine-et-Marne, 11HdtA12, fol. 32–32v.
134. Dupraz, nos. 220, 221; AD: Seine-et-Marne, 11HdtA12, fol. 66–66v.
135. Desportes, *Reims et les Rémois*, 318.

gladly and humbly personally ministered to the poorest and sickest guests of the hospital she founded. This was also true of Saint Hedwig (d. 1243), the duchess of Silesia, as well as Angela of Foligno and Margaret of Cortona, both wealthy, married women who became Franciscan tertiaries and worked in hospitals that they founded. In the early fourteenth century, Dauphine de Puimichel, who came from an aristocratic Provençal family and also had ties to the Franciscans, lived and worked for a number of years at a hospice in Apt, where she was buried. Those who promoted her cult highlighted her adoption of lowly, "vile," servant-like roles in the hospital, such as brushing out the hospital's sawdust, cleaning dishes and pots and other kitchen utensils, and sitting at the same dining table as the servants.[136] As François-Olivier Touati has shown in his study of lepers in the province of Sens, it was not uncommon during the thirteenth century for aristocratic families to place young family members in leprosaries as a pious act. Some lay aristocrats at the end of their lives chose to retire to a leprosary, where they took the religious habit.[137]

It was also increasingly common during the thirteenth century for middle-class townspeople to place their daughters in a variety of religious institutions, from Cistercian houses to hospitals. The hospital brethren, however, were not limited to aristocrats and townspeople. Some peasants also adopted the religious habit and joined the personnel of hospital communities. Ernault Blanchard, a citizen of Reims, left the city's hospital a portion of his house in his testament from 1251 and also asked that the master and rectors receive Ernault's servant, Gaultier, as a brother in the hospital.[138] A charter from 1211 records a property dispute between the hospital of Provins and the heirs of Gilles le Meunier and his wife Mabille, two serfs ("homines") who had taken the religious habit at the hospital at the end of their lives ("in fine") and had since died.[139] Had Gilles and Mabille been tenants on land acquired by the hospital and then granted the right to enter the hôtel-Dieu as *conversi* later in life? In other words, was the recruitment of *conversi* at times tied to

---

136. Jacques Cambell, O.F.M., ed., *Enquête pour le procès de canonisation de Dauphine de Puimichel, Comtesse d'Ariano (+26 novembre 1360), Apt et Avignon, 14 mai–30 octobre 1363* (Turin: Bottega d'Erasmo, 1978), 48.

137. Touati, *Maladie et société*, 337. Not all of the healthy brethren in leprosaria were ministering to the lepers, particularly given that the number of lepers in a given leprosarium was often dwarfed by the number of brothers and sisters.

138. AMC (Reims): FH-HD B40, no. 6 (Grandchamp), a "vidimus" of the testament. Ernault also bequeathed his larger horse to this servant.

139. Dupraz, B4; AD: AD: Seine-et-Marne, 11HdtA13, fol. 45v–46.

a hospital's acquisition of land the way it was for Cistercian monasteries?[140] Or is the reference to the couple's conversion "at the end" an allusion to their having made a deathbed conversion ("ad succurrendum")? Either way, in contrast to the example of the daughter of a noblewoman becoming a hospital sister, we have here an example of a peasant couple taking religious vows at the end of their lives. Some of those who joined a hospital's religious community may have been as poor as the sick poor they served.[141] Economic security was likely a common reason that some people pursued hospital work, especially single women. Moreover, in some cases hospital work itself represented a kind of survival strategy for the poor and those in need of assistance. This could even extend to those in trouble with the law. One of the sisters at the hospital of Gonesse in 1351, Johann La Morgente, who was from Paris, was known to be a fugitive.[142] Thus, as we have seen before, the boundaries between those receiving and providing care in medieval hospitals could be remarkably fluid.

Where did a hospital's personnel come from? Alain Saint-Denis has found that of the twenty-six brothers and sisters at the Hôtel-Dieu of Laon, sixteen came from the Laonnais, with most of these coming from over ten kilometers away from the city itself and some from as far as forty kilometers away.[143] Of the hospital brethren from the Laonnais, three were from the rural aristocracy, fourteen from the landed property class, and four were clerics. Of the ten brothers and sisters who came from Laon proper, six were citizens of Laon, and several of the sisters came from the wealthiest families in the city.[144] The records for Champagne's hospitals provide less information about the place of origin of the brethren, but based on where they held property that they donated, it appears that quite a few of them came from areas where the hospital made its power felt through its own property holdings and lordship. Jean de Jouy, for example, who was a brother at the hospital at Provins, had donated his house at Jouy (about twelve kilometers northwest of Provins) and part of the woods there.[145] Sister Perrota Lavenderia gave the hospital her house and garden and fourteen *arpents* of land at Sourdun,

140. Constance H. Berman, *Medieval Agriculture, the Southern French Countryside, and the Early Cistercians: A Study of Forty-Three Monasteries* (Philadelphia: American Philosophical Society, 1986), 53–60.

141. Le Blévec, "Le rôle des femmes," 184.

142. Le Grand, ed., "Les maisons-Dieu et les léproseries," 246–47.

143. Saint-Denis, *L'hôtel-Dieu de Laon*, 93.

144. Saint-Denis, *L'hôtel-Dieu de Laon*, 94–95.

145. *Obituaires de la province de Sens*, 1:950.

just five kilometers southeast of Provins.[146] Sister Theota Pometa gave land at Servolles (thirteen kilometers south), where the hospital already had a press, as well as a vineyard at Mez-de-la Madeleine (today, Sainte Colombe), just five kilometers southeast of Provins.[147] The parents of Guillaume Normans, a priest and brother at the hospital at Provins, gave some land they owned at Lizines, just ten kilometers southwest of Provins, as well as land at Viseuviliers.[148] The sister Juliana Villana gave a pasture and a rent on territory in Molinpré, which is modern-day Rouilly, just five kilometers north of Provins.[149]

We noted in chapter 3 that it was common for some hospital donors to come from a family with a history of patronizing the same hospital, and in some cases, the donor even had a relative who worked there. Some of Champagne's hospital workers likely had a prior connection to the hospital they joined, and this was true at leprosaries as well. In 1248, Ysabelle de Chevière, recognizing the donations made by her late mother, Blanche de Chevière, to the leper house of Les Deux Eaux near Troyes, decided now to "give herself to the hospital" as a *donata*, while reserving the use of her property during her lifetime.[150] Likewise, some hospital brethren made donations to a hospital many years before deciding to take the religious habit there.

It was not uncommon for several members of a family (or even multiple generations) to live in a hospital. A charter from 1214 mentions that the daughter (Emelina) and granddaughter (Maria) of a certain Evrard Blond both wore the religious habit at the hôtel-Dieu-le-Comte in Troyes.[151] Evrard had given a vineyard in dowry to his two daughters, and although a certain priest had a lifetime lease on the land, the daughters would not lose their hereditary right to the land. After the priest's death, half of the land would go to the *domus Dei*, and the other half would go to the heirs of Evrard's daughter, Agnès, who did not live in the hospital. One can only wonder how a mother and daughter both ended up working in the hospital and whether they had joined at the same time or separately.

At times, charters make it possible to determine that some hospital brothers and sisters joined the community at an early age and lived and worked

146. *Obituaires de la province de Sens*, 1:931.
147. *Obituaires de la province de Sens*, 1:937.
148. *Obituaires de la province de Sens*, 1:926.
149. *Obituaires de la province de Sens*, 1:927.
150. Harmand, *Notice*, 49.
151. AD: Aube 40H1, no. 22 (September 2014); see also 40H189 (cartulary for the hôtel-Dieu-le-Comte), fol. 61–61v (September 1214).

there for many years. Obituaries, such as the one for the hospital of Provins, also sometimes provide the number of years that a sister or brother worked at the hospital, and as we have seen with the *magistri*, these tenures were at times more than forty years in length. This continued to be true at northern French hospitals in the later Middle Ages. When the bishop delegate of Paris visited the hospital of Gonesse in 1351, he found six sisters, two of whom had already been at the hospital for thirty-three years.[152] That three of these six sisters all joined the hospital on the same day in 1349, right in the midst of the Black Death, suggests that they arrived together, perhaps in response to the massive scale of suffering that they saw around them.[153] There were also cases of *conversi* joining a hospital community quite late in life. The obituary for the hospital of Provins records a donation made by a certain Acelin for the celebration of the anniversary of his father, Robert, who had been a brother at the hospital.[154] This Robert would have presumably joined the hospital as a *conversus* later in life, evident in his grown son's donation to the hospital at the time of his death. Jacques de Hongrie, who served as sergeant to Countess Blanche, is another example. According to the hospital's obituary, he took the religious habit, becoming a *conversus* at the hospital of Provins "at the end of his life," while still married. In his testament of 1219, Jacques made bequests to a long list of religious and charitable institutions, including the brothers of Saint John of Jerusalem, the lepers of Crolebarbe (near Provins), the church of Saint-Marie Magdalene of Mez, and three other churches where his anniversaries would be celebrated, the Cistercian abbeys of Jouy and Sellières, the convent of Champ-Benoist of Provins, and the "domus Dei scolarum" of Provins if it ended up being established.[155] But in addition to these gifts, Jacques showed a special attachment to the hospital of Provins, to which he made a bequest of forty-three *arpents* of land at Sourdun. There was no evidence at this point that Jacques planned to join the hospital. By 1222, he and his wife had bought an additional forty-six *arpents*

---

152. Le Grand, ed., "Les maisons-Dieu et les léproseries," 246–47. Likewise, in her study of the hôtel-Dieu of Paris in the later Middle Ages, Christine Jéhanno cites the example of Pierre Luillier, who was received as a novice brother at the hôtel-Dieu of Paris on June 1, 1401, and then named *magister* fifty-seven years later, on August 28, 1458. Within three years of becoming *magister*, he was described as "senex et debilitatus de persona," and in 1467 he died. Martin Thoulouse was admitted to the hôtel-Dieu Paris on April 3, 1400, and he was still a brother at the hospital in 1450. See Jéhanno, "Sustenter les povres malades," 704, 707.

153. Le Grand, ed., "Les maisons-Dieu et les leproseries," 246–47.

154. *Obituaires de la province de Sens*, 1:932.

155. Dupraz, no. 446; AD: Seine-et-Marne, 11HdtA12, fol. 129v–130.

at Champrond to give to the hospital.[156] It is only in the hospital's obituary that we learn that at the end of his life, Jacques took the religious habit.[157]

Married Couples Working in Hospitals

Serving in a hospital represented one of the only ways a married couple could be part of a religious community.[158] Yet church councils held in Reims and Paris in 1213 and Rouen in 1214 prohibited married couples from living in hospitals, alleging that some married couples were joining hospital communities so as to gain immunity from secular jurisdiction even while continuing to live full married lives.[159] A number of thirteenth-century hospital statutes prohibited married couples from being received. The statutes for the hôtel-Dieu-le-Comte at Troyes, while including such a ban, also stipulated that the hospital master had the right to waive this prohibition. In fact, it was not uncommon for hospital brethren to include married couples, and this was true at leper houses as well.[160] A couple making a donation to the hôtel-Dieu of Bar-sur-Aube in 1232 reserved the right to enter the hospital as religious at some point in the future.[161] Among the sixty-four hospitals that were visited during the mid-fourteenth century by the bishop delegate of Paris, there were numerous examples of married couples, and even married *magistri*, managing hospitals. At the hospital of Longjumeau, the bishop delegate found that the hospital's *magister* did not carry the title of *frater* because he was married to one of the hospital sisters. Yet his wife, who in fact had remarried after her first husband, another hospital brother, had died, continued to carry the status of being a hospital sister.[162] At the Quinze-Vingts, the Parisian hospital for the blind founded by King Louis IX, both the master and the minister (who was the second-in-command after the master) were expected, or in some cases even required, to be married. Unlike the master, the minister lived within the hospital community, and his wife played such a vital role as a caretaker that, according to the mid-fourteenth-century

---

156. Dupraz, no. 447; AD: Seine-et-Marne, 11HdtA12, fol. 130.

157. *Obituaires de la province de Sens*, 1:943.

158. Farmer, "Leper in the Master Bedroom," 91–93.

159. De Miramon, Les *"donnés,"* 187.

160. For a case of a married couple taking the religious habit and joining the leprosary of Les Deux Eaux at Troyes, see the example of Thierry le Lorgnes and his wife Crestienne, a bourgeois couple from Troyes, in Harmand, *Notice*, 50, 144–45.

161. Arbois de Jubainville, *Histoire de Bar-sur-Aube*, 81.

162. Le Grand, ed., "Les maisons-Dieu et les léproseries," 130.

statutes, if the minister's wife died, he was expected to quickly remarry so that a new wife could help care for the blind.[163]

In March of 1220 André le Comte and his wife, who were serfs at the chapter of Saint-Étienne in Troyes, made a donation of four *jugères* of land to the hospital of Saint-Nicolas in Troyes, making known that they wished to enter the hospital and live there as *conversi*, presumably no longer leading married lives after professing vows.[164] Other professed brethren in Champagne's hospitals were (or had been) married, in some cases leaving a spouse in order to become a religious in a hospital. The obituary for the hospital of Provins indicates that one of its donors, Jacob de Luserna, made a gift for the soul of his wife, Emanjarde, who was a hospital sister.[165] So, too, did Sister Ricent give the hospital some wooded lands "with her man" ("que cum viro suo").[166] Sister Richildis, who was the mother of Odo, a priest, gave the hospital a vineyard with her spouse, Richero.[167] In noting the death of the hospital sister, Juliana, and the gift she had made, the obituary notes that she had been married to Evrard Monetarii. The use of the past tense may indicate that Evrard had since died, but in most cases hospital sisters were identified as the wives of named men.[168] It may be that these were entry gifts, made to the hospital (with their husbands) when these women were still leading secular, married lives and that once they took their vows, they ceased leading married lives. It was certainly not uncommon for female (and male) religious communities to house nuns who had once been married.[169] But the sisters' married status continued to be central to their identities right up until their deaths, at least in the context of gifts that came from the married couple.

Elsewhere in northern France, hospital brethren were at times continuing to lead married lives. The martyrological obituary for Châteaudun includes an entry in a thirteenth-century hand recording the death of Robert de Villa

---

163. Sharon Farmer, "From Personal Charity to Centralised Poor Relief: The Evolution of Responses to the Poor in Paris, c. 1250–1600," in *Experiences of Charity, 1250–1650*, ed. Anne M. Scott (Farnham, U.K.: Ashgate, 2015), 32–33.

164. AD: Aube, 43H1, No. 5 (March 1220). Interestingly, the statutes for the hospital at Troyes, promulgated in 1263, specifically prohibited the hospital from receiving a married couple. See Le Grand, ed., *Statuts d'hôtels-Dieu*, 105n2.

165. *Obituaires de la province de Sens*, 1:947.

166. *Obituaires de la province de Sens*, 1:950.

167. *Obituaires de la province de Sens*, 1:929.

168. *Obituaires de la province de Sens*, 1:951.

169. Bruce Venarde, *Women's Monasticism and Medieval Society: Nunneries in France and England, 890–1215* (Ithaca: Cornell University Press, 1997), 95–103.

Galli and his wife Asa, "brothers of this house."[170] It is striking that the charter does not refer to Asa as a sister but rather as a "frater" like her husband. At the hôtel-Dieu of Gournay, according to the archbishop of Rouen, some of the brothers were sleeping with their wives, while others lived in granges, where they managed the hospital's landed property. Since this hospital did not observe a rule, these brothers had probably never taken a vow of chastity, and so there was little the archbishop could do about what he found.[171] Although the *donati* were not generally bound by the vows that the professed brethren took, they were sometimes expected to temper their secular lives, for instance by practicing sexual moderation, if not total abstinence.[172] The *donati* living at the hôtel-Dieu of Laon had once included married couples, but in 1225 a rule was established requiring much stricter physical separation of the sexes and explicitly banning married couples from entering the hospital.[173]

The fourteenth-century Chronicle of Apt, which was produced as part of the canonization inquest for Countess Dauphine de Puimichel, recounted how her flight to the hospital of Apt, probably as a *donata*, was an expression of her desire to remain in a perpetual state of virginity. In the words of the Chronicle, the hospital was itself a "testudinem," which could mean both a protective tortoise shell or a military shed used by soldiers for protection while attacking enemy fortifications. The Chronicle described Dauphine's escape from the earthly world of matrimony to the sanctuary of the hospital where she could offer her full tearful devotion to Christ and the Virgin Mother.[174] As the Chronicle later reveals, Dauphine's husband, Elziarius de Sabran, joined her in the hospital, where they shared a room and slept in the same bed, yet ceased having sexual relations.[175] Indeed, Dauphine was reportedly careful to never sleep unless dressed, and she never touched any part of her husband's body, except when she washed his head, or when he was sick and she needed to feel his head or take his pulse.[176] Dauphine represents yet another example of how fluid the lines were separating a hospital's personnel and its sick and poor guests. According to the Chronicle, which naturally sought to underscore Dauphine's humility and apostolic piety, she

---

170. *Obituaires de la province de Sens*, 2:416.

171. *The Register of Eudes*, 319, 410.

172. De Miramon, Les *"donnés,"* 348–49.

173. Saint-Denis, *L'hôtel-Dieu de Laon*, 97.

174. Cambell, ed., *Enquête*, 34.

175. Cambell, ed., *Enquête*, 37.

176. Cambell, ed., *Enquête*, 37–38.

was known to wash the feet not only of the hospital's poor and those who were sick and deformed in the face, but her own servants as well.[177] During much of her lifetime, Dauphine apparently also suffered from various bodily illnesses, including fevers and hydropsis.[178] In short, despite the canonization inquest's emphasis on the healing miracles that Dauphine provided to others, she may have been both a care provider and the recipient of the hospital's care, and this may have been some of the impetus for her entering the hospital in the first place.

The *Donati* and Boarders

When many hospitals were first established in the twelfth century, their founders envisioned a personnel made up of both clerics and lay or semi-religious women and men. That vision, however, was challenged during the thirteenth century by episcopal reformers like Robert of Courson, who sought to regularize hospitals, making them more homogeneous, monastic-like institutions in which the personnel all observed the Augustinian Rule. Of particular concern to hospital reformers were the *donati*, who were often not professed members of a hospital's religious community and who gave their property in exchange for the hospital's spiritual and material support, often in the form of annuities.[179] Since annuities could pose a strain on the financial well-being of religious institutions, they were the object of strenuous criticism within the church even though annuitants at times provided the hospital with valuable property and services. Reformers like Jacques de Vitry and Robert de Courson criticized annuitants for essentially stealing food from the poor.[180] Article 6 of the statutes for the hôtel-Dieu-le-Comte stated that no "house bread" was to be given to anyone unless he served the hospital or was a member.[181] Additionally, a donat's entry into a hospital or monastery could raise suspicions of simony, since the donat's donation of property might be regarded as an entry fee as opposed to a "free gift." This, too, was addressed by the statutes, which warned that no one's entry into the hospital was to be connected to simoniacal money or a dishonorable pact ("turpi pacto"), although as we have seen, entry gifts were common

---

177. Cambell, ed., *Enquête*, 51–52.
178. Cambell, ed., *Enquête*, 52.
179. The effort to prevent hospitals from accepting lay *donati* can be seen in the Council of Paris in 1213 and the Council of Rouen in 1214. See de Miramon, *Les "donnés,"* 187–88.
180. De Miramon, *Les "donnés,"* 186–204, 357.
181. Le Grand, ed., *Statuts d'hôtels-Dieu*, art. 6, p. 105.

even among the professed brothers and sisters.[182] Yet hospitals continued to accept *donati*, largely as a way to increase revenue, and few hospital statutes banned the practice.[183] The cartulary for the hospital of Beauvais contains a record of a donation from Agnès, the wife of Pierre du Pressoir, a bourgeois. In 1240 she gave the hospital two houses and also asked that when she died, her clothes be sold and the money used to feed the hospital's sick poor. Agnès's donation, however, also included a stipulation that should her husband predecease her, the *magister* and brothers would provide for her so that she could live comfortably at the hospital and be given two *denarios* and two breads daily.[184] The charter indicates that Agnès's first husband had died, and having already experienced widowhood once before, she was anticipating the possibility of becoming a widow again.

Although the precise terms of a donat's relationship to a hospital varied, the *autotraditio* was the legal act by which a lay or religious man or woman (or married couple) made a gift of their person and possessions ("se et sua") to a hospital, much as an oblate did in a monastery. The donat usually reserved the lifetime use of his or her donated goods. Although donats generally did not take religious vows and thus carried a different status from the professed brethren, in some cases they were nevertheless expected to live a chaste life, and they also sometimes provided the hospital with services just as the brethren did.[185] In exchange, the donat was given a lifetime guarantee of being lodged and fed by the hospital. Some *donati* were merely boarders, at times living in a dwelling outside the main hospital building.[186] These corrodians had essentially purchased a life annuity from the hospital. Other *donati*, however, dedicated themselves to serving the poor and sick and wore clothing that was different from both that worn by lay people and that deriving from the professed religious. The acts of admission were sometimes explicit about a donat's reason for vowing herself or himself "in donatum," such as devotion toward Christ and the Virgin. In 1294, Adélaide, the widow of the butcher Pierre Castillon, gave herself and her property to the

---

182. Le Grand, ed., *Statuts d'hôtels-Dieu*, art. 2, p. 105.

183. Le Grand, "Les maisons-Dieu, leur régime," 111. Even in the late fourteenth century, the account book for the hôtel-Dieu Saint-Nicolas in Troyes included a reference to the *donati* residing there. See AD Aube, G2523, fol. 22 (account book for Saint-Nicolas in Troyes for 1379). For a transcription of this account book, see Gesret, "Un hôpital au moyen âge," 466, 468.

184. Leblond, ed., *Cartulaire*, 213.

185. In declaring their intentions to give themselves to a hospital, *donati* could be explicit about their desire not to take the religious habit. The *autotraditio* of Garnier de Frenoie, for example, made this clear to the hôtel-Dieu of Beauvais. See Leblond, ed., *Cartulaire*, 269–70.

186. Gilchrist, *Contemplation and Action*, 28.

hospital of Narbonne out of a desire to consecrate herself in the service of the poor.[187] The giving of the self was ritualized by the *donata* paying homage with bended knee and giving herself between the hands of the hospital's master or prioress. By the mid-fourteenth century, some small hospitals were made up only of *donati*. The fourteenth-century visitation records of the bishop delegate of Paris reveal that the hôtel-Dieu of Saint Brice had only a master, who was himself a *donatus*, and two female *donatae*, one of whom was married to the master.[188] By this period, it was increasingly common for most hospital clerics and brethren to carry the status of being *donati*, having given themselves and their property to the hospital upon joining the community.

In 1355, a certain Isabelle from Montier-en-Der (some sixty kilometers northeast of Troyes), who had been living in Troyes, gave herself to the hospital of Saint-Nicolas as a *donata*. Her donation charter makes clear that she already had a relationship with the hospital, and her stated reasons for joining the community included not only her respect for the "good deeds, prayers, and divine offices" performed there daily but also the significant "favors, assistance, and care" that had been extended to her in the past and that continued to be given to her day after day.[189] As part of the "serene favor and humble affection" extended to Isabelle from the master, brothers, and sisters of the hospital, she was promised the same pint of good wine and two rolls of bread given daily to the brothers and sisters of the house. But Isabelle did not wish to be constrained by the religious vows and charitable and communal duties imposed on the hospital sisters. Her charter made clear that unlike the sisters, she would have the freedom to either eat and drink with the sisters at their communal table or take her food and drink to her room, where she could keep her own furniture. Isabelle was given a private room, deep within the hospital, in an upper room where a certain Anelota, probably also a *donata*, had lived before her death. The hospital offered Isabelle room and board, a Mass of the Holy Spirit during her lifetime and a requiem Mass after her death (as well as Masses for the souls of her deceased parents and friends). In return, she turned over all of her moveable property and her house in Troyes, which was next to the hospital.

---

187. Caille, *Hôpitaux et charité*, 93–94.

188. Le Grand, ed., "Les maisons-Dieu et les léproseries," 75.

189. AD Aube 43H12, layette 31, cote A, no. 58 (July, 1355): "beneficia et oraciones ac divina officia. . . . grata, auxilia, curialitates . . . retroactis temporibus, impenderunt et adhuc de die in diem impendere non desistunt."

Just as widows may have made up a disproportionate percentage of hospital sisters, they frequently appear as *donatae*, perhaps because joining a hospital community provided a widow who could not (or did not wish to) remarry with a spiritual community, the material security of guaranteed room and board, and the promise of care should she become infirm. One of the witnesses in a fourteenth-century canonization inquest, Alsacia de Mesellano, was the widow of a wealthy draper from Apt. Following her husband's death, she seems to have had her own room in a hospital there, suggesting that she was a *donata*. Ironically, however, Alsacia became seriously injured when she fell out of one of the hospital windows. She first sought medical help from several Jewish doctors outside the hospital but finally turned to the curative spiritual powers of Dauphine de Puimichel, who was herself probably a *donata* at the hospital.[190]

Apart from those who formally gave themselves to a hospital as a donat, there were others who wished to associate themselves with a hospital in other ways. The priest, Jean "Langlois," who held a benefice in the cathedral of Saint-Pierre, is one such example. He made bequests in his will of 1274 to multiple churches and religious houses as well as a small donation to each hospital of Troyes. But Jean showed a special affection for Saint-Nicolas, donating his house to the hospital, asking that pittances be distributed on the day of his funeral, requesting burial in the hospital cemetery, and most significantly, asking to be received as a "socium."[191] This did not necessarily mean that Jean planned to move into the hospital, but he clearly was interested in obtaining a title and status that conveyed his special relationship with the house. Since the cathedral had jurisdiction over the hospital and was just across the street, it is perhaps not surprising that a cathedral canon felt a special connection to the hospital and its mission. However, Jean does not appear to have formally become a "donatus," and it is possible that the title "socius" was an honorific one that he wished to be conferred on him posthumously, denoting a "fraternitas post mortem."[192]

The *donati* were not the only boarders at Champagne's hospitals. An account book for Saint-Nicolas from 1302 refers to someone who paid 6 *l.* as annual room and board for living there.[193] A charter from Countess Blanche in 1204 reveals that the hôtel-Dieu-le-Comte built additional rooms to house

190. Cambell, ed., *Enquête*, 77.
191. AD Aube 43H12, layette 31, cote A, no. 35 (1274).
192. Saint-Denis, *L'hôtel-Dieu de Laon*, 129.
193. BnF ms lat. 9111, fol. 291 (account book for Saint-Nicolas in Troyes for 1300–01).

paid boarders.[194] This was done at the initiative of Elizande de Chappes, the daughter of the late Tuboeuf de Rosnay, and confirmed by the countess. Count Thibaut had earlier made a donation so that Elizande "could have her bread" at the hospital. Given her aristocratic background and patronage of the hospital, Elizande was probably a *donata*. She was responsible for the expansion of the hospital, namely the construction of seven rooms in front of the baths of Saint-Étienne. These new guest rooms were to house "hospites" or "albani," that is, newcomers, and although Elizande was entitled to the revenue that these rooms brought in, she wanted it to go to the hospital, specifically for food and pittances for the sick poor. In short, the hôtel-Dieu-le-Comte had a secondary function as a "for-profit" guest house or inn, which provided additional income that could be used for the sick poor. We usually think of *donati* as a potential drain on institutional finances, since this was a common complaint of medieval churchmen, but a *donata* like Elizande could help a hospital tap into invaluable social networks and bring in additional revenue, as could the paying boarders who occupied the hospital's new guest rooms. After all, revenue from hospital boarders helped pay for the sick poor.

Serfs and Servants

Anne-Marie Patault has argued that serfdom was in decline in Champagne during the later Middle Ages. Even in the thirteenth century, she suggests, there were more free rural tenants in Champagne than unfree, with much of the rural population being dependent upon lords but not classified as servile. Furthermore, the lines separating free and unfree tenants were hazy, since some serfs had a surprising amount of freedom, especially those in towns. Indeed, some serfs were even able to leave their *seigneurie*, choose their lord, leave their lord for another lord, not live on their lord's land, and buy, sell, and donate property.[195] In other words, free and unfree peasants did not necessarily belong to starkly different classes; the principal difference between them was that serfs were subject to the seigneurial *taille*—an additional symbolic rent called the "chevage"—and *mainmorte*, which meant that the serf's lord was automatically his or her heir.[196]

194. AD: Aube 40H1 (1204); Guignard, ed., *Les anciens statuts*, 97–98. See also Boutiot, *Histoire de la ville*, 319, 348–49.

195. Anne-Marie Patault, *Hommes et femmes de corps en Champagne méridionale à la fin du moyen âge* (Nancy, France: Université de Nancy-II, 1978), 143–63.

196. Patault, *Hommes et femmes*, 127–41.

Yet even if serfdom was in decline during the fourteenth century and the restrictions on serfs were gradually being loosened, in 1309 the cathedral chapter of Saint-Pierre in Troyes still possessed approximately 1,250 serfs, a staggering number, especially when one considers that this chapter had only about forty canons.[197] The number of serfs possessed by the hôtel-Dieu-le-Comte was certainly not on this scale, but the hospital continued to receive serfs as pious donations "in alms" and purchased and exchanged serfs as well.[198] The "great charter" from 1189, in which Count Henri II approved the donations to the hôtel-Dieu-le-Comte made by his father, Count Henri the Liberal, lists over forty serfs, including many families.[199] Usually a serf had little agency when he or she was given as a pious donation. In 1205, Isabelle, a lady from Raiz, responding to the pleas of her brother Guido, and with the assent of her husband, Otho, then in Constantinople, gave her serf, Dodo, a carpenter, along with his whole family and their things to the hôtel-Dieu-le-Comte in alms.[200] Because Isabelle did not have a seal of her own, her mother sealed the charter. Lord Hugues de Villemoyenne gave the same hospital his fisherman, Aubert, along with his family.[201] The knight Gaultier Damenois and his wife, Lady Oda, wishing to provide for the health of their souls, gave lordship over a certain Ermengarde in perpetual alms to the master and brothers of the *domus Dei* in April of 1241.[202] The hospital also purchased serfs. Jean de Logia, a "domicellus," sold his serf, Radulph, to the hospital for 10 *l.* and stipulated that he would assign any difference between what he paid for the serf and the serf's actual value to the hospital in alms.[203]

A common pious gift in medieval Champagne was the voluntary self-subjugation to a monastery, and with the rise of hospitals, some peasants chose to submit themselves to a hospital's lordship.[204] Such a decision could be sparked by piety, but it could also be pragmatic if the person's spouse was one of the hospital's serfs. Furthermore, just as some women and men joined a hospital's staff, taking vows with the aim of acquiring greater material

---

197. Patault, *Hommes et femmes*, 21–24, 34.

198. For examples of the purchase and exchange of serfs, see AD: Aube 40H16 (April 1228; April 1241; 1244; 1244; 1245). On the exchange of serfs, see Patault, *Hommes et femmes*, 112–14.

199. AD: Aube 40H1, no. 1 (1189).

200. Aube 40H16 (1205).

201. Aube 40H1, no. 16 (1208).

202. AD: Aube 40H16.

203. Aube 40H16 (April 1228). In 1245 another serf was sold to the hospital for only 50 *s.*, just a quarter of the sale price of the serf seventeen years earlier, so it is quite likely that these "sales" in fact represented charitable bequests, but bequests wherein the donor did receive some capital. See Aube 40H16 (1245).

204. Patault, *Hommes et femmes*, 65–66.

security (or a spiritual community), so too might some peasants have voluntarily subjugated themselves to a hospital, knowing that if and when they themselves became infirm, the hospital would care for them and make sure that all their needs were met.

In 1269 Maria, who was the widow of the late Radulph de Montealano and was married to a certain Nicolas called "Baigneo," a cleric (probably of lower orders), received her husband's permission to give herself to the master and brothers of the hôtel-Dieu-le-Comte as a "femina de corpore." Maria agreed to an "abonamentum," a fixed annual seigneurial payment of 20 *s.* so long as she lived with her husband ("in consortia"), implying that she might one day leave her husband to become a religious of the hospital, in which case she would no longer owe this due, since her status would change.[205] But what explains Maria's auto-dedition, her voluntary giving of herself to the hospital as a serf?[206] There is nothing in Maria's charter to suggest that piety motivated her. In that sense, this charter is quite different from the pious language one finds in charters where a *conversa* joined a hospital as a sister (or for that matter, when a woman gave herself as a *donata*), at least in part out of a desire to be associated with the hospital's charitable mission. But like a *donata* or a hospital sister, Maria's desire to join the hospital community probably reflected her desire for greater security. In addition, all lower-class tenants in Champagne (with the exception of "albani," that is, foreigners) had to have a lord. Moreover, Henri the Liberal had made clear that lordless tenants had to establish residency under a lord's jurisdiction within one year of moving. We do not know who had previously been Maria's lord or where she had lived. If she had married Nicolas recently, she may have only just moved to Troyes. Regardless, it is likely that economic necessity pushed her into acquiring a new tenancy and accepting the hospital as her lord. Earlier we noted an example of two serfs who were married taking religious vows at the hospital of Provins, and this happened elsewhere as well. In 1216, the cathedral chapter of Troyes made clear, probably because the issue had arisen there as well, that if any of the cathedral's serfs wished to take the religious habit so as to serve the poor of the hospital of Saint-Nicolas, they would first need the chapter's permission. Just three years later, a married couple, André "Comte" and his wife, who were serfs ("homines"), received

---

205. AD: Aube 40H16. On the "abonamentum," see Evergates, *Feudal Society*, 20.

206. For a comparable example, see the case of Marmoutier in Dominique Barthélemy, *La mutation de l'an mil a t-elle-eu lieu? Servage et chevalerie dans la France des Xe et XIe siècles* (Paris: Fayard, 1997), 57–91.

the chapter's consent to give pieces of arable, vineyard, and meadow to the poor of the hospital (they were clearly landowning serfs) and to give themselves to the house as *conversi* at some future point of their choosing.[207] We do not know whether André and his wife envisioned Saint-Nicolas merely as a retirement home or were attracted by its charitable and religious mission.

In addition to serfs, many of Champagne's hospitals had servants. The statutes for the hospitals of Provins and Troyes indicated that if more help was needed beyond what the statutory number of hospital sisters and brothers could provide, servants could be employed to provide the services needed.[208] We have already observed that female servants ("meskines") were expected to minister to the sick poor during the night, and elsewhere the statutes suggest involving servants in the serving of food in the refectory.[209] A sacerdotal Mass was to be said three times for servants who died, reflective of their status as members of the hospital community.[210] The late thirteenth-century obituary for the hospital of Beauvais listed the names of servant girls ("famulae") who had died, just as it did for its patrons and clerical and religious personnel.[211] One of the members of the hospital of Gonesse in 1351 had earlier been a servant of the bishop of Paris, and one of the sisters at this hospital was referred to as a "sister-servant" ("sororem familiarem"), suggesting that perhaps she began as a servant and subsequently became a sister.[212] Not all hospitals, however, considered servants as members of the community. Servants at the hospital at Lagny, for example, were not allowed to enter the chapel, which was restricted to the brethren and the sick poor.[213] The account book for Saint-Nicolas in Troyes for 1300–01 lists an annual expenditure of 26 *l.* "for the salaries of servants of the hospice and of the granges."[214] In 1212 Countess Blanche gave most of the collateral inheritance (in the form of land) of Savine, a poor woman ("paupercule mulieris") from Payns, to the hôtel-Dieu-le-Comte in perpetual alms.[215] There is no

---

207. Arbois de Jubainville, "Étude," 92. See also AD Aube 43H12, layette 31, cote A, no. 5.

208. Le Grand, ed., *Statuts d'hôtels-Dieu*, art. 5, p. 105. Likewise, the brothers were to sleep in their dormitory with their "familiaribus." See art. 65, p. 113.

209. Le Grand, ed., *Statuts d'hôtels-Dieu*, art. 51, p. 111.

210. Le Grand, ed., *Statuts d'hôtels-Dieu*, art. 30, p. 108.

211. See, for example, the example of a servant named "Sgau," who is described as a servant of the poor ("famula pauperum"); Leblond, ed., "L'obituaire," 354.

212. Le Grand, ed., "Les maisons-Dieu et les léproseries," 246–47.

213. Le Grand, ed., "Les maisons-Dieu et les léproseries," 214.

214. BnF ms. Lat 9111, fol. 285. The following year, 24 *l.* was spent on servants' salaries. See fol. 292v.

215. Aube 40H1, no. 18 (July 1212).

reference to Savine being a "homo de corpore," the usual term for a serf, and so she was likely one of Blanche's servants. Robert "Sorins" Normand, one of the servants of the hospital in Provins, is listed in that hospital's obituary as having given 20 *l. t.* so that the hospital could buy rents.[216] A certain Jean, who was one of the servants of a craftsman, gave the same hospital 10 *l.* to buy rents.[217]

Administrative Anxieties

The sermons preached to the personnel in hospitals reflected preachers' anxieties about the way that hospitals were administered, and this included everything from the physical state of hospitals to the interactions of women and men, from the source of the money given in alms to how those resources were used. Hospital sermons were not solely words of encouragement and comfort but also included warnings, a reflection of preachers' fears about the possibility of abuse and corruption and the urgent need for reform. Just as it was believed that there was a connection between physical and spiritual health, so did preachers view the physical state of a hospital as reflecting and contributing to the spiritual and physical health of its sick and poor guests. In commenting on the need for hospitals to have clean and well-ordered beds, Jacques de Vitry noted, "For this, indeed you ought to have male and female servants, lay brothers and sisters in hospitals so that they clean dirt and maintain clean beds. Moreover, in certain places many die from foul and corrupt air as much as from the sickness of the body itself."[218] It is noteworthy that Jacques expected both female and male servants and *conversi* to take responsibility for cleaning and maintaining the hospital beds. Jacques and other thirteenth-century reformers criticized hospitals in which almost all of the physical caring for the sick and poor was done by servants, while the brothers and sisters concerned themselves with the religious life and other matters. Jacques reminded hospital brothers and sisters that it was not only servants who were expected to visit the sick and minister to them with their own hands, lifting and carrying them, "but you yourselves" (*sed per vos ipsos*), that is, the brothers and sisters.[219] Far from avoiding the sick poor, the brothers and sisters were often commanded in their own hospital statutes (beginning

216. *Obituaires de la province de Sens,* 1:954.
217. *Obituaires de la province de Sens,* 1:952.
218. Bird, "Texts on Hospitals," 119.
219. Bird, "Texts on Hospitals," 119.

with the Order of Saint John of Jerusalem) to treat the sick and poor as "our lords."[220]

In fact, as we have seen, the division of labor in hospitals quite often was gendered, with sisters ministering to the sick and poor, while the brothers were preoccupied with the religious life, managing the hospital's temporalities, and other matters.[221] As noted earlier, Jacques de Vitry compared a group of hospital workers to the mother of Christ in that they fed and nourished Christ (just as she had) through his members.[222] This is particularly interesting given developments in Cistercian spirituality of this period, with male Cistercians expressing a desire to imitate a Jesus they conceived of as a giving, nurturing, and even lactating mother.[223] In contrast, the *vita* of Jutta of Huy, written by Hugh de Floreffe, argued that Jutta's work in a leprosarium was particularly valuable for her in allowing her to prevail over the pride and vanity that were inherent to her sex. Moreover, Hugh observed, the experience of doing works of mercy had made Jutta's soul "more manly" (*viriliter*).[224]

In the eyes of churchmen and moral reformers, the diversity of those living inside hospitals—priests and other clerics, lay brothers and sisters, servants, *donati*, and the poor and sick—posed various kinds of potential problems for religious discipline. Preaching in the large and diverse hôtel-Dieu of Paris, the secular master Ranulphe de la Houblonnière expressed concern about the many different forms of religious life represented both inside and outside the hospital. In Ranulphe's view, there were simply too many lifestyles to choose from. "The multiplicity of ways," he argued, caused confusion and deviation from "the narrow gate" and "straight way" that leads to

---

220. Le Grand, "Les maisons-dieu: Leurs statuts au XIIIe siècle," 103. A thirteenth-century handbook for archdeacons exhorted them to conduct visitations of hospitals and warn the brothers and sisters not to act like lords, but rather as the servants and ministers of the poor. See *Catalogue general des manuscrits des bibliothèques publiques des départements*, vol. 1 (Laon), ed. Félix Ravaisson (Paris: Imprimerie Nationale, 1849), 637.

221. As Daniel Le Blévec has observed, although hospital roles were sometimes gendered, they were not always so, with the division of labor varying according to the size and makeup of the hospital. See Le Blévec, "Le rôle des femmes," 171–90.

222. On de Vitry's gendered view of the physical care of the sick poor, see Farmer, "Leper," 95–6.

223. Caroline Walker Bynum, "Jesus as Mother and Abbot as Mother: Some Themes in Twelfth-Century Cistercian Writing', in *Jesus as Mother: Studies in the Spirituality of the High Middle Ages* (Berkeley, 1982), 110–68.

224. See Rawcliffe, *Leprosy*, 148–49. On preaching against female vanity, see Thomas M. Izbicki, "Pyres of Vanities: Mendicant Preaching on the Vanity of Women and Its Lay Audience," in *De Ore Domini: Preacher and Word in the Middle Ages*, ed. Thomas L. Amos, Eugene A. Green, and Beverly Mayne Kienzle (Kalamazoo, MI: Medieval Institute Publications, 1989), 211–34.

life (Matthew 7:14): "This you will see today: each one makes his own way, one through the religion of the beguines, etc., thus that there are so many forms of religious life today that man does not know in which status he might be in."[225] Speaking to a diverse audience at the hôtel-Dieu in Paris, which had a staff of over one hundred, including various kinds of clerics, brothers, sisters, female novices, and servants, Ranulphe reflected on the challenges of maintaining religious discipline in such a mixed community.[226]

Both Jacques de Vitry and Humbert of Romans acknowledged in their preaching that there were corrupt hospitals, and Humbert lamented that some of those who supposedly entered a hospital to serve the poor in fact did so "not on account of God or penance or any good intention, but only so as to have sustenance, and therefore they deserve nothing before God."[227] Nor did Humbert look kindly upon hospital brothers and sisters who moved from hospital to hospital until they found the one that most suited them and then sought to procure extra quantities of food and drink for themselves.[228] Humbert reminded his listeners why they had joined (or should have joined) a hospital community in the first place: to help and serve the sick and poor. Moral reformers generally did not hold a favorable view of the *donati*, and a thirteenth-century pastoral handbook for archdeacons recommended that archdeacons investigate whether any members of a hospital community had paid in order to be admitted.[229]

Unlike the sermons that were preached in hospitals, the anonymous thirteenth-century *Summa pastoralis* for archdeacons, which contained six chapters on how an archdeacon should conduct visitations of almshouses, was principally concerned with the kinds of pragmatic administrative issues dealt with in hospital statutes: Did the hospital have a written copy of its rules and statutes? How many brothers and sisters lived in the hospital, and was this number excessive relative to the house's resources? How were the hospital's properties managed? What was the relationship between the house's revenues and expenditures?[230] Indeed, the archdeacon's visitations were intended to ensure that the statutes were being properly observed. Occasionally, as we have seen, hospital sermons did tackle the kinds of issues addressed in statutes. In one of his sermons, Jacques de Vitry, for instance, warned his

225. Bériou, *La prédication de Ranulphe*, 30–31.
226. Coyecque, *L'hôtel-dieu de Paris*, 27.
227. Humbert, "De eruditione," 476.
228. Humbert, "De eruditione," 452.
229. Ravaisson, ed., *Catalogue*, 637. See also Miramon, *Les "donnés" au moyen âge*, 357–60.
230. Ravaisson, ed., *Catalogue*, 634–40.

listeners to ensure that the hospital be separated by gender, with the infirm men to whom the brethren ministered in one part and the women to whom the sisters or female servants ministered in another part or even a separate building. "Do not place straw near fire," he cautioned, "nor women near men."[231] At times the pastoral handbook echoed some of the criticisms found in hospital sermons about what motivated brothers and sisters to join hospitals:

> No brothers or sisters ought to be received unless they wish to or are able to serve God's poor in all patience and humility and poverty, thus that they not consider themselves lords but servants and ministers of the poor. Therefore since very many do not enter so, but in order to drink and eat and as is said vulgarly, "to have their bread well baked"— they acquire damnation and they are the cause of the destruction of almshouses because they live badly there, they enter badly with insincere intention, nor do they serve God nor the poor.[232]

Reminding archdeacons that almshouses were intended to support only the traveling poor and those with temporary illnesses, the pastoral handbook railed against almshouses that were supporting those with chronic disabilities: "For the burgesses and very many others, not having God before their eyes, almost under a certain pretext of piety, are accustomed to burden houses of this kind, placing there certain members of their family or neighbors who are physically disabled, blind, old and powerless, even when the almshouses were not founded for this but for showing hospitality for the traveling poor and especially the sick until they convalesce."[233]

Humbert of Romans bemoaned those hospitals which, "although they overflow and are enriched by alms given on account of the poor, nevertheless when the destitute come, they are not received there, and it is done to them just as the Jews did to Christ, who came among his own and they did not receive Him, their own."[234] In hospitals such as these, according to Humbert, the hospital staff were living magnificently from the alms that had been collected for the poor, while the poor were "sent away to languish in great poverty. If, moreover, the rich evangelist [Pharisee] was punished thus because he did not give from his own goods to that one, Lazarus, lying before

---

231. Bird, "Texts on Hospitals," 133.
232. Ravaisson, ed., *Catalogue*, 637–38.
233. Ravaisson, ed., *Catalogue*, 637.
234. Humbert, "De eruditione," 476.

his gate, what ought to be done about those, who with the poor lying in this house with them, do not give from the goods of their poor?"[235] In an attempt to instill fear in his listeners in another sermon, Humbert echoed words from Ecclesiasticus and the Gospel of Matthew, telling his listeners, "'Be not slow in visiting the sick,' because the Lord is going to say to those on the Day of Judgment, 'I was sick and you all did not visit me.'"[236]

On the other side of the spectrum, Jacques de Vitry expressed concern not that the brothers and sisters would exhibit insufficient charity toward the sick and poor but rather that the staff would be too indulgent with them. He cautioned the staff not to give the sick and poor whatever they wanted:

> In this, moreover, many hospitallers are delinquent, as if under the guise of piety, they walk around the beds of the sick and ask each one what they wish to eat or drink. The ignorant ones, moreover the poor and sick, ask for meat or wine according to their own appetite, although they may suffer a violent fever or another fierce illness. Whence very often many die from a diet which is contrary to the diet for that infirmity. Therefore, you ought not knowingly give foods that are bad for the sick just as you would not wish to give a sword to a madman with which he might kill himself.[237]

What all of these sermons reflect is a deeply felt anxiety about sincerity, motives, and the enormous responsibility with which hospital workers were entrusted. Preachers sought to convey to hospital audiences just how high the stakes were in the way that they carried out their charitable work. It was not merely the actions of hospital workers that mattered, but the intentionality and sincerity behind their actions.

The unease expressed by ecclesiastical reformers about the way that hospitals were being administered continued into the early fourteenth century, culminating in canon 17 (the decretal *Quia contingit*) of the Council of Vienne, summoned by Clement V in 1311. This decretal, which represented the first significant treatment of hospitals in conciliar law, directly addressed some of the perceived abuses being committed by those overseeing hospitals, including hospitals that were mismanaged; the properties and rights of hospitals being usurped; funds for the sick poor being used to create benefices for nonresident clerics, with the poor being turned away as a direct consequence;

---

235. Humbert, "De eruditione," 476.
236. Humbert, "De eruditione," 502.
237. Bird, "Texts on Hospitals," 131.

buildings being left in a state of disrepair; a dearth of inventories of hospital properties and regular bookkeeping of hospital incomes and expenditures. The overriding concern of this decretal centered not on the religious life and discipline of the hospital brethren but on protecting hospital assets and ensuring that the donations made to hospitals were being used for the poor and sick, not the personnel. *Quia contingit* was meant to serve as a reminder of the need for competent personnel to carry out the caritative function for which hospitals were founded and endowed. From the perspective of the decretal, when a hospital's personnel outnumbered its poor and sick guests, the institution had lost sight of its mission. The decretal sought to affirm the power of bishops to oversee the management of hospitals where abuses were occurring, regardless of whether the hospital was exempt from episcopal control.[238] There is evidence that in the wake of *Quia contingit*, at least some bishops implemented the decretal's injunctions and sought to exercise greater control and oversight over hospitals.[239] In the mid-fourteenth-century, as we have observed, the bishop delegate of Paris conducted visitations of dozens of hospitals and leprosaria in his diocese and recorded his detailed findings in a register.[240] One of the striking things revealed by this register is just how much control the bishops of Paris were exercising over these houses of mercy in the decades following the Council of Vienne. According to the register, it would seem that almost every cleric and lay brother and sister had needed the bishop's approval to be received by a hospital or leprosarium. The bishop delegate regularly inspected the documents recording these episcopal authorizations to ensure that all personnel were legitimate and that the staff was not increasing in size.

While some French bishops expressed concern about the lack of moral and religious discipline that might result from a hospital's autonomy or lack of external oversight, a bishop's own cathedral chapter could also serve as a disruptive force to what was supposed to be the solemn and tranquil state of a hospital. In 1322 the *magister* and the brothers and sisters of the hôtel-Dieu of Reims complained to the cathedral chapter, with which they were affiliated, about an annual custom in which choirboys and young canons from the cathedral celebrated the end of the Advent fast by congregating in the hospital on Christmas morning, following the chanting of Matins and

---

238. In the above discussion of *Quia contingit* and its importance, I am drawing on the analysis of Watson, *On Hospitals*, 295–309. For *Quia contingit*, see *Decrees of the Ecumenical Councils*, ed. Norman P. Tanner, S. J., vol. 1 (London: Sheed & Ward, 1990), 374–76.

239. Mollat, *Poor in the Middle Ages*, 181–82.

240. Le Grand, ed., "Les maisons-Dieu et les léproseries."

the Nine Lessons. The choirboys and young canons would gather around a large fire in the hospital, drinking and feasting on sausages and other foods. At the request of the hospital, the Rémois chapter agreed to put an end to this annual practice, and the hospital agreed in return to pay an annual rent to the cathedral chapter.[241]

Although some French bishops sought to reform, and in some sense, "regularize" hospitals, it was not church councils or the actions of bishops that fueled the hospital movement or the broader charitable revolution. Rather, it was propelled by the broad-based social and religious impulse of members of the laity and ecclesiastics to offer up their own property, wealth, and labor in service of the *miserabiles*. The diverse members of hospital communities—lay women and men, male and female religious, clerics, peasants, townspeople, and aristocrats—were surely motivated for different reasons, but to some extent they all came to hospitals in search of greater security, whether spiritual or material, and believed that they might find that security by participating in a community dedicated to performing the works of mercy. For some, that sense of security might have come through the realization of their apostolic aspirations to live in a caritative religious community. Still others might have obtained a sense of security by no longer living alone, instead being part of a supportive community formed around mutual assistance, where they could be assured of meals, clothes, and a bed. However, the reality surely was that many medieval hospital workers never found the security they were hoping to find. Working in a hospital, which could involve caring for those suffering from malnutrition and various kinds of mental and physical illness, carried its own risks and hardships—exposure to pathogens, abuse by violent guests or fellow brethren, the possibility that the institution might at any time shut down due to insufficient resources or be taken over by another religious house—and so hospital workers, who were charged with caring for those on the margins, must have often lived with a profound sense of their own vulnerability. Ultimately, there was not that much separating the widow who worked as a hospital sister, or the aged and frail hospital chaplain, from the sick and poor for whom they cared.

---

241. AD: Marne (Reims) 2G354 (October 1322).

❧ CHAPTER 6

The Sick Poor and the Economy of Care

In 1991, the copper heiress Huguette Clark was admitted to Beth Israel Medical Center in New York City for what was a relatively minor illness. Clark ended up staying at the hospital for twenty years, dying there in 2011 at the age of 104. The hospital had been ready to discharge Clark a few weeks after she was first admitted, but as it happened, her three Manhattan apartments, worth tens of millions of dollars, were being renovated, and she found that living at the hospital was to her liking. She did not have difficulty persuading the hospital to let her stay, although it is likely that no one anticipated that her stay would last for twenty years. Seeing an opportunity in Huguette Clark, however, the development office of Beth Israel Medical Center launched an aggressive fundraising campaign. The hospital did research on Clark to learn, in the words of one of its development officers, "an appropriate cultivation approach."[1] It showered her with gifts, including compact discs, chocolates, homemade pies, playing cards from Paris, birthday balloons, and Easter baskets. The mother of the hospital's CEO was sent to sit with Clark in her hospital room, talk about her rare doll collection, and watch *The Smurfs* with her—her favorite TV

---

1. Anemona Hartocollis, "Hospital Caring for an Heiress Pressed Her to Give Lavishly," *The New York Times*, May 29, 2013.

show—while gently broaching the subject of her will. As the hospital's law-yer put it, Beth Israel provided Mrs. Clark with "a well-attended home where she was able to live out her days in security, relative good health and comfort, and with the pleasures of human company."[2] Huguette Clark ended up giv-ing at least $4 million in donations to Beth Israel, as well as an additional bequest of one million dollars in her will, and she spent close to half a million dollars a year for room and board at the hospital.[3] Although we tend to think of the modern hospital exclusively in terms of medical care, the example of Huguette Clark is a reminder of the more distant past, when hospitals served a diversity of functions and housed a wide range of people, including those without a support network and those who used hospitals as inns, paying room and board to stay there.

In this chapter, we turn to the recipients of care in medieval hospitals. In addition to interrogating who these guests were and what kind of care they received, this chapter argues that they played a vital role in the "economy of salvation" and were not simply the passive recipients of care. While the sick poor who were admitted to hospitals were often very dependent on the physical and spiritual assistance provided to them by a hospital's per-sonnel, they also carried with them a certain kind of spiritual power as the intercessors who might assist donors and the hospital brethren in obtaining salvation. The sick poor played a central role in the triangular system of exchange involving hospital workers, benefactors, and God. As we shall see, the charitable activities of hospitals extended outside the hospital walls to the city streets, where various kinds of charitable assistance were also provided for by family members, neighbors, and other religious organizations. While continuing to focus on the example of Champagne, we will also have occa-sion to draw on examples from other regions, mostly in northern France.

The sources that medieval hospitals left behind tend to reveal very little about the kind of care the poor and sick received or even who these people were. The sources for the twelfth and thirteenth centuries are even more opaque than those for the later Middle Ages, providing more infor-mation about donors and the personnel that worked in hospitals than the guests. However, a recent archaeological excavation of a medieval parish cemetery in Troyes, among the most important medieval French urban cem-eteries that have been excavated, with almost 2,500 burials found, identified a section of the cemetery that was used by the hôtel-Dieu-le-Comte in Troyes

---

2. Hartocollis, "Hospital Caring."
3. Hartocollis, "Hospital Caring."

during the twelfth and thirteenth centuries.[4] This archaeological study of a medieval hospital cemetery along with similar studies have provided valuable information about the identities of those who lived and died in hospitals, including their gender, the age when they died, their nutritional history, and some of the pathologies from which they suffered. Some thirteenth-century textual sources also provide a glimpse into the quotidian experience of living in a hospital. Hospital statutes, for example, reveal how hospitals sought to regulate who was admitted and the expectations about the kind of care that was to be provided to them. By examining hospitals' financial account books, charters, and the testaments that were sometimes drawn up for hospital guests, it is possible to find out who spent time in hospitals and for what reasons they were there. The occasional account of a miraculous cure of someone staying in a hospital, recorded as part of a canonization inquest, also sheds light on the nature of the infirmities and disabilities of hospital guests. The miracle stories about those who did not spend time in a hospital are equally useful in what they reveal about those with infirmities and disabilities who did not seek institutional assistance. Finally, model sermons that were directed at the hospital sick and poor reflect the religious and moral messages that these people heard, messages that sought to bring them comfort and help them understand their soteriological role.

Unlike some of the earlier scholarship on poor relief and the survival strategies of the medieval poor, the evidence uncovered in this book suggests that there was less of a divide between institutional forms of support for the poor and familial or neighborly assistance. As we have seen, some people turned to a hospital for help because they had a relative who worked there or who had patronized the institution. This chapter will also demonstrate the types of caring activities in which hospitals were engaged with those not even living in a hospital. We need, in other words, to have a more expansive conception of medieval hospitals' caring activities, both inside

---

4. Cécile Paresys, Dominique Castex, Cédric Roms, Isabelle Richard, and Stéphanie Degobertière, "Un nouvel cas de sépultures multiples à Troyes, Place de la Libération (Aube, Moyen Âge)," *Bulletins et Mémoires de la Société d'Anthropologie de Paris*, n.s. 20, 1–2 (2008): 125–36. See also H. Réveillas and D. Castex, "La gestion des cimetières d'hôpitaux en période de crise épidémique: Apports des données bio-archéologiques," in *Espaces, objets, populations dans les établissements hospitaliers du Moyen Age au XXème siècle*, ed. S. Le Clech (Dijon: Presses Universitaires de Dijon, 2009), 343–64. A 2015 excavation under a Monoprix supermarket in Paris revealed a medieval cemetery belonging to the hospital of La Trinité with more than two hundred interred bodies, many in mass burial pits. It appears that some of the dead actually came from the main hôtel-Dieu of Paris near the cathedral, which during the plague epidemic had run out of burial space in its own cemetery. See "Les surprises des sous-sols du Boulevard Sébastopol à Paris: Archéologie du cimitière de la Trinité": https://www.inrap.fr/les-surprises-des-sous-sols-du-boulevard-sebastopol-paris-archeologie-du-5392.

and outside the institutional walls, including what was thought to constitute "needs" and "care." In this regard, there is much to be learned about the history of hospitals from non-textual sources, such as archaeology, which, as this chapter will show, can cast new light on the health and identities of those cared for by hospitals.

Who Was Admitted to Hospitals?

In order to understand the "economy of care" in the medieval hospitals of Champagne, we must first seek to transcend the abstract categories of the "poor" and "sick poor" so often invoked in medieval sources. Who were the women and men who were received by hospitals? Even apart from leprosaria, some hospitals in thirteenth-century France were specialized in terms of the categories of people they admitted.[5] These included, among others, the famous hospital for the blind—the Quinze-Vingts—founded in Paris by Louis IX, as well as specialized hospitals or almshouses for the elderly, pregnant women, abandoned children, unwed mothers, those afflicted with ergotism, aged clergy who were no longer able to earn a living, clerical students, pilgrims or travelers ("transeuntes"), and repentant prostitutes (Filles Dieu). A confraternity in Arras even founded a hospital in the mid-thirteenth century specifically for those suffering from burns.[6]

Although most of the hospitals in Champagne that we have been examining were fairly inclusive, accepting a wide range of people who were considered "pauperes" or "infirmi"—and even some who were neither sick nor poor—the statutes for the hôtel-Dieu-le-Comte and the hospital of Provins also placed a number of restrictions on who could be admitted. For instance, abandoned children, regarded as a parochial responsibility, were barred for fear that they would place a strain on the financial health of the hospital.[7] This was in contrast to the hospital of Nemours, which did raise abandoned children and was challenged by the parish church of Saint-Jean de Nemours

---

5. See Brodman, *Charity and Religion*.

6. Catherine Vincent, *Les confréries médiévales dans le royaume de France XIIIe–XVe siècle* (Paris: Albin Michel, 1994), 75.

7. Le Grand, ed., *Statuts d'hôtels-Dieu*, art. 89, p. 115. For the French version of the statutes for the hôtel-Dieu-le-Comte, see Guignard, ed., *Les anciens statuts*. There are thirteenth-century Latin and French versions of the statutes for both the hôtel-Dieu-le-Comte and the hospital of Provins. While the statutes for these two hospitals are almost identical, there are some slight differences. Two copies of the Provins statutes are extant, neither of which has been edited: a seventeenth-century copy of the French text (AD: Seine-et-Marne 11Hdt/A3) and a Latin copy found in Nicolas-Pierre Ythier's eighteenth-century *L'histoire ecclésiastique de Provins* (BM: Provins), Supplément à Saint Thibault.

for baptizing them.[8] The largest hospitals at Troyes and Provins were, at least theoretically, willing to take care of any orphan whose parent died in the hospital for up to ten years, something that the hospital in Vernon also did.[9] In fact, a recent archaeological excavation of the cemetery used by the hôtel-Dieu-le-Comte in Troyes has identified a significant number of children. Of 105 burials, forty-four (42%) were children. In one mass burial pit that, using radiocarbon dating, has been dated as likely from 1083 to 1125, fourteen out of the thirty-four individuals (41%) buried were children, with seven of the children between the ages of five and nine when they died, and four between the ages of ten and fourteen.[10] This is one of five mass burial pits found in the hospital cemetery, with each pit containing between nine and thirty-four bodies that were buried simultaneously or in quick succession, with the bodies sometimes being layered on top of each other, suggestive of an acute mortality crisis, such as flu, dysentery, smallpox, or famine.[11] In one mass burial pit, the smaller bodies of children filled the spaces between adults and the walls of the pit.[12] This was quite unusual, since in most cemeteries, infant and child burials were generally clustered together, separate from adult burials.[13] Among twenty-four individual burials (as opposed to mass burials) in the hospital's cemetery from the twelfth and thirteenth centuries, six (25%) were those of children.[14] While no skeletal remains of newborns and very few remains of toddlers have been found in the hospital's cemetery, it is clear that there were children in the hospital, despite the mid-thirteenth-century injunction that the hospital not receive abandoned children.[15]

At the recently excavated cemetery for the medieval hospital of St. John the Evangelist in Cambridge, where a total of 404 burials were uncovered (which is estimated to represent only 27% to 40% of the original burial population), one of the larger hospital burial sites excavated, 15.3 percent were

---

8. See Émile-Louis Richemond, *Recherche généalogiques sur la famille des seigneurs de Nemours du XIIe au XVe siècle*, vol. 1 (Fontainebleau, France: M. Bourges, 1907–08), xvi–xviii.

9. Le Grand, ed., *Statuts d'hôtels-Dieu*, art. 87, p. 115; on Vernon, see art. 13, p. 162.

10. Paresys et al., "Un nouvel cas de sépultures," 129–30.

11. There are other examples of "catastrophe cemeteries" owned by hospitals before the Black Death, including mass graves at the hospitals of the Holy Ghost at Lübeck, St. Mary Spital in London, and the Saint Esprit at Besançon. As Roberta Gilchrist and Barney Sloane put it, hospitals were perhaps seen as "natural sites for disposing of the dead of epidemics." See Roberta Gilchrist and Barney Sloane, eds., *Requiem: The Medieval Monastic Cemetery in Britain* (London: Museum of London Archaeology Service, 2005), 77.

12. Paresys et al., "Un nouvel cas de sépultures," 130.

13. Gilchrist, *Medieval Life*, 205.

14. Paresys et al., "Un nouvel cas de sépultures," 134.

15. See Cessford, "St. John's Hospital Cemetery," 86.

of children under the age of sixteen. No children under the age of five were found. This dearth of very young children in both the Cambridge and Troyes hospitals stands in sharp contrast to the peak mortality in the very young. Whereas peak mortality in most parish cemeteries of this time is generally found among the very young, the elderly, and young women of childbearing age, in the Cambridge hospital cemetery the mortality peaks among adults between the ages of twenty-six and forty-five.[16]

Among the other restrictions placed by these hospitals were statutes barring pregnant women due to the potential disruption caused by childbirth, although the hôtel-Dieu-le-Comte and the hospital of Provins were willing to accept postpartum women who needed to recover.[17] A number of other hospitals did accept pregnant women, including the hospital at Gosnay in the Pas-de-Calais, where in just one year (1335–36), six women delivered babies.[18] Perhaps because pregnant women were denied entry to the hôtel-Dieu-le-Comte, a few years after the hospital's statutes were drafted an aristocratic benefactor from Troyes had his house turned into a small hospital (that even included a chapel), housing up to six pregnant women.[19] Apart from pregnant women, no lepers were admitted in the largest hospitals of Troyes and Provins; the same was true of people with disabilities.[20] In short, like many hospitals of the time, the hôtel-Dieu-le-Comte and the hospital of Provins did not wish to accept people with chronic illnesses or permanent disabilities.[21]

Of course, poverty itself could be a chronic condition, and so one wonders how often hospitals were willing to let paupers live there indefinitely. As we have seen, it was common for thirteenth-century moralists to denounce "able-bodied" beggars. The "shame-faced poor"—those who suddenly fell on hard times—tended to elicit more sympathy because they had not always needed assistance, and it was hoped that with some short-term help, they would regain their independence. The statutes from 1297 for the hospital at Billom, in central France, for example, included a provision for the special admission of destitute people who were too ashamed to beg because they had come from noble or rich families. Interestingly, these statutes

---

16. Cessford, "St. John's Hospital Cemetery," 86.

17. Le Grand, ed., *Statuts d'hôtels-Dieu,* art. 88, p. 115.

18. Saunier, *"Le pauvre malade,"* 80–83.

19. AD: Aube 40H1 #204 (June 1270). During the later fourteenth century, the hôtel-Dieu of Beauvais rented a house for pregnant women, thereby creating a space for them while keeping them separate from the main hospital. See Leblond, "Les deux plus anciens comptes," 166.

20. Guignard, *Les anciens statuts,* art. 65, p. 62.

21. Saunier, *"Le pauvre malade,"* 58.

were composed by the Dominican cardinal, Hugues de Billom, whose own brother, Étienne, a knight, had himself fallen on hard times, forcing him to turn to others for financial assistance.[22] Thirteenth-century hospital sources most often refer to those staying at hospitals as "the poor," but it is difficult to know to what extent this was a socioeconomic designation or, with the growing sanctification of the poor, a way of conferring a heightened religious status on hospital guests—and by extension the hospital's mission. Moreover, the statutes for the hôtel-Dieu-le-Comte referred to "the poor, who are messengers of God," thus associating the hospital's guests with the figure of the suffering Christ.[23]

Many of the sick in hospitals did in fact come from the working poor. Among the people miraculously cured through a connection to the tomb of the saintly king of France, Louis IX, was a young swineherd named Moriset who suffered from a large tumor in his leg. He spent time convalescing at the hospital at Saumur; the other guests avoided him due to the foul smell of his oozing tumor.[24] When the domestic servant Amelot of Chaumont became ill at the age of thirty, her bourgeois master put her in the hospital of Saint-Denis, where she eventually died.[25] Jehanne of Serris, who was described as a poor wife and mother, was suddenly stricken with paralysis and spent one month at home, bedridden. She finally entered the hôtel-Dieu in Paris because of her husband's unwillingness "to do that which was necessary for her."[26] While at the hospital, she was taught to use crutches, which had been made by the hospital sisters. The sisters helped Jehanne get out of bed and helped her walk to the altar. Eager to return home to her husband and children, Jehanne was sent home on crutches as soon as she was able to get around by herself. As it turned out, though, even with crutches, she was unable to make it home on her own, and so her husband had to carry her. Upon returning home, Jehanne once again found that her husband was not willing to help her, so she was forced to beg for alms in front of her parish church.[27] Despite a severe physical disability, Guillot of Caux, who had migrated to Paris from Rouen, lived for at least five years without any institutional assistance. Rather, he was helped by a certain Herbert the Englishman, who lodged him for three years and gave him the services of his maidservant,

---

22. Fournier, "Les statuts de l'hôpital de Billom," 134, 138.
23. Guignard, *Les anciens statuts*, art. 6, pp. 34–35.
24. Farmer, *Surviving Poverty*, 57.
25. Farmer, *Surviving Poverty*, 100.
26. Farmer, *Surviving Poverty*, 120.
27. Farmer, *Surviving Poverty*, 88.

who helped Guillot dress, undress, and get in and out of bed. When Guillot contracted a fever and was no longer able to beg, he was finally forced to seek assistance at the hôtel-Dieu of Paris. In other words, a disability was generally not grounds for being admitted to a hospital so long as one was able to beg.[28] The one possible exception was at the Parisian hospital of the Quinze-Vingts, where there was an expectation that the blind would beg in order to earn their keep.[29]

Some donations made to hospitals were earmarked "for the use and sustenance of the poor and the sick of the said house."[30] A donation of "little pots and trays" was made, "considering how much the hospital of Saint-Étienne in Troyes does generously for the indigent and how devotedly it is dedicated to the works of mercy."[31] The cartulary for the hospital of Provins includes a record of a donation of tunics and shoes for "the poor of Christ."[32] The hospital of Saint-Nicolas in Troyes was described in a charter of 1205 as "a certain house of hospitality dedicated to and inclined toward the nourishment of the poor."[33] Other charters referred to "the poor who sleep and rise up there" and the "traveling poor" who were welcomed by the hospital brethren.[34] The thirteenth-century statutes for the hôtel-Dieu of Paris referred to the "healthy poor," living both inside and outside the hospital, who were served by the hospital's personnel.[35]

The sick in hospitals were sometimes differentiated from the other poor, with a separate space being allocated for the sick. In his testament of 1299,

---

28. Farmer, *Surviving Poverty*, 90; see also Irina Metzler, *Disability in Medieval Europe: Thinking about Physical Impairment during the High Middle Ages, c. 1100–1400* (London: Routledge, 2006), 246–50.

29. Farmer, *Surviving Poverty*, 89. See also Farmer, "From Personal Charity," 18–19. On the Quinze-Vingts, see Mark P. O'Tool, "The *povres avugles* of the Hospital of the Quinze-Vingts," in *Difference and Identity in Francia and Medieval France*, ed. Meredith Cohen and Justine Firnhaber-Baker (Farnham, U.K.: Ashgate, 2010), 157–74.

30. AD: Aube 40H1 no. 59; 40H189, fol. 27–27v (1264) (cartulary for the hôtel-Dieu-le-Comte): "ad usitationem et sustentationem pauperum et infirmorum dictus domus."

31. AD: Aube 40H1, no. 28 (1218); 40H189, fol. 65 (cartulary): "considerans quantum domus Dei beati Stephani Trecen liberaliter indigentibus est posita et operibus misericordie devote dedicata."

32. Dupraz, nos. 200, 252; AD: Seine-et-Marne, 11HdtA12, fol. 60v–61, 78v–79.

33. AD: Aube 43H12, lay 31, cote A, no. 2 (donation charter by the cathedral chapter of Saint-Pierre to the hospital of Saint-Nicolas, 1205).

34. AD: Aube 43H12, lay. 31, cote A, no. 43 (1285): "povres qui illec sont couchié et levé;" AD: Aube 43H57, lay. 38, cote H, no. 3 bis: "povres passans."

35. Le Grand, ed., *Statuts d'hôtels-Dieu*, art. 53, p. 51. Whereas the thirteenth-century statutes for the hôtel-Dieu of Paris referred to the "healthy poor" ("pauperum sanorum"), by the fifteenth century this hospital had exclusively become a place of care for the sick, no longer housing the healthy poor. Moreover, during the fifteenth century most of the sick at the hôtel-Dieu Paris were not poor beggars, but rather artisans and salaried persons who went there to recuperate from an illness. See Jéhanno, "'Sustenter les povres malades,'" 141–50.

which the dean of the cathedral of Troyes composed when he himself was physically ill, Denis de Champguyon made separate bequests of pittances "for the sick" of the hospital of Saint-Nicolas and a good feather bed "for the poor lying" there.[36] A rent was donated in 1254 to the hospital of Provins for the purchase of incense that could be burned in the chapel of the infirmary.[37] At the hôtel-Dieu-le-Comte, the sick were housed in an "infirmary" or "infirmary for the poor," separate from the space for the healthy poor ("ospital" or "salle").[38] Likewise, a charter from 1307 for the hospital of Saint-Nicolas of Troyes refers to the "infirmary for the sick," and a charter from a few years earlier mentions the "infirmary for women," suggesting that not only was there a separate space in the hospital for the sick but also that sick women were housed in a separate space from sick men.[39] From the hospital's account book for 1300–01, we know that the hospital spent 12 *s.* that year to repair the latrines used by the sick.[40] Bequests to hospitals were also sometimes specifically directed to the sick as opposed to the poor. A donation of some hens was assigned to "the weaker" and "more sick ones" at the hôtel-Dieu-le-Comte.[41]

Archaeological evidence unearthed from medieval hospital cemeteries has told widely diverging stories about the health of those who died in these institutions. At the cemetery for the hospital of Saint Mary Spital in London, for instance, the skeletal remains of 10,500 individuals have been excavated, including a significant number of pregnant women, poor women, and children.[42] One-third of the skeletal remains in this cemetery showed signs of pathology, in contrast to the typical English parish cemetery, in which only 10 percent generally show signs of disease.[43] The skeletal remains excavated from Saint Mary Spital suggest that a significant number of the sick poor received medical treatment (either inside the hospital or earlier in their lives); in one case, a fractured femur had been set and healed properly, and

36. AD: Aube G2633 (1299).

37. Dupraz, no. 87; AD: Seine-et-Marne 11Hdt A12,fol. 29v–30.

38. AD: Aube 40H189, fol. 82 (1228); Le Grand, ed., *Statuts d'hôtels-Dieu,* art. 83, pp. 114–15.

39. AD: Aube 43H12, lay 31, cote A, no. 49 (1307); BnF ms 9111, fol. 300 (account book for 1302–03).

40. BnF ms lat. 9111 (account book for the hospital of Saint-Nicolas for 1300–01), fol. 285.

41. AD: Aube 40H1, no. 19, #230 (1212): "debiliores," "magis infirmi."

42. William White, "Excavations at St Mary Spital: Burial of the 'Sick Poore' of Medieval London, the Evidence of Illness and Hospital Treatment," in *The Medieval Hospital and Medical Practice,* ed. Barbara S. Bowers (Aldershot, U.K.: Ashgate, 2007), 59–60; Christopher Thomas, Barney Sloane, and Christopher Phillpotts, *Excavations at the Priory and Hospital of St. Mary Spital, London* (London: Lavenham Press, 1997).

43. White, "Excavations," 60–62.

in another case, a fractured skull had also healed well.[44] Many of the skeletal remains also showed indications of severe disabilities, this despite the fact that it was common for hospitals to bar those with chronic disabilities.

Archaeological evidence uncovered from hospital cemeteries elsewhere in Europe, however, has raised questions about whether hospital populations were necessarily sicker than the general population. The burials found in the cemetery of the hôtel-Dieu-le-Comte in Troyes, for example, revealed evidence of common infectious diseases like tuberculosis and rickets as well as individuals with dislocated hips, bone fractures, bone loss, and so forth, but in general, the individuals buried in this hospital's cemetery show a relatively weak presence of pathology, and their conditions do not seem to differ significantly from those buried in the parish cemetery.[45] The same has been found with respect to the cemetery of the hospital of St. John the Evangelist in Cambridge. Among the 404 skeletal remains excavated there, "little evidence [has been found] for serious conditions within the cemetery that would have required particular medical care."[46] There were certainly cases of chronic conditions that would have caused pain, suffering, and even mortality, including tuberculosis, DISH (the bony hardening of ligaments that attach to the spine), inflammatory infections (especially on the lower legs), and tumors, but the prevalence of these conditions does not appear to be any higher than what one finds in other cemeteries.[47] Even in terms of the level of poverty of the hospital population, the cemetery's skeletal remains indicated a high prevalence of dental plaque concretions, usually a sign of both poor oral hygiene combined with a diet rich in carbohydrates.[48] A severely poor and malnourished population would not be likely to show signs of a carbohydrate-rich diet, perhaps affirming what at least one papal letter suggests, namely that the Cambridge hospital was known to also house "poor scholars," known to eat (and drink) a diet rich in cereals.[49]

One complicating factor in drawing conclusions about the identities of those who were cared for by a hospital based on an analysis of the burials excavated in the hospital's cemetery is the question of who was interred there. The team that excavated the Cambridge hospital's cemetery believed that the hospital's personnel (its master and brethren) and its major benefactors

---

44. White, "Excavations," 64.
45. Paresys et al., "Un nouvel cas de sépultures," 134.
46. Cessford, "St. John's Hospital Cemetery," 99.
47. Cessford, "St. John's Hospital Cemetery," 100.
48. Cessford, "St. John's Hospital Cemetery," 100.
49. Rubin, *Charity and Community*, 162.

were buried in the hospital's chapel, meaning that the cemetery population was made up exclusively of those the hospital cared for and housed.[50] There is evidence from other English hospitals, however, such as the hospitals of St. Bartholomew in London and St. John at Ely, that the personnel and the poor were buried together in "mixed" outdoor cemeteries.[51] Furthermore, if we look at monastic cemeteries during the twelfth and thirteenth centuries, while it is true that noble patrons preferred to be buried in monastic churches, middle-ranking patrons and even those who were members of the knightly class tended to be buried in cemeteries, together with the monastic brethren.[52] In other words, we cannot assume that those populating hospital cemeteries are only representative of the poor and sick of these institutions, since a hospital's personnel and even some of its donors may well have also been interred there. In some cases, a hospital's poor and sick were buried in a cemetery belonging to another religious institution. The hôtel-Dieu of Reims, for example, which was a dependent of the cathedral chapter, did not have its own cemetery during the thirteenth and fourteenth centuries. It used the cemetery of the Augustinian abbey of Saint-Denis in Reims (which also had a dependent hospital), located between the abbey's church and the Dominican convent, to bury its poor and sick, a practice that at various points the abbey sought to bring to a halt.[53]

While the poor in thirteenth-century hospitals were at times differentiated from the sick, they were also often lumped together as the "povres malades" ("sick poor"). Apart from serving as an economic or religious designation, poverty could also signify what was perceived by others as a physical and psychological weakness or impairment. A "pauper" might be considered poor by virtue of being distressed or in a dependent position, and in this way, any number of categories of people were at times considered "pauperes" regardless of

---

50. Cessford, "St. John's Hospital Cemetery," 62. Gilchrist confirms that those buried in hospital churches tend to show signs of dental disease, suggestive of a sweet diet, DISH (often associated with obesity), and were generally taller than those buried in outdoor cemeteries, perhaps indicative of better nutrition. All of this points to a burial population of higher economic status. See Gilchrist, *Contemplation and Action*, 30.

51. Gilchrist and Sloane, eds., *Requiem*, 61.

52. Gilchrist and Sloane, eds., *Requiem*, 61–62. As Gilchrist and Sloane point out, a minority of those buried in monastic cemeteries during this period were lay, with most of the laity buried in parish cemeteries. Nonetheless, apart from monastic cemeteries, the cemeteries of hospitals and friaries were becoming increasingly popular burial sites for the laity.

53. Desportes, *Reims et les Rémois*, 547 and note 43. In 1349, at the height of the Black Death, the canons of Saint-Denis in Reims appealed to the pope to authorize the consecration of a new cemetery for the burial of the sick poor from the hôtel-Dieu of Notre Dame, which did not have its own cemetery, and which had long relied on Saint-Denis's cemetery. AD: Marne (Reims), 54H53 (23 October 1349), bull of Clement VI.

their social class. As Mark O'Tool has shown, most of the "poor blind" housed at the hospital of the Quinze-Vingts in Paris were not actually poor; instead, they came from the middling and lower levels of the Parisian bourgeoisie. Yet in contemporary terms, their blindness rendered them poor, and the same was true for any disability or illness during the high Middle Ages.[54]

Despite the ubiquitous references in hospital sources to "the pauperes"—a kind of blanket term used to refer to those who were admitted to hospitals—not all hospital guests were poor, and not all of them were even necessarily sick. The statutes for the hôtel-Dieu-le-Comte and the hospital of Provins refer to those spending the night at the hospital while on "worldly business." These guests were not required to attend Matins like the sick poor.[55] There is also evidence that the hôtel-Dieu-le-Comte was renting out hospital guest rooms to traveling merchants. When the nobleman Guy de Dampierre gave one of his servants to this hospital in 1208, he did so with the intention that the servant would help the hospital brothers house their "guests" ("hospites") on "market days and beyond," almost certainly a reference to merchant guests who stayed at the hospital.[56] The account book from 1300–01 for the hospital of Saint-Nicolas in Troyes records that the hospital received 6 l. that year for the room and board of a certain Michel de Froiderive, whom the account books for subsequent years continue to list as a paying boarder.[57] The account books also refer to certain rooms as the "camer[e] hospitum," which most likely housed the *donati* or other higher-class guests who may have been paying for their stays.[58] According to the account book for 1383, the hospital had a room for guests ("chambre aux hostes") in addition to thirty-eight beds in the "ospital" and "l'anfermerie."[59] It was common for hospitals elsewhere in northern France to house various kinds of boarders. When the archbishop of Rouen visited the hospital at Gournay, he found that it was accustomed to receiving healthy travelers, including the royal sergeants who were charged with overseeing the nearby Lyons forest. Although the archbishop did not object to the hospital's providing hospitality to these guests, he insisted that they sleep with the sick.[60]

54. O'Tool, *"Povres Avugles,"* 157–73.

55. Le Grand, ed., *Statuts d'hôtels-Dieu,* art. 33, p. 109.

56. AD: Aube 40H1, no. 15 (March, 1208): "Ita quod fratres domus supradicte ponent et deponent ad libitum suum in nundinis et extra nundinas hospites."

57. BnF ms lat. 9111, fol. 291b: "a Michelino de Frigid Rippa de summa sex librarum pro victu suo unius anni."

58. BnF ms lat. 9111, fol. 285v.

59. AD: Aube G3395, fol. 1.

60. *The Register of Eudes,* 471.

Testaments that were written while testators were lying sick at the hospital at Laon also reveal the wide-ranging social and geographic origins of its guests.[61] They included priests from the city and from rural parishes, some of whom used the hospital as a retirement home, as well as elite townspeople, rich merchants, rural landowners who came to the hospital from far away and returned home after recovering from an illness, minor artisans, peasants, and even the occasional member of the mid-level aristocracy.[62] The knight Pierre de Mortiers, for example, brought his gravely ill son to the hospital of Laon, where he ended up dying.[63] Another knight thanked the same hospital for the care it had provided to his father.[64] As we noted in chapter 3, some of the hospital donors who expressed gratitude for a hospital's care may well have spent time there themselves in convalescence. In such cases, one wonders whether a hospital might have viewed certain sick guests as potential benefactors, a faint echo of the story of Huguette Clark, with which we began this chapter.

Some of the stories of miraculous cures that were recorded as part of medieval canonization inquests involved individuals who had spent time convalescing at a hospital, since it was common for those awaiting a cure at a shrine to spend time at a hospital. The accounts of the events leading up to these miraculous cures also provide a window into the social class of the sick in hospitals as well as the kinds of infirmities from which they suffered. A disabled sixteen-year-old who was allegedly cured by visiting Elizabeth of Hungary's tomb at Marburg spent four weeks in 1232 at the hospital that Elizabeth herself had founded, making daily visits to the saint's tomb, before finally receiving a cure.[65] A thirteen-year-old boy with severe kyphosis, a contorted neck, bones protruding from his thighs, and legs that were twisted around each other, spent eleven weeks awaiting a cure at Elizabeth's tomb, all the while living at the hospital.[66] As Irina Metzler has pointed out, the shrines that were the sites of such miraculous cures themselves functioned as "quasi-hospitals," with those overseeing the shrines providing physical assistance to those who came in search of a cure.[67] Even though the cure was generally

---

61. Saint-Denis, *L'hôtel-Dieu de Laon,* 117.

62. Saint-Denis, *L'hôtel-Dieu de Laon,* 117–18. Daniel Le Blévec, in contrast, has argued that when the wealthy became sick, they did not come to hospitals but were treated at home. See Le Blévec, *La part du pauvre,* 778.

63. Saint-Denis, *L'hôtel-Dieu de Laon,* 118.

64. Saint-Denis, *L'hôtel-Dieu de Laon,* 118.

65. Metzler, *Disability,* 246.

66. Metzler, *Disability,* 249.

67. Metzler, *Disability,* 169.

linked in the minds of many to the disabled person's visits to the saint's tomb, it could take weeks before there were any signs of physical improvement, and during this period of waiting, the disabled person often spent time convalescing at a nearby hospital.[68] In one of the miracles associated with the Countess Dauphine de Puimichel, the judge mayor of Provence, who happened to be visiting Apt, was admitted to the hospital there after being stricken with head pain. This pain recurred every year for ten years during the winter months. None of the treatments he received from doctors (including a royal doctor) worked, but when the Countess Dauphine came to the hospital where he was residing, she was miraculously able to cure him.[69]

The sick who were cared for by medieval hospitals were sometimes members of the hospital's own religious community. As we saw in the last chapter, some women and men may have joined a hospital community in part because it offered them greater security than living alone, particularly when they became too infirm to be self-sufficient. In one of the miracles associated with Saint Louis of Toulouse, a certain hospital sister from Marseille reportedly lived for more than eight years in the hospital, suffering great pain from a fistula in her eyes. She consulted with doctors and was given many medicines, but no remedy was found until she turned to Saint Louis of Toulouse, who was reported to have miraculously cured her.[70] In the section of an account book for the hospital of Saint-Nicolas in Troyes for 1388–89, a certain Jehan le Capitain is listed as having both been one of the hospital's renters and someone who was often employed by the hospital, making barrels for wine ("relieur de vins"). Most interesting for our purposes, however, is that Jehan is recorded in the hospital's account book as having "died a poor man in the 'ospital' of the 'ostel.'"[71] In short, one of the hospital's own workers had died a poor man in the hospital's infirmary. Agnès la Galoise, on the other hand, who was probably a *donata* at the same hospital, lived, according to the account book for 1382, in her own room, high up in the "ostel," even after becoming sick. When she died in August of 1389, the hospital went to the expense of buying her a coffin, reflective of her higher social status, and the cathedral's bell ringer dug a pit in which to bury her. At her death, she still owned a house in Troyes, which the hospital sold, along with her bed

---

68. Metzler, *Disability*, 256.

69. Cambell, O.F.M., ed., *Enquête*, 367–68.

70. "Processus canonizationis et legendae variae Sancti Ludovici, O.F.M.," *Analecta Franciscana*, vol. 7 (1951): 295.

71. AD: Aube G2530, fol. 10v: "a esté mors povres homs en l'ospital de l'ostel"; Gesret, "Soustenir les povres," 213.

CHAPTER 6

...nted them with a rare opportunity for spiritual conversion and redemp-
...n Humbert's discussion of how to preach to the sick in hospitals, he
...d all would-be preachers to remember that their listeners would likely
...er and impatient. He therefore recommended that preachers address
...k pleasantly, usefully, and comfortingly, and that the preachers find
...o teach their sick listeners to be patient.[91] (In a sermon on how to
...o lepers, he advised preachers never to refer to leprosy in front of
...rs but rather only to speak about their condition in the most gen-
...ns so as to avoid upsetting them.)[92] According to Humbert, the sick
...o be persuaded that God did not inflict illness on them out of hatred,
...an enemy would, but rather out of a father's sense of love.
...bert advised preachers who might address sick audiences in hospitals
...he ways that illness can foster moral virtue and serve as a restraint
...on the kinds of bad habits regularly committed while in a state of
...th. Drawing on the Book of Ecclesiasticus 31:2, Humbert pointed
...grievous sickness returns the soul sober, since it restricts it from
...hts just as sobriety does."[93] An infirmity, he argued, provides an
...y for the purgation of sin and conversion from bad habits. Hum-
...layed with the word purgatio, suggesting that by being physically
...their capacity to sin, the sick would later be spared the suffer-
...gatory and Hell, since they had experienced their purgatory on
...Humbert was echoing Gregory the Great's explanation in the
...lis of illness being sent by God as a "purification of the present
...umbert put it plainly, "So therefore it is evident that sickness is
...od than health, since it guards from many sins, and it makes
...m sins."[95] The sick, he went on, need to be reminded of the
...l in 2 Corinthians 12:9, "Gladly will I glory in my sicknesses."
...group of lepers, Jacques de Vitry also stressed the ways that
...ities served a moral and religious purpose: "In equal measure,
...ished by the whip of infirmity, is not able to attack you much
...ragance."[96] Indeed, Jacques went so far as to suggest that the
...cked a person's flesh with infirmities, the more God cared for

...e eruditione praedicatorum, 1.2.92, in Maxima bibliotheca, ed. de la Bigne, 502.
...rosy, 338.
...e eruditione praedicatorum, 1.2.92, in Maxima bibliotheca, ed. de la Bigne, 502.
...n and François-Olivier Touati, Voluntate Dei leprosus: Les lépreux entre conversion
...e et XIIIème siècles (Spoleto: Centro Italiano di Studi Sull'alto Medioevo, 1991),
...his phrase, see also Touati, Maladie, 195–6.
...eruditione praedicatorum, 1.2.92, in Maxima bibliotheca, ed. de la Bigne, 502.
...e, 123n160.

and other property.[72] There were also cases of someone who was sick, decid-ing to join a hospital's religious community after being restored to health.[73]

In addition to taking in boarders, the hospital of Saint-Nicolas in Troyes also took in clerical students who were studying at Troyes, functioning, in that regard, like the houses of "Bons Enfants" in Reims and other cities.[74] The students received lodging at the hospital in a separate space, referred to as the "calamité." In exchange for being housed there, they were expected to perform occasional services for the hospital, such as traveling to collect rents from the hospital's tenants.[75] In 1307 a testamentary bequest was made to the hospital with the purpose of buying charcoal for the clerical students living there.[76] Some of these clerical students, who may have been studying with the cathedral cantor, stayed at the hospital for several years, and their names repeatedly appear in the hospital's annual account books. Jaquinot, a "povre clerc" who was staying at "la calmité de l'ostel" of Saint-Nicolas in 1381–82, was still living there in 1383–84.[77] Likewise, the foundation charter for the hospital at Tonnerre repeatedly refers to the "quatre enfants clercs," essentially choirboys who assisted the hospital's chaplains and master.[78]

The Meaning of Care

When we think of the care that the poor and sick received in medieval hos-pitals, we tend to think of the way that their physical needs were met by being bathed and given food, clothing, a bed, and so forth. Yet "sacramental medicine" was at the very heart of what medieval hospitals did.[79] Canon 22 of the Fourth Lateran Council asserted that sickness was a form of divine punishment for sin and therefore required spiritual healing before any kind

72. AD: Aube G2524 (1381–82), fol. 28v, G2525, fol. 28 (1382–83), G2530, fol. 23 (1388–89); Ges-ret, "Soustenir les povres," 218, 244, 246.

73. Henderson, Renaissance Hospital, 216.

74. AD: Aube 43H12 lay. 1, cote A, no. 49 (Nov. 1307). On the "Bons Enfants" in general, see Reitzel, "Medieval Houses," 179–207.

75. AD: Aube G2523, fol. 43 (account book for 1383–84). Gesret, "Soustenir les povres," 213–14.

76. AD: Aube 43H12, lay 31, cote A, no. 49 (1307): "clericis scolaribus in dicta domo residentibus [...] pro carbonibus emendis"; Gesret, "Soustenir les povres," 214.

77. AD: Aube G 2524, fol. 24 (account book of 1381–82); G 2526, fol. 43 (account book for 1383–84); Gesret, "Soustenir les povres," 213–14.

78. Challe, Histoire du comté, 206.

79. Peregrine Horden, "A Non-Natural Environment: Medicine without Doctors and the Medi-eval European Hospital," in The Medieval Hospital and Medical Practice, ed. Barbara S. Bowers (Alder-shot, U.K.: Ashgate, 2007), 133–45. See also Elma Brenner, "The Care of the Sick and the Needy in Twelfth- and Thirteenth-Century Rouen," in Society and Culture in Medieval Rouen, 911–1300, ed. Leonie V. Hicks and Elma Brenner (Turnhout, Belgium: Brepols, 2013), 339–68.

of physical healing.[80] In fact there were no separate medical and religious categories during the high Middle Ages, with spiritual medicine considered an integral part of medicine writ large. Christ was considered the preeminent "medicus." By the thirteenth century, many hospitals had a central infirmary hall that opened up onto the chapel on the east end so that those who were not well enough to get out of bed could nonetheless fully participate in religious services, with the corpus Christi carried to them in bed.[81] The chaplains and choirboys of the hospital at Tonnerre were enjoined to sing the Mass and canonical hours in a loud enough voice that the sick could hear from their beds.[82] The dean of the cathedral at Laon referred to the hospital as "the house where each day the Son is sacrificed to the Father," an indication of the value he placed on the daily celebration of the Mass there.[83] In addition to the celebration of the Mass, at many hospitals the canonical hours were recited and other sacraments administered. The sacrament of penance was regarded as particularly important, since it was thought to bring about the purification of the confessee and thus help in that person's convalescence. Moreover, when new guests were first received, they first had to confess their sins to a priest and then have their head and feet bathed, which was itself considered a religious, purifying act.[84] Physical healing was thought to depend on penance and sacerdotal mediation more generally.

The inextricable connection between spiritual and physical healing lay at the heart of the medieval hospital's mission. As Peregrine Horden has observed, the liturgy, sacraments, religious offices, and relics were all considered as central to hospital care.[85] The Fourth Lateran Council of 1215 made plain that spiritual health should be prioritized over physical medicine, since there was no possibility of physical healing without sacramental

---

80. Tanner, ed., *Decrees*, 1:245–46.

81. As Lindy Grant has shown, this model of a hospital with an integrated infirmary hall and chapel only became the norm during the thirteenth century, replacing the model found in twelfth-century hospital foundations, such as at Angers, Le Mans, and Laon, where the chapel and infirmary hall were separate spaces. See Lindy Grant, "The Chapel of the Hospital of Saint-Jean at Angers: Acta, Statutes, Architecture, and Interpretation," in *Architecture and Interpretation: Essays for Eric Fernie*, ed. Jill A. Franklin, T. A. Heslop, and Christine Stevenson (Woodbridge, U.K.: Boydell & Brewer, 2013), 306–14.

82. Challe, *Histoire du comté*, 207.

83. Saint-Denis, *L'hôtel-Dieu de Laon*, 106.

84. Le Grand, *Statuts d'hôtels-Dieu*, art. 73, p. 113; Saint-Denis, *L'hôtel-Dieu de Laon*, 103.

85. Peregrine Horden has also called attention to the ways in which a hospital's physical environment (gardens, sounds, etc.) was believed to play a role in bodily and spiritual healing. See Horden, "Religion as Medicine: Music in Medieval Hospitals," in *Religion and Medicine in the Middle Ages*, ed. Peter Biller and Joseph Ziegler (York, 2001), 135–54. See also Christopher Page, "Music and Medicine in the Thirteenth Century," in *Music as Medicine: The History of Music Therapy Since Antiquity*, ed. Peregrine Horden (Aldershot, U.K.: Ashgate, 2000), 109–19.

---

medicine.[86] Drawing on a tradition that stretched (and particularly the homilies and *Liber pastoralis* was common for thirteenth-century preachers to to nourishing food and life-saving medicine. This function of preaching carried particular resonan pitals, where preaching was a regular occurren important part of the care that was provided to and Mary Rouse have pointed out, by the thirt acquired a "quasi-sacramental status."[87] Indee of Romans, who composed model sermons f claimed that whereas the sacraments could someone already prepared to receive them, pr vert listeners, to move them to faith, and t sacraments. In one of his sermons, he lame to church, heard sermons, or knew anyth tion. Rather, in their anger at being poor, t stressed how important it was for the poor tenets of the Christian faith and confess ar In another sermon, he observed that the *simplices*, rarely heard talk about God—an word of God.[89] Humbert ended his serr ing that although he could not offer the able to offer them a spiritual (and ther the word of God. What the sick in hosp not money or even physical healing bu ing.[90] Humbert's words were more th they reflected a sincere belief in the for listeners who were afflicted with

One of the principal themes of was that physical misery and suffe served an important divine purpo upbraid their sick audiences for those afflicted with illness that the

---

86. Tanner, ed., *Decrees* 1:245–46.

87. Richard H. Rouse and Mary A. Ro *ulus florum" of Thomas of Ireland* (Toronto

88. Humbert, *De eruditione praedicate* also Murray, "Religion," 298–99.

89. Humbert, *De eruditione praedica*

90. Humbert, *De eruditione praedica*

that person's soul: "Man is struck in body so that he may be restored and illuminated in conscience."[97]

In his *ad status* sermons "to lepers and the abject," the Franciscan Guibert de Tournai stressed the way that physical infirmity represented a divine test:

> Let those who have been tested not say, "God hates us and has abandoned us." For a knight does not hate the horse on whom he presses spurs, nor the craftsman the iron that he pounds vigorously, nor the vine-dresser the bunch of grapes from which he elicits wine by pressing and trampling with his feet, nor the fuller the cloth which he strikes with a pole, nor the pelterer the hide which he strikes with a rod, nor God the man whom he attacks with the whip of infirmity or temptation.[98]

Guibert went on to argue that God only tests friends and that he does so in order that they might be cleansed, humiliated, and then crowned. Being tempted and humiliated leads to greater self-understanding, including a recognition of one's fragility and dependence on divine grace for the strength to resist temptation. "Just as the continuation of health and prosperity are a sign of divine reprobation," Guibert suggested, "so temptation and infirmity of the body are a sign of love."[99] Guibert exhorted his audience not to pity themselves or interpret their misfortune as a sign of divine anger. Instead, he reminded them, "The true mother loves her sick son with more tenderness and assists him with greater care."[100] In another sermon addressed to lepers and the abject, Guibert sought to reassure his listeners that if they endured their afflictions patiently, their sickness would render them martyrs, and they would not have to experience another purgatory.[101] In adumbrating the virtues of bodily infirmities, he pointed out the ways that illness promotes humility and spiritual repentance. Whereas the "spoiled and healthy" think little about death, since it is at their backs, "you," Guibert commended his audience, "truly [have death] before your face."[102] Thus, Guibert and other preachers sought to comfort the sick, telling them that instead of despairing, they should rejoice that their suffering on earth prepared them spiritually for salvation in the world to come.

---

97. Touati, *Maladie*, 199. See also Rawcliffe, *Leprosy*, 57.

98. Guibert de Tournai, sermon 2, in Bériou and Touati, *Voluntate Dei leprosus*, 138.

99. Guibert, sermon 2, in Bériou and Touati, *Voluntate Dei leprosus*, 139. Guibert makes this same point in Sermon 3, in *Voluntate Dei*, ed. Bériou and Touati, 151.

100. Guibert, sermon 2, in Bériou and Touati, *Voluntate Dei leprosus*, 139–40.

101. Guibert, sermon 3, in Bériou and Touati, *Voluntate Dei leprosus*, 150.

102. Guibert, sermon 3, in Bériou and Touati, *Voluntate Dei leprosus*, 152.

Apart from what was thought to be the spiritual medicine provided by preaching, in some cases hospitals contained relics that were also thought to have the power to heal those who were sick. The hospital of Saint-Mary Magdalene in Rouen, for example, had relics that had been given by King Louis IX and delivered by Archbishop Eudes Rigaud.[103] To the archbishop's horror, he once found while visiting this hospital that stalls had been erected, both along the chapel wall and at the entrance to the hospital, where various items, such as hoods, were being sold. Eudes found it "unseemly" and "improper" for the hospital and its chapel to function as a market.[104] The hospitals at Champlain, Corbeil, and Pontoise all claimed to possess pieces of the true cross, while the hospital of Longjumeau maintained that it had the tooth of Saint Lawrence.[105] The hospital at Corbeil claimed to have the relics of Saints Rustique, Catherine, and Eustache as well as oil from the tomb of Saint Nicolas.[106] Saint Louis participated in the translation of relics to the hospital for the blind, the Quinze-Vignts, in Paris.[107] In addition to their curative powers, relics were also valuable in bringing pilgrims and potential donors to a hospital.[108] Marguerite of Burgundy bequeathed her relics to her executors for the benefit of the hospital that she had founded in Tonnerre, and it is possible that these relics had already been placed in the hospital during her lifetime.[109] While it is not known if any of Champagne's hospitals possessed relics of their own, there were important relics in both Provins—notably, the relics of Saint-Ayoul—and Troyes, where the abbey of Saint-Loup housed the relics of Bishop Lupus of Troyes. In Troyes, thanks in part to the efforts of Count Henri the Liberal, the chapter of Saint-Étienne allegedly possessed the relics of Saint Altinus and Saint Potentianus (the third-century bishop of Sens), a piece of the shroud of Christ, a fragment of the prophet Elijah's arm, a tooth of Lazarus, two teeth of Saint Geneviève, and the relics of Saint Étienne as well as relics associated with Thomas Becket, fragments of the Cross, a dish from the Last Supper, and the skull, bones, and teeth of Saint Anthony.[110] Some of these had been purchased by Count Henri, and others had been brought back from the Fourth Crusade by

---

103. *The Register of Eudes*, 687.

104. *The Register of Eudes*, 570.

105. Le Grand, ed., *Les maisons-Dieu et les léproseries*, cxxvii.

106. Le Grand, ed., *Les maisons-Dieu et les léproseries*, cxxvii.

107. Anne E. Lester, "Saint Louis and Cîteaux Revisited: Cistercian Commemoration and Devotion during the Capetian Century, 1214–1314," in *The Capetian Century, 1214–1314*, ed. William Chester Jordan and Rebecca Phillips (Turnhout, Belgium: Brepols, 2017), 33n1.

108. *The Register of Eudes*, 687.

109. Courtenay, "The Hospital of Notre Dame des Fontenilles, 90–91.

110. Evergates, *Henry the Liberal*, 67, 140.

Bishop Garnier de Traînel. By the fourteenth century, the chapter had more than 240 reliquaries; one can imagine that pilgrims visiting Saint-Étienne might have stayed at the neighboring hospital.[111] The sick or disabled living in the hospital might also have visited these relics, which were just across the street, in the hope of being cured.

In addition to relics, some of the religious images that appeared in hospitals and hospital chapels conveyed the connection between penance and healing. Marcia Kupfer, for example, has studied the pictorial program of a crypt inside the Romanesque collegiate church of Saint-Aignan, south of Blois.[112] The canons of this church likely oversaw several local hospitals, and Kupfer argues that the crypt's pictorial focus on the relationship between physical healing and the divine forgiveness of sin bolstered the notion that the canons were the indispensable mediators between the sick on the one hand, and the saints and God on the other. In one scene, three paupers with crutches in their hands petition for grace and offer votive gifts and prayers at the feet of Christ and the apostles, who offer them blessings. As the hospitals at Tonnerre, Laon, and Angers illustrate, it was common for thirteenth-century hospitals to cover certain walls with frescoes and painted hangings.[113] Paintings such as the boss in the chapel of the hospital at Angers, which was decorated with the Agnus Dei, may have served not only to reinforce the idea of the works of mercy as penance and valuable preparation for the Last Judgment, as discussed in chapter 1, but also to strengthen the spirits of the sick poor. The devotional images found in hospitals, whether in paintings or sculpted reliefs on portals, were also probably meant to play a therapeutic role. As was often the case, visual imagery reinforced central themes in sermons that were preached in hospitals, such as the idea that physical adversity served as a divine test.

Although it was relatively rare for there to be physicians working in hospitals during this period, there are some scattered references to the presence of physicians in twelfth- and thirteenth-century hospitals in Champagne.[114]

111. Evergates, *Henry the Liberal*, 68, 128.

112. Marcia Kupfer, *The Art of Healing: Painting for the Sick and the Sinner in a Medieval Town* (University Park: Pennsylvania State University Press, 2003).

113. Alain Saint-Denis, "Soins du corps et médecine contre la souffrance à l'hôtel-Dieu de Laon au XIIIe siècle," *Médiévales* 8 (1985): 38; Christian Davy, *La peinture murale romane dans les pays de la Loire: L'indicible et le ruban plissé* (Laval: Société d'Archéologie et d'Histoire de la Mayenne, 1999), 326–29.

114. On the presence of canons at the cathedral of Laon who were also doctors, and their possible connections to the hospital, which was overseen by the cathedral chapter, see Saint-Denis, *L'hôtel-Dieu*, 109–14.

As noted in the last chapter, a "physicus" (physician) appears both in the martyrological obituary for the hospital of Provins and as a witness in 1281 and 1283 in the hospital's cartulary.[115] One of the earliest mentions of a practicing physician in a French hospital was at the leprosary of Les Deux Eaux, near Troyes, in 1151.[116] It was also observed in the last chapter that "Magister Herbertus medicus," who held a prebend at the chapter of Saint-Étienne in 1199 and whose prebend Thibaut III gave to the poor of the hospital, might have been the same Magister Herbertus who was serving as the *magister* of the hôtel-Dieu-le-Comte in 1206.[117] Troyes and Provins, in other words, appear to have been unusual in having practicing physicians already in the twelfth and thirteenth centuries, perhaps due to the fact that Troyes was internationally known as a center for medical studies during this period, with its medical school considered the equal of those in Auxerre, Paris, and Chartres.[118] Some of the most famous doctors and medical academicians lived in the province of Sens, including Aldobrandino of Siena, who lived in Troyes. In his influential *Régime du corps*, which he wrote in 1256, Aldobrandino wrote extensively about bodily hygiene and the relationship between diet and health, subjects that were of great relevance for the care of the sick in contemporary hospitals. At the very least, Aldobrandino took interest in the hospitals of his adopted city of Troyes, bequeathing his own house to the hospital of Saint-Antoine.[119] But it is also quite possible that Aldobrandino had spent time sharing his medical expertise in this or other Troyen hospitals. There are also records of two other doctors making pious bequests to the leprosary of Les Deux Eaux outside Troyes: a certain Gauthier in 1220 and Perrinet in 1269.[120] In the 1389/90 account book for Saint-Nicolas of Troyes, there is a reference to a sick hospital brother being visited by a certain Master D—— the Jew, who received 10 *s.* from the hospital; this may record a Jewish doctor coming to the hospital to treat a sick brother.[121]

While hospital statutes made no reference to the relatively rare presence of physicians, they did display an interest in how the sick and poor were treated by the hospital's personnel. The statutes for the hôtel-Dieu-le-Comte

---

115. *Obituaires de la province de Sens*, 1:943; Dupraz, nos. 431, 353; AD: Seine-et-Marne, 11HdtA12, fol.106, 125–26. See Touati, *Maladie et société*, 457–58. See Jacquart, *Le milieu médical*, 127–37, 73.

116. Jacquart, *Le milieu médical*, 128. See also Harmand, ed., *Notice*, 93.

117. AD: Aube 40H189, fol. 75v, 82; Guignard, ed., *Les anciens statuts*, xvii.

118. Touati, *Maladie et société*, 458.

119. Saunier, "Le pauvre malade," 168. See also *Le régime du corps de maître Aldebrandin de Sienne: Texte français du XIIIe siècle*, ed. Louis Landouzy and Roger Pépin (Paris: H. Champion, 1911).

120. Boutiot, *Histoire de la ville de Troyes*, 315.

121. AD Aube G2531, fol. 25; Gesret, "Soustenir les povres," 245.

and the hospital of Provins made clear that the sick poor ought to be treated as "the lords of the house" and "served with nobility and pity and true compassion."[122] Nine of the hospital statutes composed between 1200 and 1270 and edited by Léon Le Grand contain references to the sick being treated as the "lords of the house," a phrase that seems to have originated with the statutes for the Hospital of Saint John of Jerusalem.[123] The foundation charter for the hospital at Tonnerre indicated that the master and mistress of the hospital were expected to take an oath of fidelity in caring for the institution's affairs, including being focused on treating the poor with compassion.[124] The rule for the hospital of Montreuil-sur-Mer enjoined the brethren to serve the sick with affection daily. Elsewhere, the statutes enjoined the hospital community to "refresh daily [the sick inmates] as a kind of lord with humility and devotion."[125] In founding the hôtel-Dieu of Château-Thierry in 1305, Jeanne of Navarre drafted statutes that were explicit about the proper treatment of the sick, referred to as "the noble members of Christ."[126] The statutes enjoined the hospital brethren to never leave the sick unattended.

The statutes for the hôtel-Dieu-le-Comte in Troyes threatened anyone who complained about the sick or who lost their patience with them with a penance of bread and water for three days.[127] There is no discussion in the statutes about specific treatment regimens for the sick, although there is a passing reference that suggests that rings and precious stones were sometimes worn as a superstitious healing remedy for illness, a practice that the author of the statutes seems not to have minded.[128] The statutes did address the need to provide special treatment to those in the infirmary who were the most gravely sick and to ensure that the food portions were smaller for the healthy than for the sick. The sick were to be served their meals before the brothers unless a brother was going out for worldly business and was therefore pressed for time.[129] The sick could have whatever food they desired, so long as it was procurable and not harmful.[130] Apart from these questions

---

122. Le Grand, ed., *Statuts d'hôtels-Dieu*, p. 104.

123. Le Grand, ed., *Statuts d'hôtels-Dieu*; Saunier, *"Le pauvre malade,"* 37n138.

124. Challe, *Histoire du comté*, 208.

125. Le Grand, ed., *Statuts d'hôtels-Dieu*, art. 73; Saunier, *"Le pauvre malade,"* 37.

126. Brown, "La mort," 132–34. Jeanne made a testamentary bequest of 1,000 l. to the hôtel-Dieu of Paris, and she also gave 1,000 l. each year to the hospital she founded at Château-Thierry. She left the oversight of this hospital to the future counts of Champagne.

127. Le Grand, ed., *Statuts d'hôtels-Dieu*, art. 85, p. 115.

128. Le Grand, ed., *Statuts d'hôtels-Dieu*, art. 16, p. 107.

129. Le Grand, ed., *Statuts d'hôtels-Dieu* art. 80, p. 114.

130. Le Grand, ed., *Statuts d'hôtels-Dieu* art. 81, p. 114.

related to diet, the statutes expressed concern that the sick poor might be taunted and therefore sought to protect them.[131]

In the thirteenth-century pastoral handbook for archdeacons, one section was devoted to the kinds of questions that an archdeacon, conducting a visitation of a hospital, should ask about the care of the poor.[132] During a visitation of a hospital, an archdeacon was enjoined to interrogate not only the *magister*, the clerics, and the brethren but the poor themselves. Did the poor confess? Did they regularly receive the Eucharist? Was extreme unction ministered at a suitable time and place? Were the poor given a proper burial? Were the poor suitably cared for and honored by the hospital's brethren? Were their feet and other parts of their body washed? Did the hospital turn too many poor people away or force them to leave the hospital too soon? Did a hospital with sufficient resources and space receive insufficient numbers of sick poor? Many of these questions relating to the treatment of the hospital poor were in fact pursued during the visitations of Archbishop Eudes Rigaud of Rouen. While visiting the hospitals and monastic houses of Normandy, he sought to ensure that the needs of the sick were provided for, and this included spiritual and physical needs. At the hospital of Saint-Mary Magdalene in Rouen, Eudes criticized the *magister* for not preaching with sufficient frequency to the infirm.[133] Preaching was a regular component of the archbishop's own visitations at hospitals. He reproached the staff of hospitals in which confession and the celebration of the Mass were happening irregularly.[134] But the archbishop also showed concern about the physical care of the sick, particularly that the sick be given an adequate diet.[135] At the Benedictine abbey of La Trinité-du-Mont in Rouen, he wanted the sick to have access to a physician.[136] At the hospitals of Gournay and Neufchâtel, he found that the sick were not well provided for. In particular, he criticized the prior of the hospital at Neufchâtel for allegedly never visiting the sick. Eudes even expressed concern that the house where the sick were housed was about to collapse.[137] In general, the archbishop worried that temporal goods that had been given to hospitals as alms were being used by the hospital personnel to the detriment of the sick poor. At the hospital of Saint-Mary

---

131. Le Grand, ed., *Statuts d'hôtels-Dieu* art. 83–85, pp. 114–15.

132. The *Libellus pastoralis* is found in Ravaisson, ed., *Catalogue*, 592–649.

133. *The Register of Eudes*, 645.

134. *The Register of Eudes*, 468–69.

135. The archbishop also showed concern about the diet given to the sick at monasteries. See *The Register of Eudes*, 356–57.

136. *The Register of Eudes*, 489.

137. *The Register of Eudes*, 462.

Magdalene in Rouen, the archbishop sent away a *donatus* so that the hospital's resources would be preserved for those most in need of assistance.[138]

Unlike the lepers living in a leprosarium, whose condition was considered permanent and who were therefore expected to live out their lives there, the sick living in hospitals were regarded as transient figures whose stays would be temporary. The thirteenth-century statutes for the hospitals at Vernon and Pontoise stipulated that once the sick had recovered, they would be given seven additional days before being released.[139] The hôtel-Dieu at Château-Thierry gave its sick guests at least ten days after their recovery before leaving.[140] An account book for the hospital in Gosnay in 1335–36 indicates that there were eight sick guests there that year, and they remained at the hospital anywhere from one to twenty-six weeks; six pregnant women who were there that year all stayed for a month.[141] The statutes for the hospital of Saint-Pol permitted postpartum women to convalesce at the hospital for three weeks or more if needed.[142] There is almost no textual evidence that would make it possible to determine the mortality rate for thirteenth-century hospitals; however, archaeological evidence for the hospital of St. Mary Spital in London suggests a mortality rate during the thirteenth century of just under 7 percent.[143] Evidence for the later Middle Ages suggests that, with the vagaries of epidemic disease and war, hospital mortality rates varied a great deal depending on the hospital and the year.[144]

Although the experience of living in a hospital would surely have varied, not all medieval hospitals were sordid, miserable places. It was common for hospitals to be built adjacent to rivers or even natural springs, as was the case with the hôtel-Dieu at Angers, which developed a sophisticated system for channeling water from various sources into and out of the hospital for sanitation and hygiene.[145] This hospital also owned a laundry house on the river where it washed sheets and clothes.[146] From statutes and charter evidence from various hospitals, it is clear that a good deal of attention was paid to the comfort of the sick poor, and this included the comfort of their beds. Some

---

138. *The Register of Eudes*, 469.

139. Le Grand, ed., *Statuts d'hôtels-Dieu*, 138, 161.

140. Brown, "La mort," 135.

141. Saunier, *"Le pauvre malade,"* 80–83.

142. Le Grand, ed., *Statuts d'hôtels-Dieu*, art. 32, p. 124.

143. Thomas, Sloane, and Phillpotts, *Excavations*, 39–40.

144. Saunier, *"Le pauvre malade,"* 198–203.

145. François Comte, "Hygiène hospitalière à Saint-Jean d'Angers (Maine-et-Loire, France): Adduction et évacuation des eaux du XIIe au XIIIe siècle," in *L'hydraulique monastique: milieux, réseaux, usages*, ed. Léon Pressouyre and Paul Benoît (Paris: Créaphis, 1996), 437–53.

146. Grant, "The Chapel of the Hospital of Saint-Jean," 310.

beds had mattresses, sheets, feather quilts, or wool covers with fur for the winter months, with the sick getting special pillows and cushions.[147] Obtaining sufficient firewood for heating the interior of hospitals during the winter months was also a concern, evident in the frequent donations of wood for heating purposes. The high windows of the hospital at Tonnerre, which is one of the largest and best-preserved medieval hospital buildings, illustrate how the importance of good air circulation was considered in the design.[148] Even today, one can see the beam sockets in the walls from the wooden galleries that ran above both sides of the beds, along the full length of the infirmary, providing easy access to adjust the opening of the windows and also making it possible for the sisters to observe the infirm in their beds. As Lynn Courtenay describes the hospital at Tonnerre, "the building provided an environment in which profuse light, exchange of air, and good acoustical space for liturgical prayer were created to facilitate the spiritual and physical care provided by the hospital staff."[149]

Hospital account books indicate that the diet inside hospitals was quite varied. The diet at Saint-Nicolas in Troyes, for instance, included meat, fish, almonds, onions, peas, beans, peppers, Swiss chard, eggs, bread, and wine. Many of the foodstuffs that were consumed did not have to be purchased, since they were cultivated by the hospital. Based on the records of the hospital's purchases, the bread that was being consumed was made with relatively little wheat and maslin but instead was mostly made with rye and barley, suggestive of an inferior, black bread.[150] The account book for 1302–03 shows that the hospital bought a *setier* of wheat specifically so that it could be "ground for the sick."[151] Archaeological evidence has also been suggestive about the use of herbal medicines in medieval hospitals.[152]

Although sources rarely provide much information about how the sick poor in hospitals spent their time, it is clear that they were not merely the passive recipients of institutional assistance.[153] These guests were expected to play a vital role in praying for the souls of the hospitals' benefactors (and their relatives). Admittedly, the sick and poor in hospitals were not considered

---

147. Saint-Denis, *L'hôtel-Dieu de Laon*, 104.

148. Saint-Denis, *L'hôtel-Dieu de Laon*, 103

149. Courtenay, "The Hospital of Notre Dame des Fontenilles," 102.

150. Gesret, "Soustenir les povres," 228.

151. BnF ms lat. 9111, fol. 297v.

152. Gilchrist, *Contemplation and Action*, 35.

153. Miri Rubin, "Imagining Medieval Hospitals: Considerations on the Cultural Meaning of Institutional Change," in *Medicine and Charity before the Welfare State*, ed. Colin Jones and Jonathan Barry (London: Routledge, 1991), 24–25.

part of the religious communities of their hospitals in the manner of the lepers living in leprosaria, who took religious vows and wore habits. However, the hospital poor were clearly assisting in chapel services.[154] The hospitals of the Order of Saint John of Jerusalem had a prayer, dating at least as early as the late twelfth century, that was to be recited by "the sick lords" of the hospital, asking God to bless the hospital and its brethren, its donors, the church and its clergy, Christian pilgrims, Christian princes, barons, knights, and all who suffer. Every night, after Compline, the clerics belonging to the Order were to form a procession through the hospital's "palace of the sick" and implore the sick to perform a long litany of specific prayers, with each verse beginning, "Seigneurs maladies, priez. . . ."[155] While hospitals belonging to the Trinitarian Order seem to have had a similar custom, it is unclear whether the sick poor in other hospitals in the Latin West recited prayers from such a formulary.[156] Nevertheless, there was a widespread belief that the intercessory prayers of the poor and sick were powerful. The bourgeois Laonais Jean Tieger made a donation to his city's hospital with the hope of benefiting from "the prayers that are said by the poor for the benefactors, day and night."[157] Even beyond their participation in the religious life, the *pauperes* at times carried particular responsibilities, such as caring for the hospital garden. In some cases, they might even receive a small salary for performing such tasks.[158] Count Henri I gave the poor of the hospital of Provins the right to collect firewood in the forests around Provins, so it was not only the hospital personnel doing these kinds of jobs.[159] A twelfth-century carpenter named Adwyn, who was disabled in his hands and feet, spent time making various wooden objects while convalescing at a hospital in Smithfield, London. As Irina Metzler has suggested, the making of these wooden crafts might have been a way to pass time engaged in a hobby but might also have served as a form of physical therapy, as the carpenter regained strength in his hands.[160] He might also have been selling the wooden crafts he made in the hospital. A bone flute and tuning peg found at the almshouse of St. Bartholomew, Bristol, which housed a significant number of elderly people,

154. Saint-Denis, *L'hôtel-Dieu de Laon*, 107.

155. Léon Le Grand, "La prière des malades dans les hôpitaux de l'Ordre de Saint-Jean de Jérusalem," *Bibliothèque de l'École des Chartes* 57 (1896): 325–38.

156. Le Grand, "La prière des malades," 329.

157. Saint-Denis, *L'hôtel-Dieu de Laon*, 106.

158. Nicole Gonthier, "Les hôpitaux et les pauvres à la fin du moyen âge: L'exemple de Lyon," *Le Moyen Age* 34, no. 2 (1978): 302.

159. Arbois de Jubainville, *Histoire des ducs*, vol. 3, no. 410 (1190), p. 398.

160. Metzler, *Disability*, 106.

suggests that one of the leisure activities in which they engaged was playing (and listening to) music.[161] Thimbles and bone needles found at St. Mary Spital in London indicate that nurses and hospital guests were engaged in needlework and sewing.[162]

Charitable Assistance outside of Hospitals

The limited number of beds in medieval hospitals could never begin to fully meet the needs of the large number of sick and poor during the thirteenth century, with as much as 10 percent of the typical urban population made up of beggars.[163] Yet hospitals were not necessarily the first place to which the sick poor turned for assistance. In fact, far from turning people away, there is evidence that some hospitals were operating below capacity.[164] Twice a week, the hospital at Angers sent out hospital brothers into the city streets to find and transport to the hospital any weak or sick individuals who might need assistance, perhaps a sign that this hospital was hardly overwhelmed with people clamoring to be admitted.[165] Nor were hospitals the only or even necessarily the principal providers of charitable assistance. It was common for testators to make bequests to the poor of a particular parish, as the chaplain of Saint-Pierre in Provins did in 1267, and it is often not clear what kind of institutional mechanisms there were for distributing such poor relief.[166] In some regions of Europe, confraternities and guilds played an active role in distributing food, clothing, and coins to the urban poor, and by the later Middle Ages, parishes had become increasingly active in the administration of poor relief.[167]

Many of the urban poor were far more reliant upon various forms of assistance that they received from family, friends, and neighbors than upon organized, institutional forms of charity. Sharon Farmer has shown how critical informal charity was to the survival of many of the medieval poor, disabled, and sick. Contrary to what was once thought, supportive kinship networks

---

161. Gilchrist, *Medieval Life*, 146.

162. Gilchrist, *Medieval Life*, 146.

163. Geremek, *Margins*, 194.

164. Brodman, *Charity and Welfare*, 72.

165. Le Grand, ed., *Statuts d'hôtels-Dieu*, art. 5–6, pp. 23–24.

166. Dupraz, no. 426; AD: Seine-et-Marne, 11HdtA12, fol. 124–124v.

167. Catherine Vincent, *Des charités bien ordonnées: Les confréries en Normandie de la fin du XIIIᵉ siècle au début du XVIᵉ siècle* (Paris: Éditions Rue d'Ulm, 1988), 159–67; André Vauchez, "Assistance et charité en occident, XIII–XVᵉ siècles," in *Domanda e consumi: Livelli e strutture nei secoli (XIII–XVIIIᵉ)*, ed. by V. Barbagli Bagnoli (Florence: Olschki, 1978), 153. On confraternities in Reims, see Desportes, *Reims et les Rémois*, 336–37, 366–67.

even in northern Europe extended beyond the nuclear household in providing family members with a safety net.[168] Yet as Farmer has demonstrated, the likelihood of receiving help from friends and neighbors often depended upon the gender, social class, and physical condition of the person in need as well as on the social class of the friend or neighbor. Modest artisans and the working poor, for example, tended to be more likely to offer care to those in need than elites were. There is still more to learn about why some in need of assistance turned to a hospital, whereas others received help from family or friends. As we observed with the stories about the beneficiaries of healing miracles, some poor people with illnesses and disabilities were helped both by neighbors or family members and by hospitals, often turning to hospitals when their family or friends could no longer support them. In short, choosing where to turn for assistance was not simply an either/or proposition between familial and institutional help.

In many regions of thirteenth-century Europe, including Champagne, hospitals played a significant role in providing "outdoor" poor relief in addition to their provision of charity to their own poor.[169] The poor of Laon, for example, regularly came to the hospital entrance to receive food, even though they never actually set foot inside the hospital.[170] At the time of the fair of Saint Rémi, the hospital brothers of the hôtel-Dieu-le-Comte distributed 20 s. in pittances to the poor on the outskirts of the town of Saint Augustine, just south of Troyes.[171] The hospital of Tonnerre's foundation charter instructed the hospital's mistress to distribute any unused food or wine to poor prisoners and other poor people in the city.[172] The curate of Fontenay made a donation to the hospital of nearby Louviers in 1315 that included bedding and land, and in exchange, he asked the hospital brothers and sisters to distribute a full pot of beans to the parish poor every Friday from All Saints' Day in the autumn to Pentecost in the late spring.[173]

---

168. Farmer, *Surviving Poverty*, 26–27; Horden, "Household Care and Informal Networks: Comparisons and Continuities from Antiquity to the Present," in *The Locus of Care: Families, Communities, Institutions, and Provision of Welfare Since Antiquity*, ed. Peregrine Horden and Richard Smith (London: Routledge, 1998), 21–67.

169. Gonthier, "Les hôpitaux et les pauvres," 185–86; Brodman, *Charity and Welfare*, 18. As Brodman shows, an almshouse in Girona distributed 130,000 loaves of bread to the street poor each year, with as many as 2,500 individuals receiving bread daily from the hospital.

170. Saint-Denis, *L'hôtel-Dieu de Laon*, 102.

171. AD: Aube 40H1, no. 38 (December 1232): "in exitibus ville de S. Augustinus dictis pauperibus assignatis." This gift came from the mother of Guillaume, lord of Lisines and maréchal of Champagne, a member of the Villehardouin family, who made the bequest while on her deathbed.

172. Challe, *Histoire du comté*, 208.

173. Le Grand, ed., *Les maisons-Dieu et les léproseries*, 49.

Hospitals also frequently oversaw the disbursements of food, clothing, and coins to the city poor at a wealthy person's funeral. One testator from Bar-sur-Aube made clear that the distributions, which were to be made on the first, third, and seventh day following his death, were to be given to "the poorest of the poor" ("minutis pauperibus").[174] In his testament of 1257, Count Thibaut V made bequests to a number of hospitals, ranging from the 400 *l*. he left for all the hospitals of Provins and Troyes to the 60 *l*. he left for the hospital of Sézanne and 50 *l*. for the hospital of Meaux. Yet all of these donations were dwarfed by the 1,000 *l*. that he left for the poor commoners of Champagne to purchase clothing and shoes on the feast of Saint Rémi (January 13) following his death.[175] It is possible that the hôtel-Dieu-le-Comte oversaw this distribution. In his testament of 1299, the dean of Saint-Pierre of Troyes, Denis de Champguyon, left somewhere between 20 *s*. and 60 *s*. to each hospital of Troyes as well as a furnished bed for the hospital of Saint-Nicolas. He left much larger sums, however, to feed the poor of various cities: on the day of his burial, he assigned 20 *l. t.* to feed the poor of Troyes, and apart from the day of his burial, he allocated 50 *l*. to feed the poor of Champguyon, 100 *l*. to feed the poor of Troyes, 25 *l*. to feed the poor of Sainte-Syre, and 25 *l*. to feed the poor of Vallant.[176] Denis clearly regarded the scale of need as far greater outside hospitals than inside, and yet it is possible that hospitals oversaw these distributions.

Hospitals may have employed tokens in the distribution of outdoor poor relief. We know that from as early as the late thirteenth century, tokens, usually made of lead (but also copper and tin) were used to help with the distribution of charity.[177] These tokens served as a substitute form of currency and allowed for the deferred payment of a meal or clothing. As William Courtenay has pointed out, these medieval tokens have most often been found in riverbeds near the hubs of both charitable and commercial activity. In Paris, for example, medieval tokens were found in the Seine River, just below the site of the hôtel-Dieu, near the Pont au Change, the bridge where moneychangers, goldsmiths and others had shops.[178] Courtenay has argued that these tokens, which were connected to commercial activity, are evidence of a shift from alms distributed in kind to the monetization of alms, a means of simplifying charity and exerting greater control over it.[179] During

---

174. AD: Aube 3H336 (1255 testament of Pierre the Jew of Bar-sur-Aube).
175. Evergates, *Feudal Society*, 70–72.
176. AD: Aube G2633 (1299).
177. Courtenay, "Token Coinage."
178. Courtenay, "Token Coinage," 277.
179. Courtenay, "Token Coinage," 285–86.

the fourteenth and fifteenth centuries, tokens became increasingly popular means of administering charity.

As noted earlier, the sisters from Saint-Nicolas in Troyes sometimes left the hospital to care for sick cathedral canons in their residences. Sisters from the hôtel-Dieu in Paris also cared for some of the wealthier sick in their homes.[180] It was also possible for those who were wealthier to have access to medical care without leaving their homes. Moreover, six of the sixteen propertied beneficiaries of cures in the "Miracles of Saint Louis" consulted physicians in their homes in and around the Paris region.[181] In Champagne, the testament of the squire, Guyot d'Engente, included a bequest of 5 s. to Master Jean de Fontisuenna, a "physicus," "for the service he extended to me."[182] If this physician provided some kind of medical service for Jean, it was in all likelihood not performed inside a hospital.[183] Furthermore, most medical practitioners at this time were not even physicians or surgeons. As Cornelius O'Boyle has put it, "medical care provided by those who called themselves physicians and surgeons bore little relation to the medical care more usually experienced by the great majority of people in the Latin West."[184] In short, the fact that it was relatively rare for physicians to be working in hospitals certainly does not mean that there was therefore no medical care there.

There were a variety of ways that hospitals provided assistance to nonresidents. At times, for example, hospitals provided charitable financing to individuals through economic transactions, such as selling or exchanging property with them. In 1214, for example, the hôtel-Dieu-le-Comte bought a piece of land from Jean de Banlieue-sur-Barberey at La Chapelle, near the enclosure of the hospital. However, this was not an ordinary purchase by the hospital, since Jean was a leper, and according to the charter that recorded the transaction, "he was forced by nudity and poverty" to sell the hospital land that he had inherited.[185] The hospital promised Jean a lifetime rent of four measures of coarse wool ("burello"), presumably for clothing, every two years. But was this the only payment that the leper received for his land, and if not, was it a charitable addition to another form of payment? Was the

---

180. Jéhanno, "'Sustenter les povres malades,'" 141.

181. Farmer, *Surviving Poverty*, 54.

182. AD: Aube 3H336 (December 1273): "pro servicio michi impenso."

183. Among the many religious houses that received bequests in Guyot's testament, no mention is made of any hospital, except for a small bequest for the leprosary of Bar-sur-Aube.

184. Cornelius O'Boyle, "Surgical Texts and Social Contexts: Physicians and Surgeons in Paris, c. 1270 to 1430," in *Practical Medicine from Salerno to the Black Death*, ed. Luis García-Ballester et al. (Cambridge: Cambridge University Press, 1994), 158. See also Jacquart, *Le milieu médical*, 246–47.

185. AD: Aube 40H189, fol. 36 (1214).

hospital taking pity on Jean by paying him more than the market value of the land? Or rather, was the hospital taking advantage of Jean's desperate plight and paying him less than his land was worth? The hospital could not admit Jean, since its statutes barred lepers from being received, but the hospital could provide him with the material he needed for warm clothing, while also acquiring a new piece of land near the hospital.

In addition to selling or exchanging property below its market value, another way that hospitals could provide financial assistance was through counter-gifting. As we saw in chapter 3, counter-gifts served to strengthen the relationship between a donor and a hospital. But a counter-gift, especially in the form of money, could also function as a source of liquid funds for a donor in need. Even when a donation to a hospital was cast as a pious gift, in some cases it may have represented a donor's attempt to secure an immediate cash payment in the form of a counter-gift. In such a case, a hospital was able to simultaneously serve a charitable function by providing a cash payment to someone in need, while also making a long-term investment through the acquisition of new properties.

The granting of life annuities to donors could represent a form of charitable assistance. In 1245 four brothers and two sisters gave the hôtel-Dieu-le-Comte in Troyes some rooms "in perpetual alms," and the hospital, "considering the generosity and kindness of these brothers and sisters," promised Contessa, one of the donors, a lifetime annuity of bread and clothing.[186] It is not clear why the hospital conferred a life annuity on this one sister, but she was likely in need of special assistance. In short, this annuity seems to have been a form of charity. There is no indication that Contessa lived in the hospital, but through her gift (and that of her siblings), she became another one of the hospital's many dependents and participated in the hospital's network of gift exchanges.

Medieval hospitals engaged in the lending of money both as a form of poor relief and as a way to advance institutional interests. Miri Rubin has found evidence that the Hospital of St. John the Evangelist in Cambridge was serving as a supplier of credit during the thirteenth century. Among the recipients of its loans were pilgrims and those needing to pay off existing debts to Jews. As Rubin points out, from a medieval hospital's perspective, "Freeing Christians from Jewish moneylenders was an act of piety and charity."[187] The loans granted by hospitals were often hidden under the guise of a fee farm,

186. AD: Aube 40H189 fol. 79v (1245).
187. Rubin, *Charity and Community*, 224.

in which the borrower leased land to the hospital for a short period in return for a cash rent that, unlike a genuine fee farm, had to be paid in full up front. Moreover, the land was merely pledged as a way of securing what was in fact a loan.[188] During the later Middle Ages, a hospital such as Saint-Nicolas in Troyes at times even provided loans to aristocrats in need. In 1471, Jean Pavye, a squire and lord of Villechétif, gave the hospital an annual rent of 23 s. t. to acquit himself of a loan he had contracted from the institution.[189] That same year, Jean made another small donation to the hospital for his "love for the master, brothers and sisters of the hôtel-Dieu Saint-Nicolas of Troyes, and also since they have now given me ten golden écus to help with my affairs and have given me some wheat and oats of their own free will."[190] It had become part of this hospital's charitable function to help an indebted lord.

Conclusion

The growing visibility of the urban poor during the twelfth and thirteenth centuries was tied to the significant migration of peoples from rural to urban areas, and more generally, the explosive growth of urban populations. In addition, the frequent dispersal of families during this period meant that many of the new arrivals to urban areas did not have a local familial support system, and in that sense, they were living on the edge. This was particularly true for those who were unmarried. The lack of familial support was felt especially acutely by clerics, whether or not they were migrants, since they generally never married and did not have children who could support them when they became elderly or were ill. Many rural women who never married or were widowed migrated to urban centers like Troyes, Provins, and Bar-sur-Aube, in search of work as domestic servants, and they too largely went without local familial support.[191] We have seen examples of several female domestic servants who were migrants and who fell on hard times, eventually ending up in a hospital. During the mid-twelfth century, Count Henri the Liberal actively encouraged people from outside Champagne to immigrate, with the promise of better tenurial conditions. Indeed, new residents of Troyes, Provins, and Bar-sur-Aube were given up to one year to choose

---

188. Rubin, *Charity and Community*, 222.

189. AD: Aube 43H13, lay. 32, cote B, no. 14b (July 20, 1471); Gesret, "Soustenir les povres," 352.

190. AD: Aube 43H13, lay. 32, cote B, no. 14a (November 7, 1471); Gesret, "Soustenir les povres," 352: "pour l'amour que [j'ay] aux maistre, freres et seurs de l'ostel Dieu Saint Nicolas dudit Troyes et aussi qu'ilz m'ont baillié presentement dix escus d'or pour secourir a mes affaires, du froment et de l'avoine de leur volonté."

191. Farmer, *Surviving Poverty*, 23–32.

their own lords, but without the support and protection of a lord, they were in some ways even more vulnerable.[192]

Even apart from migration, however, Christopher Dyer has underscored the enormous vulnerability of medieval village life, where it was easy to suddenly slide into poverty for any number of reasons, from life cycle poverty, to nuclear poverty (such as when the elderly were not looked after by family), to poverty that was due to environmental factors.[193] Dyer has rightly argued that quite often there was not much of a gulf separating almsgivers and the recipients of those alms, an observation that resonates with studies showing that in many countries today the poorest give the highest proportion of their income to charity.[194] In medieval Europe as well, the givers and recipients often came from the same socioeconomic class, and they themselves could see how easy it was for the working poor or even the non-poor to quickly become dependent upon others. Poverty was not necessarily a permanent state, and a significant percentage of the population experienced poverty at least periodically. With its fairs and thriving commercial economy, Champagne brought in an unusual number of transients, including merchants and migrants who came in search of employment. It is possible that the county developed a reputation for its charitable wealth, which was visible most dramatically in the counts' benefaction of religious houses and hospitals. As we have seen, Champagne's culture of charity extended beyond its aristocratic circles to include a wide variety of bourgeois townspeople. The broad, popular support for those in need of assistance may have made the county an attractive place to settle.

This chapter has highlighted that the medieval hospital's "economy of care" reached beyond the sick and the poor and extended well beyond the hospital's walls. What constituted hospital care is clearly more complex than often imagined, since these institutions sought to relieve many different forms of need, from material and bodily to social and spiritual. A hospital's care of its sick and poor could include hearing confessions, celebrating Mass, providing access to local relics, preaching, providing the sick poor with a bed, giving them sufficient food and drink, and helping them with their various physical needs. But was a hospital "caring" for an aristocratic widow when it received her as a *conversa*? Even apart from her social class, as a *conversa* she was technically considered a member of the hospital's personnel and its religious community, not one of its sick poor. Yet she may have joined

---

192. Evergates, *Henry the Liberal*, 139.
193. Dyer, "Poverty and Its Relief."
194. Ken Stern, "Why the Rich Don't Give to Charity," *The Atlantic*, April 2013.

the hospital in search of the security that came with being part of such a community. Did a hospital's hiring of a poor maidservant constitute "care"? What about a hospital's granting an indebted donor a much-needed loan (or counter-gift) of cash in return for his donation of a rent in perpetuity?

Hospitals were of course not willing or able to respond to all of society's pressing needs. Hospital administrators had to decide what constituted "legitimate" needs and whether the institution could accommodate those needs. It is difficult to gauge how successful medieval hospitals were in providing relief to those in need of assistance, but the diversity of the recipients of assistance and the wide-ranging forms that that assistance could take should make us reject any lingering Foucauldian notions that medieval hospitals were repressive, disciplining institutions that stripped their "inmates" of freedom and dignity. Moreover, hospital statutes make clear that in principle the sick poor were expected to be treated as the lords of the house. They were to be given life-saving sacramental medicine in addition to attentive physical care, food, drink, and a bed. Hospital benefactors regarded the intercessory prayers of the sick poor as critical for their own hopes of salvation, and they often donated pittances of food or drink for distribution. While the medieval sick and poor had a limited number of relief options open to them, they were by no means forced into hospitals, and most of the sick and poor in thirteenth-century Europe never even set foot in a hospital. When they did, it was usually for a limited time. Most importantly, though, the boundaries separating a hospital's personnel from those who received assistance were often remarkably permeable, as were the boundaries separating a hospital's donors from the recipients of care. A hospital's sick poor, its personnel, and its benefactors were in many ways all bound up together in a social and spiritual web of mutual need, dependency, and assistance.

Epilogue

When the thirteenth-century cardinal and moralist Jacques de Vitry singled out the hospital of Provins as one of only a few exemplary hospitals that he considered "hospitals of piety" and "houses of good reputation," one wonders how well acquainted he was with this institution and its practices.[1] Since the brethren of the Provinois hospital followed the Augustinian Rule and took vows, it appeared to be the type of religious community that Jacques favored. Yet as noted in chapter 5, at least some of the hospital sisters were receiving life annuities from family and friends, something Jacques surely would have frowned upon. Other brethren were making entry gifts.[2] There were tensions between the religious ideals articulated by churchmen like Jacques de Vitry about the way that hospitals were expected to be run and the pragmatic realities of administering these complex charitable institutions, with their manifold functions and diverse residents and personnel all living under the same roof. Reformers like Jacques criticized hospitals for accepting *donati*, who were permitted to receive room and board without taking vows. The reality, however, was that the *donati* at times brought in valuable resources that could be used

---

1. Bird, "Texts on Hospitals," 112–13.
2. Bird, "Medicine for Body and Soul," 105–6.

to serve the poor and sick. Some of the *donati* were married couples, and some hospital administrators were also married. Recognizing the advantages in allowing married couples to manage hospitals, Robert of Courson argued that married couples could enter a hospital together but had to remain chaste and live in separate quarters.[3] Other churchmen, however, viewed marriage as fundamentally incompatible with the expectation that members of a hospital community should take religious vows and follow the Augustinian Rule.

There were also divergent visions on where hospitals would find the resources to support their mission and how they should use those resources. Jacques de Vitry castigated as wicked those hospitals that were founded by merchants ("mercatores") and artisans ("caupones"). Yet the hospital of Provins, a comital foundation that Jacques praised, was very much the beneficiary of the patronage of shopkeepers, artisans, drapers, and merchants.[4] The hospital owned a number of houses in Provins that were used for commercial purposes and served as a powerful landlord and creditor in the region, with hundreds of tenants and serfs who cultivated its landed properties. As it was located just a stone's throw away from the town's bustling commercial market, the site of commercial transactions and moneylending, much of the hospital's ability to carry out its caritative function rested on the privileges it received from the counts and the income generated from commerce. Jacques de Vitry opposed hospitals' practice of "investing" alms, which he viewed as a form of hoarding. Instead, he argued that hospitals should immediately distribute any alms they received directly to the poor.[5] Yet as chapter 4 demonstrated, several of Champagne's larger hospitals, including the hospital at Provins, were powerful landlords and major players in the urban economy, managing their assets with an eye toward long-term economic growth.

In addition to the manifold ways that charitable institutions benefited from commerce—whether from their own commercial activities or those of their patrons—the increased commercialization of late twelfth- and thirteenth-century society, particularly in a region like Champagne, may have contributed to the idea of a moral economy, including the obligation of charitable

---

3. I am relying here on Watson's exposition of Courson's discussion of hospitals in his unpublished *Summa*. See Watson, *On Hospitals*, 268–71.

4. Bonenfant-Feytman, "Les organisations hospitalières," 42

5. In this regard, Jacques's critique anticipated some of the criticisms in our own day of some U.S. hospitals' multi-billion-dollar endowments; investments in high-risk stocks, emerging markets, and venture capital; and in the case of some for-profit hospitals, the payment of large dividends to shareholders while charging patients ever more for rooms, diagnostic tests, and medical treatments.

giving and service. As Lawrin Armstrong has shown in his study of Gerard of Siena, the Augustinian master of theology at Paris, the scholastic preoccupation with economic questions during this period very much centered on justice, charity, and the common good. Moreover, the starting premise for medieval scholastic discussions of the economic order was a moral one, namely that "human needs take precedence over profit."[6] Already in the late twelfth and early thirteenth centuries, Peter the Chanter and members of his circle, which included Jacques de Vitry, were taking up the same types of questions that Gerard of Siena would address a century later, including the moral status of usury and whether charitable giving constituted an appropriate restitution for usurious profits. As part of this notion of a Christian moral economy, it was often pointed out that commerce could (and did) result in the social and economic exploitation of others, creating greater social and economic divisions and inequalities. Medieval moralists who denounced accepting tainted or illicit profits as charitable gifts pointed to the irony that exploitative business practices were harming the poor only for the perpetrators to then give alms derived from those very business practices to the same poor they had just harmed.[7] This medieval critique of the use of almsgiving as an expiatory tool has echoes in some of the modern critiques of philanthrocapitalism as philanthropic posturing, with the stated desire "to do well and do good" merely serving as "an apparatus of justification."[8]

The twelfth- and thirteenth-century social conditions that created a conducive environment for the flourishing of commerce were also advantageous for fostering charity and pious giving more generally. Moreover, some scholars have argued that a key ingredient to the success of Champagne's

---

6. Lawrin Armstrong, *The Idea of a Moral Economy: Gerard of Siena on Usury, Restitution, and Prescription* (Toronto: University of Toronto Press, 2016), 12, 26. See also Langholm, *Economics in the Medieval Schools*; Henri Dubois, "Le pouvoir économique du prince," in *Les princes et le pouvoir au moyen âge: Actes du XXIIIe Congrès de la Société des Historiens Médiévistes de l'Enseignement Supérieur Public de Brest, 1992* (Paris: Publications de la Sorbonne, 1993); Joel Kaye, "Monetary and Market Consciousness in Thirteenth and Fourteenth Century Europe," in *Ancient and Medieval Economic Ideas and Concepts of Social Justice*, ed. S. Todd Lowry and Barry Gordon (Leiden: Brill, 1998), 376–403.

7. In his *Summa* (XI.II), Robert of Courson addressed what a cleric ought to do if he discovered that a church had been built with the profits from usury. See Kennedy, "Content of Courson's *Summa*," 90; Watson, *On Hospitals*, 268.

8. In his examination of the dark underbelly of philanthrocapitalism, Anand Giridharadas sought to uncover "the connection between these elites' social concern and predation, between the extraordinary helping and the extraordinary hoarding." One of the many examples of this "apparatus of justification" cited by Anand Giridharadas are the millions of dollars that the Sackler family has donated to universities and art museums based on revenues deriving from the opioid industry. See Anand Giridharadas, *Winners Take All: The Elite Charade of Changing the World* (New York: Knopf, 2018), 7, 176–83, 268.

international trade fairs was the creation of a climate of trust through the law merchant courts, which enforced contracts and maintained social cohesion by publicizing the names of merchants known to have violated their word.[9] These courts sought to ensure that merchants knew about each other's past behavior, and this served as a deterrent against the temptation to cheat. The trade fairs could not have functioned efficiently without this trust, which the sociologist Robert Putnam has called the essence of social capital.[10] Social networks and relationships that were marked by trust, cooperation, and reciprocity were as vital to commerce as they were to the dynamic relationships between hospitals and their personnel, their donors, and their sick and poor guests. By the fourteenth and fifteenth centuries, that climate of trust and sense of community had largely been replaced by a heightened suspicion of vagrants and beggars. As a result of the economic downturn of the early fourteenth century, there was less surplus capital to be used for charitable provision. In addition, there seems to have been a decline in confidence that religious institutions would actually use the alms they received to help the poor. Consequently, as Francine Michaud has noted for Provence, testators increasingly channeled bequests directly to the poor themselves.[11]

During the twelfth and thirteenth centuries, however, the traditional notion of an economy of salvation took on new meaning in an increasingly commercial context. The works of mercy were cast as the virtuous antidote to the vice of avarice. Jessalynn Bird has noted that even Jacques de Vitry, who otherwise denounced any hint of a hospital or other religious institution being corrupted or secularized, employed "mercantilistic imagery familiar to the artisan, burgher and noble classes" in his sermons to hospitallers so as to reassure them that "their charitable work converts transitory riches into heavenly treasure and earns them participation in the Church's prayers and masses and eternal life, in contrast to the merciless, whom Christ will condemn at the last judgment."[12] The medieval Franciscan embrace of religious poverty (one of many medieval religious movements to do so) represented a radical rejection of the love of money and the inexorable desire for gain. Yet over the course of the thirteenth and early fourteenth centuries, Franciscans,

---

9. Paul R. Milgrom, Douglass C. North, and Barry R. Weingast, "The Role of Institutions in the Revival of Trade: The Law Merchant, Private Judges, and the Champagne Fairs," *Economics and Politics* 2, no. 1 (March 1990): 1–23; Munro, "'New Institutional Economics.'"

10. Robert D. Putnam, "The Prosperous Community: Social Capital and Public Life," *American Prospect* 13 (Spring 1993): 35–42; Robert D. Putnam, *Making Democracy Work: Civic Traditions in Modern Italy* (Princeton: Princeton University Press, 1993).

11. Michaud, "Le pauvre transformé," 278–81.

12. Bird, "Medicine for Body and Soul," 100–101.

Dominicans, and Augustinians paradoxically took a leading role in justifying questionable economic practices by arguing that almsgiving was a way to render wealth virtuous. The concept of a Christian moral economy, dedicated to the common good as opposed to private profit, thus in some ways emerged as an outgrowth of the new profit economy, helping foster greater charitable giving and service. Thirteenth-century preaching, vernacular treatises on the virtues and vices, penitential and confessional texts, and visual imagery all served to teach the Christian laity and clergy how to perform the works of mercy properly, underlining the enormous salvific power of these works and how they could function as a form of penance. Helping the stranger or needy neighbor was regarded as a pious, penitential act that earned one spiritual redemption, thereby potentially shortening one's time in Purgatory. Religious ambivalence about the new profit economy, in other words, in fact stimulated almsgiving and charitable service.

Historically, the dynamic interplay between charity and commerce, including the idea of charity as restitution, has by no means been confined to medieval Europe. In American history, for instance, there has long been a tradition of charitable activity and the market being intertwined.[13] Nineteenth-century charitable society relied on commercial activity to raise funds, with Bible societies, for example, innovating with mass-market techniques. During the Civil War, the Sanitary Commission, which was established to support sick and wounded Union soldiers, set up and staffed hospitals. Unlike the older Christian Commission, which represented an older, evangelical tradition that catered to wounded soldiers' spiritual needs, relied on unpaid volunteers, and encouraged sentimental attachments between gift-givers and individual soldiers, the Sanitary Commission was highly bureaucratic, favoring a professionalized, salaried staff and a more disciplined environment within its hospitals. Anticipating the scientific charity movement that emerged later in the decade, the Sanitary Commission was enormously successful in raising funds through the fairs that it sponsored.[14] Later in the nineteenth century, the business magnate and philanthropist Andrew Carnegie laid out a new doctrine of benevolence in "The Gospel of Wealth" (1889), which criticized the kind of indiscriminate charity long associated with the Catholic Middle Ages while taking up the question of how to ensure, in an

---

13. Kathleen D. McCarthy, *American Creed: Philanthropy and the Rise of Civil Society, 1700–1865* (Chicago: University of Chicago Press, 2003); Benjamin Soskis, "The Problem of Charity in Industrial America, 1873–1915" (PhD dissertation, Columbia University, 2010).

14. George M. Frederickson, *The Inner Civil War: Northern Intellectuals and the Crisis of the Union*, 2nd ed. (Urbana: University of Illinois Press, 1993), 98–112.

age of industrialization and growing economic inequalities, that one's private wealth would have the maximum impact in advancing the public good. The Standard Oil magnate John D. Rockefeller, who was much reviled in his day, committed himself early on to the principles of Christian stewardship, accumulating as much property and wealth as he could in order to give it away. As Peter Dobkin Hall has written, "Big business and private wealth underwrote the growth of universities, libraries, hospitals, museums, social-welfare organizations, professional societies, and private clubs."[15] In this regard, there was even a direct link between both Rockefeller and Carnegie and the region of Champagne, which has been the focus of this book. When the city of Reims lay in ruins following World War I, Rockefeller contributed a significant sum for the restoration of the city's famed Gothic cathedral. Today, the street leading up to the parvis of the cathedral and the former site of the medieval hôtel-Dieu is named "rue Rockefeller." It was the Carnegie Endowment, meanwhile, that put up the funds during the 1920s for the city of Reims to build a new municipal library, which to this day bears the Carnegie name.

During the nineteenth and early twentieth centuries, American philanthropy was not just the beneficiary of economic development; it also helped fuel that economic development. Kathleen McCarthy has shown that from the early nineteenth century, American philanthropic nonprofit organizations, in which women often played a formative role, engaged in commercial activities, provided mechanisms for the accumulation and liquification of capital in a cash-scarce economy, and served as employers and "engines for economic development."[16] Evangelical churches also played a pronounced role in promoting market values, and these churches "created a nonprofit machinery that provided a foundation for the economic success of their adherents."[17] It was no coincidence that the regions of the United States that experienced the most robust economic growth, namely the northeast and the mid-Atlantic, were also the ones with the most extensive voluntarist institutions.

The evidence from medieval Europe (or the nineteenth- and twentieth-century United States) by no means suggests that profit economies, by themselves, spur greater social cohesion and altruistic behavior. Indeed, as modern and particularly contemporary history has borne out, it is very often

---

15. Peter Dobkin Hall, *Inventing the Nonprofit Sector and Other Essays on Philanthropy, Voluntarism, and Nonprofit Organizations* (Baltimore: Johns Hopkins University Press, 1992), 39.

16. McCarthy, *American Creed*, 205–6.

17. Hall, *Inventing the Nonprofit Sector*, 35.

an unrestrained "free market" that is responsible for the widening of social and economic inequalities, resulting in greater social dislocation, desperation, and material want. Premodern religious charity, however, was far more intricately connected to economic developments than is generally acknowledged. At various points during the last five hundred years, "traditional charity," often associated with the Middle Ages, has come under assault, whether from Enlightenment *philosophes* or Gilded Age benefactors, who promoted "scientific charity" or philanthropy, which they regarded as more effective, rational (in being targeted to specific groups and causes), and impersonal (and thereby less paternalistic).[18] Even in today's new Gilded Age, the nonprofit sector has become increasingly commercialized and business practices have been fully incorporated into the charitable realm. Philanthrocapitalism, meanwhile, is premised on the notion that philanthropy must harness the profit motive and the power of the market to achieve social good, in contrast to traditional charitable giving, long maligned for being intrinsically anti-market.[19] This book has challenged some of these long-held assumptions about how premodern charity differed from modern philanthropy by elucidating the ways that charity was becoming commercialized, both in practice and in the religious imagination during the first great age of European commerce.

Whether in the context of medieval Christian hospitals or nonprofit hospitals in the twenty-first century United States, the mixing of commercial and charitable imperatives can have an effect on the essential nature of institutions. For decades, regulatory stipulations in the United States required nonprofit hospitals to devote a certain percentage of their spending on the poor and the public good in the form of "charity care." Since the passage of the Affordable Care Act, however, the number of uninsured patients in the United States has dropped significantly, and as a result, hospitals are responsible for paying for far less free and reduced-cost care. How much "charity

18. Jeremy Beer, *The Philanthropic Revolution: An Alternative History to Charity* (Philadelphia: University of Pennsylvania Press, 2015); Benjamin Soskis, "Both More and No More: The Historical Split Between Charity and Philanthropy," Hudson Institute, October 15, 2014, available at www.hudson.org/research/10723-both-more-and-no-more-the-historical-split-between-charity-and-philanthropy. Both Beer and Soskis are critical of bureaucratic, corporatized philanthropy, which they view as having abandoned the personalist and localist ethic of more traditional forms of charity.

19. On philanthrocapitalism, see Matthew Bishop and Michael Green, *Philanthrocapitalism: How Giving Can Save the World* (London: A & C Black, 2010). Critics of philanthrocapitalism almost seem to echo Jacques de Vitry in casting doubt on the sincerity of philanthrocapitalists' motives, arguing that they are "using giving as a fig leaf to hide embarrassing or dodgy business activities, to exploiting tax loop holes, to boosting social status out of overweening vanity." See Bishop and Green, *Philanthrocapitalism*, 31.

care" are hospitals now providing as a condition for their tax-exempt status? And what constitutes that "charity care"? Long before hospitals became coopted by "big business," becoming the embodiment of the "for-profit" sector, including those hospitals that are ostensibly "not-for-profit," indeed from the time of their medieval origins as Christian charitable and religious institutions, hospitals were inextricably tied to markets and the expanding profit economy while also serving as sites of evangelical devotion and discipline. During a period of urban transformation, which created greater prosperity for some but also increasing poverty and insecurity for many others, the medieval hospital opened up new opportunities for social reciprocity and mutual assistance. For those with various kinds of needs, the hospital served as a source of physical, social, and material support in this earthly world, with all of its vagaries and vulnerabilities. In addition, though, the medieval hospital held out the promise of spiritual redemption in the world to come.

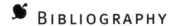 # BIBLIOGRAPHY

Unpublished Sources

AD: Aisne H-dépot 19

AD: Aube G2633; G1275; 40H189 (cartulary for HD-le-Comte de Troyes); 40H1; 43H4; 43H12; 40H16; HD33; 43H8; G3394; G3395; G2525; G2524; G2530; G2531; 3H336; HD 33/50; G2669; HD33/209; 43H57

AD: Marne (Reims), 2G454; 54H23; 54H53

AD: Seine-et-Marne, 11HdtA12 ("grand cartulaire" for the HD Provins); 11HdtA13 ("petit cartulaire" for the HD Provins); 11Hdt B177–182 (censiers for the HD Provins); 11Hdt/B1; 11Hdt/C5 (martyrological obituary); 11Hdt/E6; 9Hdt/ B103; 9Hdt/B19; H suppl. B83; 9Hdt/B75; 11Hdt/A3

AMC (Reims): FH-HD B62; FH-HD B50; FH-HD B54; FH-FG, A6; FH-HD B40

BM Provins, mss 85, 266, 267, 298

Paris, BnF ms lat. 15941, 9111

Printed Source Material

Augustine. "Sermon 123." In *Patrologia Latina*, edited by J. P. Migne. Paris: 1865. 38:684–86.

Benton, John and Michel Bur, eds. *Recueil des actes d'Henri le Libéral, comte de Champagne (1152–1181)*. Paris: Boccard, 2009.

Bird, Jessalynn. "Texts on Hospitals: Translation of Jacques de Vitry, *Historia Occidentalis* 29, and Edition of Jacques de Vitry's Sermons to Hospitallers." In *Religion and Medicine in the Middle Ages*, edited by Joseph Ziegler and Peter Biller, 109–34. York: York University Press, 2001.

Caesarius of Heisterbach. *Dialogus miraculorum*. Edited by Josephus Strange. 2 vols. Cologne: J. M. Heberle, 1851; repr. Ridgewood, NJ: Gregg Press, 1966.

Cambell, O.F.M., Jacques, ed. *Enquête pour le procès de canonisation de Dauphine de Puimichel, Comtesse d'Ariano (+26 novembre 1360), Apt et Avignon, 14 mai–30 octobre 1363*. Turin: Bottega d'Erasmo, 1978.

Camuzat, Nicholaus. *Promptuarium sacrarum antiquitatum Tricassinae diocesis*. V. Moreau, 1610.

Conciliorum oecumenicorum generaliumque decreta: Editio critica, ed. A. García y García. Vol. 2.1 (869–1424). Turnhout, Belgium: Brepols, 2013.

Cossé-Durlin, Jeannine, ed. *Cartulaire de Saint-Nicaise de Reims*. Paris: CNRS, 1991.

de Jubainville, Henri Arbois, ed. "Étude sur les documents antérieurs à l'année 1285, conservés dans les archives des quatre petits hôpitaux de la ville de Troyes." *Mémoires de la Société Académique de l'Aube* vol. 21 (vol. 8, 2nd ser.) (1857): 49–116.

de la Marche, Lecoy, ed. *Anecdotes historiques, légendes et apologues, tirés du recueil inédit d'Étienne de Bourbon, dominicain du XIIIe siècle.* Paris: Librairie Renouard, 1877.

Depoin, Joseph, ed. *Cartulaire de l'hôtel-dieu de Pontoise.* Pontoise, France: Société historique du Vexin, 1886.

Desportes, Pierre, ed. *Testaments Saint-Quentinois du XIVe siècle.* Paris: CNRS Éditions, 2003.

Drossbach, Gisela, and Gerhard Wolf, eds. *Caritas im Schatten von Sankt Peter: Der Liber Regulae des Hospitals Santo Spirito in Sassia: Eine Prachthandschrift des 14. Jahrhunderts.* Regensburg, Germany: Verlag Friedrich Pustet, 2015.

Dupraz, Dominique. "Les cartulaires de l'Hôtel-Dieu de Provins: Édition critique." Thesis, L'École Nationale des Chartes. Paris, 1973.

Evergates, Theodore, ed. *The Cartulary of Countess Blanche of Champagne.* Toronto: University of Toronto Press, 2010.

——. *Feudal Society in Medieval France: Documents from the County of Champagne.* Philadelphia: University of Pennsylvania Press, 1993.

Frenken, Goswin, ed. *Die Exempla des Jacob von Vitry: Ein Beitrag zur Geschichte der Erzählungsliteratur des Mittelalters.* Munich: C. H. Beck, 1914.

Frère Laurent. *La somme le roi.* Edited by Edith Brayer and Anne-Françoise Leurquin-Labie. Paris: Société des Textes Français Modernes, 2008.

Gaposchkin, M. Cecilia, and Sean L. Field, eds. *The Sanctity of Louis IX: Early Lives of Saint Louis by Geoffrey of Beaulieu and William of Chartres.* Translated by Larry F. Field. Ithaca: Cornell University Press, 2013.

The Good Wife's Guide (Le Ménagier de Paris): A Medieval Household Book. Translated and edited by Gina L. Breco and Christine M. Rose. Ithaca: Cornell University Press, 2009.

Guignard, Philippe, ed. *Les anciens statuts de l'Hôtel-Dieu-le-Comte de Troyes.* Troyes, France: A. Guignard, 1853.

Guillaume d'Auvergne. *Sermones de communi sanctorum et de occasionibus.* Edited by Franco Morenzoni. *Corpus Christianorum. Continuatio Mediaevalis,* vol. 230C. Turnhout, Belgium: Brepols, 2013.

——. *Sermones de tempore.* Edited by Franco Morenzoni. *Corpus Christianorum, Continuatio Mediaevalis,* vol. 230. Turnhout, Belgium: Brepols, 2010.

Guillaume de Saint-Pathus. *Les miracles de Saint Louis.* Edited by Percival B. Fay. Paris: H. Champion, 1931.

——. *Vie de Saint Louis.* Edited by H. François-Delaborde. Paris: Alphonse Picard, 1899.

Humbert of Romans. "De eruditione praedicatorum." In *Maxima bibliotheca veterum partum.* Vol. 25. Edited by Marguerin de la Bigne (Lyon, 1677): 456–567.

Innocent III. *Libellus de eleemosyna.* In *Patrologia Latina,* edited by J. P. Migne. Paris: 1855. 217:752–62.

Jacques de Vitry. *The Exempla or Illustrative Stories from the Sermones Vulgares of Jacques de Vitry.* Edited by Thomas Frederick Crane. London, 1890; repr. New York, 1971.

——. *The Life of Marie d'Oignies.* Translated by Margot H. King. Edited by Margot H. King and Miriam Marsolais. Toronto: Peregrina, 1993.

——. *Vita de Marie de Oignies, Supplementum.* Edited by R. Huygens. *Corpus Christianorum, Continuatio Mediaevalis,* vol. 252. Turnhout, Belgium: Brepols, 2012.

Jean de Joinville. *Vie de Saint Louis.* Edited by Jacques Monfrin. Paris: Dunod, 1995.

Kennedy, V. L. "The Content of Courson's *Summa." Mediaeval Studies* 9 (1947): 81–107.

Kushelevsky, Rella, ed. and trans. *Tales in Context: Sefer ha-ma'asim in Medieval Northern France.* Detroit: Wayne State University Press, 2017.

Landouzy, Louis, and Roger Pépin. *Le régime du corps de maître Aldebrandin de Sienne: Texte français du XIIIe siècle.* Paris: H. Champion, 1911.

The Life and Afterlife of St. Elizabeth of Hungary: Testimony from Her Canonization Hearings. Translated by Kenneth Baxter Wolf. New York: Oxford University Press, 2011.

Leblond, Victor, ed. "Les deux plus anciens comptes de l'hôtel-Dieu de Beauvais (1377–1380)." *Bulletin philologique et historique (jusqu'à 1715) du Comité des travaux historiques et scientifiques* (1914): 163–344.

Le Grand, Léon, ed. "Les maisons-Dieu et les léproseries du diocèse de Paris au milieu du XIVe siècle, d'après le registre de visites du délégué de l'évêque (1351–69)." *Mémoires de la Société de l'Histoire de Paris et de l'Ile-de-France* 24 (1897): 61–365.

——. *Statuts d'hôtels-Dieu et de léproseries: Recueil de textes du XIIe au XIVe siècle.* Paris: Picard, 1901.

Lognon, Auguste, ed. *Documents relatifs au comté de Champagne et de Brie, 1172–1361.* 3 vols. Paris: Imprimerie Nationale, 1901–14.

Magna vita sancti Hugonis: The Life of St. Hugh of Lincoln [by Adam of Eynsham]. Edited by D. L. Douie and D. H. Farmer. 2nd ed. 2 vols., Oxford, 1985.

Matfre Ermengaud. *Le breviari d'amor.* Edited by Peter T. Ricketts. Leiden: Brill, 1976.

The Middle English "Weye of Paradys" and the Middle French "Voie de Paradis:" A Parallel-Text Edition. Edited by F. N. M. Diekstra. Leiden, The Netherlands: Brill, 1991.

Morlet, M. T., and M. Mulon, eds. "Le censier de l'Hôtel-Dieu de Provins." *Bibliothèque de l'École des Chartes* 134 (1976): 5–84.

Mulder-Bakker, Anneke B., ed. *Living Saints of the Thirteenth Century: The Lives of Yvette, Anchoress of Huy; Juliana of Cornillon, Author of the Corpus Christi Feast; and Margaret the Lame, Anchoress of Magdeburg.* Translated by Jo Ann McNamara. Turnhout, Belgium: Brepols, 2011.

Nicolaus de Lyra. *Postilla super totam Bibliam.* Strasbourg, 1492; repr. Munich, 1971.

Nusse, C. "Charte de fondation d'un Hôtel-Dieu à Barre." *Annales de la Société historique et archéologique de Château-Thierry* 48 (1874): 191–92.

Peter the Chanter. *Summa de sacramentis et animae consilii.* Edited by Jean-Albert Dugauquier. Leuven, Belgium: Nauwelaerts, 1954.

——. *Verbum abbreviatum: Textus conflatus.* Edited by Monique Boutry. Corpus Christianorum, vol. 196. Turnhout, Belgium: Brepols, 2004.

"Processus canonizationis et legendae variae Sancti Ludovici, O.F.M." *Analecta Franciscana* 7. Quaracchi, Italy: Fratri Collegii S. Bonaventurae, 1951.

Prou, Maurice, and Jules d'Auriac, eds. *Actes et comptes de la commune de Provins de l'an 1271 à l'an 1330.* Provins, France: Briard, 1933.

Ravaisson, Félix, ed. *Catalogue général des manuscrits des bibliothèques publiques des départements.* Vol. 1 (Laon). Paris: Imprimerie Nationale, 1849.

Recueil des historiens de la France: Obituaires de la province de Sens. Vol. 1, Part 2: *Diocèses de Sens et de Paris.* Edited by Auguste Molinier and Auguste Longnon. Paris: Imprimerie Nationale, 1902.

The Register of Eudes of Rouen. Translated by Sydney M. Brown. Edited by Jeremiah O'Sullivan. New York: Columbia University Press, 1964.

Richard, Jules-Marie, ed. *Cartulaire de l'hôpital Saint-Jean-en-l'Estrée d'Arras.* Paris: H. Champion, 1888.

Rigoli, Luigi, ed. *Volgarizzamento dell'Esposizione del Paternostro fatto da Zucchero Bencivenni.* Florence: Academia della Crusca, 1828.

Saint Bonaventure. *Sermones dominicales.* Edited by Jacques-Guy Bougerol. Grottaferrata, 1977.

Stein, Henri. "Cartulaire de l'hôtel-Dieu de Crecy-en-Brie." *Bulletin de la conférence d'histoire et d'archéologie du diocèse de Meaux* 2 (1899): 136–45.

Stephani de Borbone. *Tractatus de diversis materiis praedicabilibus.* Edited by Jacques Berlioz. *Corpus Christianorum. Continuatio Mediaevali,* vol. 124A. Turnhout, Belgium: Brepols, 2015.

Tanner, S.J., Norman P., ed. *Decrees of the Ecumenical Councils.* 2 vols. London: Sheed and Ward, 1990.

Teulet, Alexandre, et al., eds. *Layettes du trésor des chartes.* 5 vols. Paris, 1863–1909.

Thomas Aquinas, *Summa theologica.* Translated by the Fathers of the English Dominican Province. New York: Benziger Bros., 1947.

Thomas of Chobham. *Sermones.* Edited by Franco Morenzoni. *Corpus Christianorum. Continuatio Mediaevalis,* vol. 82A. Turnhout, Belgium: Brepols, 1993.

——. *Summa de arte praedicandi.* Edited by Franco Morenzoni. *Corpus Christianorum. Continuatio Mediaevalis,* vol. 82. Turnhout, Belgium: Brepols, 1988.

Varin, Pierre, ed. *Archives administratives de la ville de Reims: Collection de pièces inédites.* Paris: Crapelet, 1839.

Vincent of Beauvais, *Bibliotheca mundi, seu Speculi maioris Vincentii Burgundi.* Douai, 1624.

Secondary Sources

Aladjidi, Priscille. "L'idéal politique du roi 'père des pauvres.'" In *Une histoire pour un royaume (XIIe–XVe siècle): Actes du colloque Corpus Regni, organisé en hommage à Colette Beaune,* edited by Anne-Hélène Allirot, Murielle Gaude-Ferragu, and Gilles Lecuppre, 88–101. Paris: Perrin, 2010.

Ancelet-Hustache, Jeanne. *Gold Tried by Fire: St. Elizabeth of Hungary.* Chicago: Franciscan Herald Press, 1963.

Anderson, Gary A. *Charity: The Place of the Poor in the Biblical Tradition.* New Haven: Yale University Press, 2013.

Anderson, Mark Alan. "Hospitals, Hospices, and Shelters for the Poor in Late Antiquity." PhD dissertation, Yale University, 2012.

Angenendt, Arnold. "Donationes Pro Anima: Gift and Countergift in the Early Medieval Liturgy." In *The Long Morning of Medieval Europe: New Directions in Early Medieval Studies,* edited by Jennifer R. Davis and Michael McCormick, 131–54. London: Routledge, 2017.

Armstrong, Lawrin. *The Idea of a Moral Economy: Gerard of Siena on Usury, Restitution, and Prescription.* Toronto: University of Toronto Press, 2016.

Arnoux, Mathieu. *Des clercs au service de la réforme: Études et documents sur les chanoines réguliers de la province de Rouen.* Turnhout, Belgium: Brepols, 2000.

Aufauvre, Amédée, and Charles Fichot. *Les monuments de Seine-et-Marne: Description historique et archéologique et reproduction des édifices religieux, militaires et civils du département.* Paris, 1858.

Babeau, Albert. "L'hôtel-Dieu Saint-Bernard de Troyes." *Annuaire administratif, statistique et commercial du département de l'Aube* 80 (1906): 31–47.

Bain, Emmanuel. *Église, richesse et pauvreté dans l'occident médiéval: L'exégèse des Évangiles aux XIIe–XIIIe siècles.* Turnhout, Belgium: Brepols, 2014.

Baldwin, John W. *Masters, Princes, and Merchants: The Social Views of Peter the Chanter and His Circle.* 2 vols. Princeton: Princeton University Press, 1970.

Barber, Malcolm. "The Charitable and Medical Activities of the Hospitallers and Templars." In *A History of Pastoral Care,* edited by G. R. Evans, 148–68. London: Cassell, 2000.

Barnhouse, Lucy C. "The Elusive Medieval Hospital: Mainz and the Middle Rhine Region." PhD dissertation, Fordham University, 2017.

Baron, Françoise. "Les possessions hors les murs de l'Hôtel-Dieu de Provins au XIIIe siècle." *Bulletin de la Société d'histoire et d'archéologie de l'arrondissement de Provins* 130 (1976): 45–57.

Barthélemy, Dominique. *La mutation de l'an mil a t-elle-eu lieu? Servage et chevalerie dans la France des Xe et XIe siècles.* Paris: Fayard, 1997.

Baudin, Arnaud, Ghislain Brunel, and Nicolas Dohrmann, eds. *L'économie templière en Occident: Patrimoines, Commerce, Finances: Actes du colloque international (Troyes— Abbaye de Clairvaux, 24–26 octobre 2012).* Langres, 2013.

Bautier, Robert-Henri. "Les aumônes du roi aux maladreries, maisons-Dieu et pauvres établissements du royaume: Contribution à l'étude du réseau hospitalier et de la fossilisation de l'administration royale de Philippe Auguste à Charles VII." In *Assistance et assistés jusqu'à 1610. Actes du 97e congrès des Sociétés savantes, Nantes 1972,* 37–106. Paris: Bibliothèque Nationale, 1979.

——. "Les foires de Champagne: Recherches sur une évolution historique." In *La Foire,* vol. 5 of *Recueils de la Société Jean Bodin,* 97–147. Brussels: Editions de la Librairie Encyclopédique, 1953.

Beck, Patrice, Philippe Bernardi, and Laurent Feller, eds. *Rémunérer le travail au moyen âge: Pour une histoire sociale du salariat.* Paris: Picard, 2014.

Beer, Jeremy. *The Philanthropic Revolution: An Alternative History to Charity.* Philadelphia: University of Pennsylvania Press, 2015.

Bériou, Nicole. *L'avènement des maîtres de la Parole: La prédication à Paris au XIIIe siècle.* 2 vols. Paris: Institut d'Études Augustiniennes, 1998.

——. "L'esprit de lucre entre vice et vertu: Variations sur l'amour de l'argent dans la prédication du XIIIe siècle." In *Actes des congrès de la Société des historiens médiévistes de l'enseignement supérieur public* 28, no. 1 (1997): 267–87.

——. *La prédication de Ranulphe de la Houblonnière: Sermons aux clercs et aux simples gens à Paris au XIIIe siècle.* 2 vols. Paris: Études Augustiniennes, 1987.

——. "Le vocabulaire de la vie économique dans les textes pastoraux des frères mendiants au XIIIe siècle." In *L'economia dei conventi dei frati minori e predicatori fino alla metà del Trecento: Atti del XXXI Convegno internazionale, Assisi, 9–11 ottobre 2003,* 151–86. Spoleto, Italy: Centro italiano di studi sull'alto Medioevo, 2004.

Bériou, Nicole, and Jacques Chiffoleau, eds. *Économie et religion: L'expérience des ordres mendiants (XIIIe–XVe siècle)*. Lyon: Presses Universitaires de Lyon, 2009.

Bériou, Nicole, and François-Olivier Touati. *Voluntate Dei leprosus: Les lépreux entre conversion et exclusion aux XIIème et XIIIème siècles*. Spoleto, Italy: Centro Italiano di Studi Sull'alto Medioevo, 1991.

Berlovitz, Yaffa. "Seven Good Years." *Sippur Okev Sippur: Encyclopedia of the Jewish Story*. Vol. 1. Edited by Yoav Elstein, Avidov Lipsker, and Rella Kushelevsky. Ramat-Gan, Israel: Bar Ilan University Press, 2004.

Berman, Constance H. "Distinguishing between the Humble Peasant Lay Brother and Sister, and the Converted Knight in Medieval Southern France." In *Religious and Laity in Western Europe, 1000–1400: Interaction, Negotiation, and Power*, edited by Emilia Jamroziak and Janet Burton, 263–86. Turnhout, Belgium: Brill, 2006.

——. *Medieval Agriculture, the Southern French Countryside, and the Early Cistercians: A Study of Forty-Three Monasteries*. Philadelphia: American Philosophical Society, 1986.

Bertelsmeier-Kierst, Christa, ed. *Elisabeth von Thüringen und die neue Frömmigkeit in Europa*. Frankfurt: Peter Lang, 2008.

Bertrand, Paul. *Commerce avec dame pauvreté: Structures et fonctions des couvents mendiants à Liège (XIIIe–XIVe siècles)*. Geneva: Droz, 2004.

Bijsterveld, Arnoud-Jan. "The Medieval Gift as Agent of Social Bonding and Political Power: A Comparative Approach." In *Medieval Transformations: Texts, Power, and Gifts in Context*, edited by Esther Cohen and Mayke B. De Jong, 123–56. Leiden: Brill, 2001.

Bird, Jessalynn. "Medicine for Body and Soul: Jacques de Vitry's Sermons to Hospitallers and Their Charges." In *Religion and Medicine in the Middle Ages*, edited by Joseph Ziegler and Peter Biller, 91–108. York: York Medieval Press, 2001.

——. "The Religious's Role in a Post-Fourth Lateran World: Jacques de Vitry's *Sermones ad status* and *Historia occidentalis*." In *Medieval Monastic Preaching*, edited by Carolyn Muessig, 209–29. Leiden: Brill, 1998.

Bishop, Matthew, and Michael Green. *Philanthrocapitalism: How Giving Can Save the World*. London: A & C Black, 2010.

Blampignon, Émile-Antoine. *Bar-sur-Aube*. Paris: Picard, 1900.

Bolton, Brenda. "Hearts Not Purses? Pope Innocent III's Attitude to Social Welfare." In *Innocent III: Studies on Papal Authority and Pastoral Care*, 123–45. Aldershot, U.K.: Variorum, 1995.

Bonenfant-Feytmans, Anne-Marie. "Les organisations hospitalières vues par Jacques de Vitry (1225)." *Annales de la Société belge d'histoire des hôpitaux* 18 (1980): 17–45.

Botana, Federico. *The Works of Mercy in Italian Medieval Art, c.1050–c.1400*. Turnhout, Belgium: Brepols, 2012.

Bouchard, Constance Brittain. *Holy Entrepreneurs: Cistercians, Knights, and Economic Exchange in Twelfth-Century Burgundy*. Ithaca: Cornell University Press, 1991.

——. *Sword, Miter, and Cloister: Nobility and the Church in Burgundy, 980–1198*. Ithaca: Cornell University Press, 1987.

Bourquelot, Félix. *Études sur les foires de Champagne: Sur la nature, l'étendue et les règles du commerce qui s'y faisait aux XIIe, XIIe et XIVe siècles*, 2nd ser., vol. 5 of *Mémoires présentés par divers savants à l'Académie des Inscriptions et Belles-Lettres de l'Institut Impérial de France*. Paris: Le Portulan, 1865.

——. *Histoire de Provins*. Paris, 1839; repr. 2004.

Boutiot, Théophile. *Histoire de la ville de Troyes et de la Champagne méridionale*. Troyes, France: Dufey-Robert, 1870.

Bove, Boris. "Vie et mort d'un couple de marchands-drapiers parisiens d'après les testaments de Jeanne et Étienne Haudri (1309, 1313)." *Paris et Ile-de-France 52* (2001): 19–81.

Brasher, Sally Mayall. *Hospitals and Charity: Religious Culture and Civic Life in Medieval Northern Italy*. Manchester: Manchester University Press, 2017.

Brenner, Elma. "The Care of the Sick and the Needy in Twelfth- and Thirteenth-Century Rouen." In *Society and Culture in Medieval Rouen, 911–1300*, edited by Leonie V. Hicks and Elma Brenner, 339–68. Turnhout, Belgium: Brepols, 2013.

——. *Leprosy and Charity in Medieval Rouen*. Woodbridge, U.K.: Boydell and Brewer, 2015.

Britnell, Richard H., and Bruce M. S. Campbell. *A Commercialising Economy: England 1086 to c. 1300*. Manchester: Manchester University Press, 1995.

Brodman, James W. *Charity and Religion in Medieval Europe*. Washington, DC: Catholic University of America Press, 2009.

——. *Charity and Welfare: Hospitals and the Poor in Medieval Catalonia*. Philadelphia: University of Pennsylvania Press, 1998.

——. *Ransoming Captives in Crusader Spain: The Order of Merced on the Christian-Islamic Frontier*. Philadelphia: University of Pennsylvania Press, 1986.

Brown, Elizabeth A. R. "La mort, les testaments et les fondations de Jeanne de Navarre, reine de France (1273–1305)." In *Une histoire pour un royaume (XIIe–XVe siècle). Actes du colloque Corpus Regni organisé en hommage à Colette Beaune*, edited by Anne-Hélène Allirot, 124–41. Paris: Perrin, 2010.

Brown, Peter. *Through the Eye of a Needle: Wealth, the Fall of Rome, and the Making of Christianity in the West, 350–550 AD*. Princeton: Princeton University Press, 2012.

——. *The Ransom of the Soul: Afterlife and Wealth in Early Western Christianity*. Cambridge: Harvard University Press, 2015.

Bruckner, Matilda Tomaryn. *Narrative Invention in Twelfth-Century French Romance: The Convention of Hospitality (1160–1200)*. Lexington, KY: French Forum Publishers, 1980.

Buhrer, Eliza. "From *Caritas* to Charity: How Loving God Became Giving Alms." In *Poverty and Prosperity in the Middle Ages and the Renaissance*, edited by Cynthia Kosso and Anne Scott, 113–28. Turnhout, Belgium: Brepols, 2012.

Bulst, Neithard, and Karl-Heinz Spieß, eds. *Sozialgeschichte mittelalterlicher Hospitäler*. Ostfildern, Germany: Jan Thorbecke Verlag, 2007.

Bur, Michel. "Les 'autres' foires de Champagne." In *La Champagne médiévale: Recueil d'articles*, edited by Michel Bur, 499–514. Langres, France: Dominique Guéniot, 2005.

——. "Le comte de Champagne dans le diocèse de Reims au XIIe siècle." In *La Champagne médiévale: Recueil d'articles*, edited by Michel Bur, 239–56. Langres, France: Dominique Guéniot, 2005.

——. "Meaux dans l'histoire de la Champagne du Xe au XIIe siècle." In *La Champagne médiévale: Recueil d'articles*, edited by Michel Bur, 443–51. Langres, France: Dominique Guéniot, 2005.

———. "Note sur quelque petites foires comtales de Champagne." In *La Champagne médiévale: Recueil d'articles,* edited by Michel Bur, 485–97. Langres, France: Dominique Guéniot, 2005.

———. "Remarques sur les plus anciens documents concernant les foires de Champagne." In *La Champagne médiévale: Recueil d'articles,* edited by Michel Bur, 463–84. Langres, France: Dominique Guéniot, 2005.

Burgess, Clive. "Late Medieval Wills and Pious Conventions: Testamentary Evidence Reconsidered." In *Profit, Piety, and the Professions in Later Medieval England,* edited by Michael Hicks, 14–33. Gloucester: A. Sutton, 1990.

Bynum, Caroline Walker. "Jesus as Mother and Abbot as Mother: Some Themes in Twelfth-Century Cistercian Writing." In *Jesus as Mother: Studies in the Spirituality of the High Middle Ages,* 110–68. Berkeley: University of California Press, 1982.

Caille, Jacqueline. *Hôpitaux et charité publique à Narbonne au moyen âge.* Toulouse: Privat, 1977.

Carraz, Damien. *L'ordre du Temple dans la basse vallée du Rhône (1124–1312): Ordres militaires, croisades et sociétés méridionales.* Lyon: Presses Universitaires de Lyon, 2005.

———. "Présences et dévotions féminines autour des commanderies du Bas-Rhône (XIIe–XIIIe siècle)." In *Les orders religieux militaires dans le Midi (XIIe–XIVe siècle),* vol. 41, *Cahiers de Fanjeaux,* 71–99. Toulouse: Privat, 2006.

———. "Templars and Hospitallers in the Cities of the West and the Latin East (Twelfth to Thirteenth Centuries)." *Crusades* 12 (2013): 103–20.

Carrière, Victor. *Histoire et cartulaire des Templiers de Provins.* Paris: Champion, 1919.

Cavallo, Sandra. *Charity and Power in Early Modern Italy: Benefactors and Their Motives in Turin, 1541–17.* Cambridge: Cambridge University Press, 1995.

———. "The Motivations of Benefactors: An Overview of Approaches to the Study of Charity." In *Medicine and Charity Before the Welfare State,* edited by Colin Jones and Jonathan Barry, 46–62. London: Routledge, 1991.

Ceccarelli, Giovanni. "'Whatever' Economics: Economic Thought in Quodlibeta." In *Theological Quodlibeta in the Middle Ages: The Thirteenth Century,* edited by Christopher Schabel, 475–506. Leiden: Brill, 2006.

Cessford, Craig. "The St. John's Hospital Cemetery and Environs, Cambridge: Contextualizing the Medieval Urban Dead." *Archaeological Journal* 172, no. 1 (2015): 52–120.

Challe, Ambroise. *Histoire du comté de Tonnerre.* Auxerre, France: Imprimerie de Gustave Perriquet, 1875.

Chapin, Elizabeth. *Les villes de foires de Champagne, des origines au début du XIVe siècle.* Paris: H. Champion, 1937.

Chiffoleau, Jacques. *La comptabilité de l'au-delà: Les hommes, la mort et la religion dans la région d'Avignon à la fin du moyen âge (vers 1320–vers 1480).* Rome: École Française de Rome, 1980.

———. "Pour une économie de l'institution ecclésiale à la fin du moyen âge." *Mélanges de l'École française de Rome* 96, no.1 (1984): 247–79.

Cohn Jr., Samuel K. *The Cult of Remembrance and the Black Death: Six Renaissance Cities in Central Italy.* Baltimore: Johns Hopkins University Press, 1992.

Comte, François. "Hygiène hospitalière à Saint-Jean d'Angers (Maine-et-Loire, France): Adduction et évacuation des eaux du XIIe au XIIIe siècle." In *L'hydraulique monastique: milieux, réseaux, usages*, edited by Léon Pressouyre and Paul Benoît, 437–53. Paris: Créaphis, 1996.

Courtenay, Lynn T. "Les chartes de Marguerite de Bourgogne: Une étude préliminaire." In *Les établissements hospitaliers en France du moyen âge au XIXe siècle: Espaces, objets et populations*, edited by Sylvie Le Clech-Charton, 31–52. Dijon, France: Éditions Universitaires de Dijon, 2010

——. "The Hospital of Notre Dame des Fontenilles at Tonnerre: Medicine as Misericordia." In *The Medieval Hospital and Medical Practice*, edited by Barbara S. Bowers, 77–106. Aldershot, U.K.: Ashgate, 2007.

——. "Seigneurie et charité: L'exercise du patronage de Marguerite de Bourgogne, comtesse de Tonnerre." In *Les établissements hospitaliers en France du Moyen Âge au XIXe siècle: Espaces, objets et populations*, edited by Sylvie Le Clech-Charton, 13–30. Dijon, France: Éditions Universitaires de Dijon, 2010.

Courtenay, William J. "Token Coinage and the Administration of Poor Relief in the Later Middle Ages." *Journal of Interdisciplinary History* 3 (1972 / 73): 275–95.

Coyecque, Ernest. *L'hôtel-Dieu de Paris au moyen âge: L'histoire et documents*. Paris: H. Champion, 1889.

Cusato, O.F.M., Michael. "Two Uses of the *Vita Christi* Genre in Tuscany, c. 1300: John de Caulibus and Ubertino da Casale Compared. A Response to Daniel Lesnick, Ten Years Hence." *Franciscan Studies* 57 (1999): 131–48.

——. "Where Are the Poor in the Writings of Angelo Clareno and the Spiritual Franciscans?" In *Angelo Clareno Francescano: Atti del XXXIV Convegno internazionale, Assisi, 5–7 ottobre 2006*, 123–65. Spoleto, Italy: Centro Italiano Di Studi Sull'alto Medioevo, 2007.

Daniell, Christopher. *Death and Burial in Medieval England*. London: Routledge, 1997.

Davies, Wendy, and Paul Fouracre, eds. *The Languages of Gift in the Early Middle Ages*. Cambridge: Cambridge University Press, 2010.

Davis, Adam J. *The Holy Bureaucrat: Eudes Rigaud and Religious Reform in Thirteenth-Century Normandy*. Ithaca: Cornell University Press, 2006.

——. "Preaching in Thirteenth-Century Hospitals." *Journal of Ecclesiastical History* 36, no. 1 (March 2010): 72–89.

——. "The Social and Religious Meaning of Charity in Medieval Europe." *History Compass* 12, no. 12 (December 2014): 935–50.

Davis, Adam J., and Bertrand Taithe. "From the Purse and the Heart: Exploring Charity, Humanitarianism, and Human Rights in France." *French Historical Studies* 34, no. 3 (Summer 2011): 413–32.

Davy, Christian. *La peinture murale romane dans les pays de la Loire: L'indicible et le ruban plissé*. Laval, Canada: Société d'Archéologie et d'Histoire de la Mayenne, 1999.

de Jubainville, Henri d'Arbois. *Histoire de Bar-sur-Aube sous les comtes de Champagne, 1077–1284*. Paris: Auguste Durand, 1859.

——. *Histoire des ducs et des comtes de Champagne*. 6 vols. Paris: Auguste Durand, 1859–66.

de Melin, Joseph Roserot. *Le diocèse de Troyes des origines à nos jours*. Troyes, France: Imprimerie de la Renaissance, 1957.

de Miramon, Charles. *Les "donnés" au moyen âge: Une forme de vie religieuse laïque (v. 1180–v.1500).* Paris: Cerf, 1999.

——. "Quatre notes biographiques sur Guillaume de Champeaux." In *Arts du langage et théologie aux confins des XIe et XIIe siècle,* edited by I. Rosier-Catach, 45–82. Turnhout, Belgium: Brepols, 2011.

De Spiegeler, Pierre. *Les hôpitaux et l'assistance à Liège (Xe–XVe siècles): Aspects institutionnels et sociaux.* Paris: Société d'édition "Les Belles Lettres," 1987.

Delmaire, Bernard. *Le diocèse d'Arras de 1093 au milieu du XIVe siècle: Recherches sur la vie religieuse dans le nord de la France au moyen âge.* Arras, 1994.

——. "Hôpitaux urbains et hôpitaux ruraux en Artois entre le XIIe et XIVe siècle." *Histoire médiévale et archéologie* 17 (2004): 221–40.

Delmas, Sophie. "*La Summa de abstinentia* attribuée à Nicolas de Biard: Circulation et réception." In *Entre stabilité et itinérance: Livres et culture des ordres mendiants, XIIIe–XVe siècle,* 303–27. Turnhout, Belgium: Brepols, 2014.

Derville, Alain. *L'agriculture du Nord au moyen âge: Artois, Cambrésis, Flandre Wallonne.* Paris: Presses Universitaires du Septentrion, 1999.

Desportes, Pierre. *Reims et les Rémois aux XIIIe et XIVe siècles.* Paris: Picard, 1979.

Dietrich-Strobbe, Irène. "Sauver les riches: La charité à Lille à la fin du moyen âge." Thesis, l'Université Paris-Sorbonne, 2016.

Drossbach, Gisela. *Christliche Caritas als Rechtsinstitut: Hospital und Orden von Santo Spirito in Sassia (1198–1378).* Paderborn, Germany: Schöningh, 2005.

Drossbach, Gisela, ed. *Hospitäler in Mittelalter und früher Neuzeit: Frankreich, Deutschland und Italien: Eine vergleichende Geschichte.* Munich: R. Oldenbourg Wissenschaftsverlag, 2007.

Dubois, Henri. "Le pouvoir économique du prince." In *Les princes et le pouvoir au moyen âge: Actes du XXIIIe congrès de la Société des historiens médiévistes de l'enseignement supérieur public de Brest, 1992,* 229–46. Paris: Publications de la Sorbonne, 1993.

Duby, Georges. *L'économie rurale et la vie des campagnes dans l'Occident médiéval (France, Angleterre, Empire, IXe–XVe siècles). Essai de synthèse et perspectives de recherches.* Paris: Aubier, 1962.

Dyer, Christopher. "The Experience of Being Poor in Late Medieval England." In *Experiences of Poverty in Late Medieval and Early Modern Europe,* edited by Anne M. Scott, 20–39. Aldershot, U.K.: Ashgate, 2012.

——. "Poverty and Its Relief in Late Medieval England." *Past and Present* 216 (2012): 41–78.

Edwards, Jeremy, and Sheilagh Ogilvie. "What Lessons for Economic Development Can We Draw from the Champagne Fairs?" *Explorations in Economic History* 49 (2012): 131–48.

Elliott, Dyan. *Spiritual Marriage: Sexual Abstinence in Medieval Wedlock.* Princeton: Princeton University Press, 1993.

Epstein, Steven. *Wills and Wealth in Medieval Genoa, 1150–1250.* Cambridge: Harvard University Press, 1984.

Evergates, Theodore. *The Aristocracy in the County of Champagne.* Philadelphia: University of Pennsylvania Press, 2007.

——. *Feudal Society in the Bailliage of Troyes Under the Counts of Champagne, 1152–1284.* Baltimore: Johns Hopkins University Press, 1975.

——. *Henry the Liberal*. Philadelphia: University of Pennsylvania Press, 2016.

——. "Nobles and Knights in Twelfth-Century France." In *Cultures of Power: Lordship, Status, and Process in Twelfth-Century Europe*, edited by Thomas Bisson, 11–35. Philadelphia: University of Pennsylvania Press, 1995.

Farmer, Sharon. "From Personal Charity to Centralised Poor Relief: The Evolution of Responses to the Poor in Paris, c. 1250–1600." In *Experiences of Charity, 1250–1650*, edited by Anne M. Scott, 17–42. Farnham, U.K.: Ashgate, 2015.

——. "The Leper in the Master Bedroom: Thinking Through a Thirteenth-Century Exemplum." In *Framing the Family: Narrative and Representation in the Medieval and Early Modern Periods*, edited by Diane Wolfthal and Rosalynn Voaden, 79–100. Tempe: Arizona Center for Medieval and Renaissance Studies, 2005.

——. "Persuasive Voices: Clerical Images of Medieval Wives," *Speculum* 61, no. 3 (July 1986): 517–43.

——. *Surviving Poverty in Medieval Paris: Gender, Ideology, and the Daily Lives of the Poor*. Ithaca: Cornell University Press, 2002.

Firey, Abigail. "'For I Was Hungry and You Fed Me': Social Justice and Economic Thought in the Latin Patristic and Medieval Christian Traditions." In *Ancient and Medieval Economic Ideas and Concepts of Social Justice*, edited by S. Todd Lowry and Barry Gordon, 333–70. Leiden: Brill, 1998.

Forey, Alan. "The Charitable Activities of the Templars." *Viator* 34 (2003): 109–41.

Fossier, Robert. "La puissance économique de l'abbaye de Clairvaux au XIIIe siècle." In *Histoire de Clairvaux, Actes du Colloque 1990*, 73–83. Bar-sur-Aube, France: Association Renaissance de l'Abbaye de Clairvaux, 1991.

Fournier, Pierre-François. "Les statuts de l'hôpital de Billom (Puy-de-Dôme)." In *Assistance et assistés jusqu'à 1610. Actes du 97ᵉ Congrès National des Sociétés Savantes, Nantes, 1972*, 129–46. Paris: Bibliothèque Nationale, 1979.

Frederickson, George M. *The Inner Civil War: Northern Intellectuals and the Crisis of the Union*. 2nd ed. Urbana: University of Illinois Press, 1993.

Galinsky, Judah. "'Hazkarat Nishamot' (i.e. 'Yizkor'), 'Poskim al ha-Zeddaka,' and the Funding of Communal Activities in Medieval Ashkenaz." Unpublished paper.

——. "Jewish Charitable Bequests and the Hekdesh Trust in Thirteenth-Century Spain." *Journal of Interdisciplinary History* 35, no. 3 (2005): 423–40.

Galvin, Michael. "Credit and Parochial Charity in Fifteenth-Century Bruges." *Journal of Medieval History* 28, no. 2 (2002): 131–54.

Gaposchkin, M. Cecilia. *The Making of Saint Louis: Kingship, Sanctity, and Crusade in the Later Middle Ages*. Ithaca: Cornell University Press, 2008.

Génestal, Robert. *Rôle des monastères comme établissements de credit étudié en Normandie du XIe à la fin du XIII siècle*. Paris, 1901.

Genicot, Léopold. "L'évolution des dons aux abbayes dans le comté de Namur du Xe au XIVe siècle." In *XXXe Congrès de la Fédération archéologique et historique de Belgique, Bruxelles, 28 Juillet–2 Août 1935: Annales*, 133–48. Brussels, 1936.

Geremek, Bronislaw. *The Margins of Society in Late Medieval Paris*. Cambridge: Cambridge University Press, 1987.

Gesret, Julie. "Un hôpital au moyen âge: L'hôtel-Dieu Saint-Nicolas de Troyes du XIIIe au XVe siècle, "soustenir les povres." PhD dissertation, École des Chartes, Paris, 2003.

Gilchrist, Roberta. *Medieval Life: Archaeology and the Life Course*. Woodbridge: Boydell Press, 2012.

Gilchrist, Roberta, and Barney Sloane, eds. *Requiem: The Medieval Monastic Cemetery in Britain*. London: Museum of London Archaeology Service, 2005.

Giridharadas, Anand. *Winners Take All: The Elite Charade of Changing the World*. New York: Knopf, 2018.

Godding, Philippe. "La pratique testamentaire en Flandre au XIIIe siècle." *Revue d'histoire du droit* 58, no. 3 (1990): 281–300.

Goetz, Jennifer L., Dacher Keltner, and Emiliana Simon-Thomas. "Compassion: An Evolutionary Analysis and Empirical Review." *Psychological Bulletin* 136 (2010): 351–74.

Gonthier, Nicole. "Les hôpitaux et les pauvres à la fin du moyen âge: L'exemple de Lyon." *Le Moyen Age* 34, no. 2 (1978): 279–308.

Goodich, Michael. "Ancilla Dei: The Servant as Saint in the Late Middle Ages." In *Women of the Medieval World: Essays in Honor of John H. Mundy*, edited by Suzanne F. Wemple and Julius Kirshner, 119–36. Oxford: Basil Blackwell, 1985.

Grant, Lindy. "The Chapel of the Hospital of Saint-Jean at Angers: Acta, Statutes, Architecture, and Interpretation." In *Architecture and Interpretation: Essays for Eric Fernie*, edited by Jill A. Franklin, T. A. Heslop, and Christine Stevenson, 306–14. Woodbridge, U.K.: Boydell & Brewer, 2013.

———. "Royal and Aristocratic Hospital Patronage in Northern France in the Twelfth and Early Thirteenth Centuries." In *Laienadel und Armenfürsorge im Mittelalter*, 105–14. Edited by Lukas Clemens, Katrin Dort, and Felix Schumacher. Trier, Germany: Kliomedia, 2015.

Gray, Alyssa M. "Redemptive Almsgiving and the Rabbis of Late Antiquity." *Jewish Studies Quarterly* 18, no. 2 (2011): 144–84.

Guest, Gerald B. "A Discourse on the Poor: The Hours of Jeanne d'Evreux." *Viator* 26 (1995): 153–80.

Hall, Peter Dobkin. *Inventing the Nonprofit Sector and Other Essays on Philanthropy, Voluntarism, and Nonprofit Organizations*. Baltimore: Johns Hopkins University Press, 1992.

Harding, Vanessa. "Burial Choice and Burial Location in Later Medieval London." In *Death in Towns: Urban Responses to the Dying and the Dead, 100–1600*, edited by Steven Bassett, 119–35. London: Leicester University Press, 1992.

Harmand, Auguste. "Notice historique sur la léproserie de la ville de Troyes," *Mémoires de la Société Académique de l'Aube* 14 (1848): 429–669.

Henderson, John. *The Renaissance Hospital: Healing the Body and Healing the Soul*. New Haven: Yale University Press, 2006.

Holladay, Joan A. "The Education of Jeanne d'Evreux: Personal Piety and Dynastic Salvation in her Book of Hours at the Cloisters." *Art History* 17, no. 4 (December 1994): 585–611.

Horden, Peregrine. "Cities Within Cities: Early Hospital Foundations and Urban Space." In *Stiftungen zwischen Politik und Wirtschaft: Ein Dialog zwischen Geschichte und Gegenwart*, edited by Sitta von Reden, 157–76. Munich, 2015.

———. "A Discipline of Relevance: The Historiography of the Later Medieval Hospital." *Social History of Medicine* 1 (1988): 359–74.

———. "Household Care and Informal Networks: Comparisons and Continuities from Antiquity to the Present." In *The Locus of Care: Families, Communities, Institutions, and Provision of Welfare Since Antiquity*, edited by Peregrine Horden and Richard Smith, 21–67. London: Routledge, 1998.

———. "How Medicalised Were Byzantine Hospitals?" In *Hospitals and Healing from Antiquity to the Later Middle Ages*, edited by Peregrine Horden, 213–35. Aldershot, U.K.: Ashgate, 2008.

———. "A Non-Natural Environment: Medicine Without Doctors and the Medieval European Hospital." In *The Medieval Hospital and Medical Practice*, edited by Barbara S. Bowers, 133–45. Aldershot, U.K.: Ashgate, 2007.

———. "Religion as Medicine: Music in Medieval Hospitals." In *Religion and Medicine in the Middle Ages*, edited by Peter Biller and Joseph Ziegler, 135–54. York: York Medieval Press, 2001.

Howell, Martha C. *Commerce Before Capitalism in Europe, 1300–1600*. Cambridge: Cambridge University Press, 2010.

Hunt, Lynn Avery. *Inventing Human Rights: A History*. New York: Norton, 2007.

Huyskens, Albert. *Quellenstudien zur Geschichte der Hl. Elisabeth Landgräfin von Thüringen*. Marburg, U.K.: Elwert, 1908.

Imbert, Jean, ed. *Histoire des hôpitaux en France*. Toulouse: Privat, 1982.

———. *Les hôpitaux en droit canonique (du décret de Gratien à la sécularisation de l'administration de l'Hôtel-Dieu de Paris en 1505)*. Paris: J. Vrin, 1947.

Izbicki, Thomas M. "Pyres of Vanities: Mendicant Preaching on the Vanity of Women and Its Lay Audience." In *De Ore Domini: Preacher and Word in the Middle Ages*, edited by Thomas L. Amos, Eugene A. Green, and Beverly Mayne Kienzle, 211–34. Kalamazoo, MI: Medieval Institute Publications, 1989.

Jacquart, Danielle. *Le milieu médical du XIIe au XVe siècle*. Geneva: Droz, 1981.

Jeanne, Damien. "Le roi charitable: Les politiques royales envers les établissements d'assistance de la Normandie centrale et occidentale, XIIIe–XVe siècle." In *Une histoire pour un royaume, XIIe–XVe siècle: Actes du colloque Corpus Regni, organisé en hommage à Colette Beaune*, edited by Anne-Hélène Allirot and Colette Beaune, 119–55. Paris: Perrin, 2010.

Jéhanno, Christine. "Entre le chapitre cathédral et l'hôtel-Dieu de Paris: Les enjeux du conflit de la fin du moyen âge." *Revue Historique* 313, no. 3 (2011): 527–60.

———. "'Sustenter les povres malades:' Alimentation et approvisionnement à la fin du moyen âge: L'exemple de l'hôtel-Dieu de Paris." Doctoral thesis, Paris I, 2000.

Jones, Colin. *Charity and Bienfaisance: The Treatment of the Poor in the Montpellier Region 1740–1815*. New York: Cambridge University Press, 1982.

Jordan, Erin. "Exploring the Limits of Female Largesse: The Power of Female Patrons in Thirteenth-Century Flanders and Hainaut." In *Women and Wealth in Late Medieval Europe*, edited by Theresa Earenfight, 149–70. New York: Palgrave, 2010.

Kaye, Joel. *Economy and Nature in the Fourteenth Century: Money, Market Exchange, and the Emergence of Scientific Thought*. Cambridge: Cambridge University Press, 2009.

———. "The Impact of Money on the Development of Fourteenth-Century Scientific Thought," *Journal of Medieval History* 14 (1988): 251–70.

——. "Monetary and Market Consciousness in Thirteenth and Fourteenth Century Europe." In *Ancient and Medieval Economic Ideas and Concepts of Social Justice*, edited by S. Todd Lowry and Barry Gordon, 376–403. Leiden: Brill, 1998.

Kemp, Simon. "Quantification of Virtue in Late Medieval Europe." *History of Psychology* 21, no. 1 (2018): 33–46.

Kerr, Julie. *Monastic Hospitality: The Benedictines in England, c. 1070–c. 1250*. Woodbridge, Suffolk: Boydell Press, 2007.

Keyser, Richard L. "Gift, Dispute, and Contract: Gift Exchange and Legalism in Monastic Property Dealings, Montier-la-Celle, France, 1100–1350." PhD dissertation, Johns Hopkins University, 2001.

——. "La transformation de l'échange des dons pieux: Montier-la-Celle, Champagne, 1100–1350." *Revue historique* 305, no. 4 (2003): 793–816.

——. "The Transformation of Traditional Woodland Management: Commercial Silviculture in Medieval Champagne." *French Historical Studies* 32, no. 3 (2009): 353–84.

Kupfer, Marcia. *The Art of Healing: Painting for the Sick and the Sinner in a Medieval Town*. University Park: Pennsylvania State University Press, 2003.

Lacomme, Thomas. "Gager sa dette avec le mobilier liturgique: Thibaud IV de Champagne, l'abbaye de Saint-Denis et la collégiale Saint-Étienne de Troyes (XIIIe siècle)." *Éditions du CRINI* 9 (2017).

Lalore, Charles. *Liste des prieurés, commanderies et hôpitaux de l'ancien diocèse de Troyes, d'après le pouillé de l'évêque de 1761*. Troyes, 1886.

Langholm, Odd. *Economics in the Medieval Schools: Wealth, Exchange, Value, Money and Usury According to the Paris Theological Tradition, 1200–1500*. Leiden: Brill, 1992.

——. *The Merchant in the Confessional: Trade and Price in the Pre-Reformation Penitential Handbooks*. Leiden: Brill, 2003.

Laqua, Benjamin. *Bruderschaften und Hospitäler während des hohen Mittelalters: Kölner Befunde in westeuropäisch-vergleichender Perspektive*. Stuttgart: Anton Hiersemann, 2011.

Le Blévec, Daniel. "Les moines et l'assistance: L'exemple des pays du Bas-Rhône (XIIe–XIIIe siècles)." In *Moines et monastères dans les sociétés de rite Grec et Latin*, edited by Jean-Loup Lemaitre, Michel Dmitriev, and Pierre Gonneau, 335–45. Geneva: Droz, 1996.

——. "Le rôle des femmes dans l'assistance et la charité." In *La femme dans la vie religieuse du Languedoc (XIIIe–XIVe s.)*, vol. 23, *Cahiers de Fanjeaux*, 171–90. Toulouse: Privat, 1988.

——. "Fondations et œuvres charitables au moyen âge." In *Fondations et œuvres charitables au moyen âge*, edited by Jean Dufour and Henri Platelle, 7–22. Paris: Éditions du CTHS, 1999.

——. "Maladie et soins du corps dans les monastères cisterciens." In *Horizons marins, itinéraires spirituels: Mélanges offerts à Michel Mollat*, vol. 1: *Mentalités et sociétés*, 171–82. Paris: Publications de la Sorbonne, 1987.

——. *La part du pauvre: L'assistance et charité dans les pays du Bas-Rhône du XIIe siècle au milieu du XVe siècle*. Rome: École Française de Rome, 2000.

Le Clech-Charton, Sylvie. *L'hôtel-Dieu de Tonnerre: Métamorphose d'un patrimoine hospitalier, XIIIe–XXe siècle*. Langres, France: Éditions Dominique Guéniot, 2012.

Le Goff, Jacques. *The Birth of Purgatory*. Translated by Arthur Goldhammer. Chicago: University of Chicago Press, 1984.

——. *Money and the Middle Ages: An Essay in Historical Anthropology*. Translated by Jean Birrell. Cambridge: Polity Press, 2012.

——. *Saint Louis*. Translated by Gareth Evan Gollrad. South Bend: Notre Dame University Press, 2009.

——. "Temps de l'Église et temps du marchand." *Annales* 15, no. 3 (May-June 1960): 417–33.

Le Grand, Léon. "Les maisons-Dieu: Leurs statuts au XIIIe siècle." *Revue des questions historiques* 60 (1896): 95–134.

——. "La prière des malades dans les hôpitaux de l'Ordre de Saint-Jean de Jérusalem." *Bibliothèque de l'École des Chartes* 57 (1896): 325–38.

Lehrer, Jonah. "Kin and Kind: A Fight About the Genetics of Altruism." *The New Yorker*, March 5, 2012.

Lenoble, Michel. "Le site de l'ancien hôtel-Dieu de Troyes." *La vie en Champagne* 38, no. 414 (November 1990): 3–18.

Lester, Anne E. "Cares Beyond the Walls: Cistercian Nuns and the Care of Lepers in Twelfth- and Thirteenth-Century Northern France." In *Religious and Laity in Western Europe, 1000–1400: Interaction, Negotiation, and Power*, edited by Janet Burton and Emilia Jamroziak, 197–224. Turnhout, Belgium: Brepols, 2006.

——. *Creating Cistercian Nuns: The Women's Religious Movement and Its Reform in Thirteenth-Century Champagne*. Ithaca: Cornell University Press, 2011.

——. "Saint Louis and Cîteaux Revisited: Cistercian Commemoration and Devotion During the Capetian Century, 1214–1314." In *The Capetian Century, 1214–1314*, edited by William Chester Jordan and Rebecca Phillips, 17–42. Turnhout, Belgium: Brepols, 2017.

Leurquin-Labie, Anne-Françoise. "La *Somme le roi*: De la commande royale de Philippe III à la diffusion sous Philippe IV et au-delà." In *La moisson des lettres: L'invention littéraire autour de 1300*. Edited by Hélène Bellon-Méguelle et al., 195–212. Turnhout, Belgium: Brepols, 2011.

Lindbeck, Kristen H. *Elijah and the Rabbis: Story and Theology*. New York: Columbia University Press, 2010.

Little, Lester K. *Religious Poverty and the Profit Economy in Medieval Europe*. Ithaca: Cornell University Press, 1978.

Longère, Jean. "Pauvreté et richesse chez quelques prédicateurs durant la seconde moitié du XIIe siècle." In *Études sur l'histoire de la pauvreté*, edited by Michel Mollat, vol. 1, 255–73. Paris: Publications de la Sorbonne, 1974.

Luttrell, Anthony. "Les femmes hospitalières en France méridionale." In *Les ordres religieux militaires dans le Midi (XIIe–XIVe siècle)*. Vol. 41, *Cahiers de Fanjeaux*, 101–13. Toulouse: Privat, 2006.

Luttrell, Anthony, and Helen J. Nicholson, eds. *Hospitaller Women in the Middle Ages*. Aldershot, U.K.: Ashgate, 2006.

Magnani, Eliana, ed. *Don et sciences sociales: Théories et pratiques croisées*. Dijon: Editions de l'Université de Dijon, 2007.

——. "Le pauvre, le Christ et le moine: La correspondance de rôles et les cérémonies du *mandatum* à travers les coutumiers du XIe siècle." In *Les clercs, les fidèles et les saints en Bourgogne médiévale*, edited by Vincent Tabbagh, 11–26. Dijon: Editions universitaires de Dijon, 2005.

Mauss, Marcel. *The Gift: The Form and Reason for Exchange in Archaic Societies.* Translated by W. D. Halls. Foreword by Mary Douglas. New York: Norton, 2000.

Mazel, Florian. "Amitié et rupture de l'amitié: Moines et grands laïcs provençaux au temps de la crise grégorienne (milieu XIe–milieu XII siècle)." *Revue historique* 633, no, 1 (2005): 53–95.

McCarthy, Kathleen D. *American Creed: Philanthropy and the Rise of Civil Society, 1700–1865.* Chicago: University of Chicago Press, 2003.

McLaughlin, Megan. *Consorting with the Saints: Prayer for the Dead in Early Medieval France.* Ithaca: Cornell University Press, 1994.

McNamer, Sarah. *Affective Meditation and the Invention of Medieval Compassion.* Philadelphia: University of Pennsylvania Press, 2010.

Merlo, G. G. *Esperienze religiose e opere assistenziali nei secoli XII et XIII.* Turin, 1987.

Mesqui, Jean. *Provins: La fortification d'une ville au moyen âge.* Geneva: Droze, 1979.

Metzler, Irina. *Disability in Medieval Europe: Thinking About Physical Impairment during the High Middle Ages, c. 1100–1400.* London: Routledge, 2006.

Michaud, Francine. "Le pauvre transformé: Les hommes, les femmes et la charité à Marseille du XIIIe siècle jusqu'à la peste noire." *Revue historique* 311, no. 2 (2009): 243–90.

Michelin, Jules, and Claude Léouaon Le Duc. *État des bienfaiteurs de l'hôtel-Dieu de Provins.* Provins, France: A. Vernant, 1887.

Milgrom, Paul R., Douglass C. North, Barry R. Weingast. "The Role of Institutions in the Revival of Trade: The Law Merchant, Private Judges, and the Champagne Fairs." *Economics and Politics* 2, no. 1 (March 1990): 1–23.

Miller, Tanya Stabler. *The Beguines of Medieval Paris: Gender, Patronage, and Spiritual Authority.* Philadelphia: University of Pennsylvania Press, 2014.

Miller, Timothy S. *The Birth of the Hospital in the Byzantine Empire.* Baltimore: Johns Hopkins University Press, 1985.

——. "The Knights of Saint John and the Hospitals of the Latin West." *Speculum* 53, no. 4 (October 1978): 709–33.

Miller, Timothy S., and John W. Nesbitt. *Walking Corpses: Leprosy in Byzantium and the Medieval West.* Ithaca: Cornell University Press, 2014.

Mischlewski, Adalbert. *Un ordre hospitalier au moyen âge: Les chanoines réguliers de Saint-Antoine-en-Viennois.* Grenoble: Presses Universitaires de Grenoble, 1995.

Mollat, Michel, ed. *Études sur l'histoire de la pauvreté: Moyen âge–XVIe siècle.* 2 vols. Paris: Publications de la Sorbonne, 1974.

——. "L'hôpital dans la ville au moyen âge en France." *Société française d'histoire des hôpitaux* 47 (1983): 6–17.

——. *The Poor in the Middle Ages: An Essay in Social History.* Translated by Arthur Goldhammer. New Haven: Yale University Press, 1986.

Montaubin, Pascaul. "Le déménagement de l'Hôtel-Dieu d'Amiens au XIIIe siècle: Un hôpital dans les enjeux urbanistiques." In *Hôpitaux et maladreries au moyen âge: Espace et environnement. Actes du colloque international d'Amiens-Beauvais, 22, 23, et 24 novembre 2002,* edited by Pascal Montaubin, 51–86. Amiens, France: Centre d'Archéologie et d'Histoire Médiévales des Établissements Religieux, 2004.

Munro, John H. "The 'New Institutional Economics' and the Changing Fortunes of Fairs in Medieval and Early Modern Europe: The Textile Trades, Warfare, and Transaction Costs." *Vierteljahrschrift fur Sozial- und Wirtschaftsgeschichte* 88 (2001): 1–47.

Murard, Jean. "L'ordre des Trinitaires ou des Mathurins à Troyes, Bar-sur-Seine et la Gloire-Dieu." *Mémoires de la Société Académique de l'Aube* 129 (1995): 37–56.

Murray, Alexander. "Piety and Impiety in Thirteenth-Century Italy." *Studies in Church History* 8 (1972): 83–106.

——. "Religion Among the Poor in Thirteenth-Century France: The Testimony of Humbert de Romans." *Traditio* 30 (1974): 285–324.

Murray, James M. *Bruges, Cradle of Capitalism, 1280–1390.* Cambridge: Cambridge University Press, 2005.

Nelli, René. "L'aumône dans la littérature occitane: Le 'Breviari d'amor' de Matfre Ermengau." In *Assistance et charité, Cahiers de Fanjeaux* 13 (1978): 51–56.

Neveux, François. "Naissance et développement des hôtels-Dieu en Normandie (XIIe–XIVe siècle)." In *Hôpitaux et maladreries au moyen âge: Espace et environ-ment. Actes du colloque international d'Amiens-Beauvais, 22, 23 et 24 novembre 2002,* edited by Pascal Montaubin, 241–54. Amiens, France: Centre d'Archéologie et d'Histoire Médiévales des Établissements Religieux, 2004.

Newhauser, Richard. "Justice and Liberality: Opposition to Avarice in the Twelfth Century." *Virtue and Ethics in the Twelfth Century.* Edited by Richard Newhauser and István P. Bejczy, 295–316. Leiden: Brill, 2005.

Nicholas, David. *The Growth of the Medieval City: From Late Antiquity to the Early Four-teenth Century.* London: Longman, 1997.

Nutton, Vivian. Review of Timothy S. Miller's *The Birth of the Hospital in the Byzan-tine Empire. Medical History* 30 (1986): 218–21.

O'Boyle, Cornelius. "Surgical Texts and Social Contexts: Physicians and Surgeons in Paris, c. 1270 to 1430." In *Practical Medicine from Salerno to the Black Death,* edited by Luis García-Ballester et al., 156–85. Cambridge: Cambridge University Press, 1994.

O'Tool, Mark P. "The *povres avugles* of the Hospital of the Quinze-Vingts." In *Differ-ence and Identity in Francia and Medieval France,* edited by Meredith Cohen and Justine Firnhaber-Baker, 157–74. Farnham, U.K.: Ashgate, 2010.

Page, Christopher. "Music and Medicine in the Thirteenth Century." In *Music as Med-icine: The History of Music Therapy Since Antiquity,* edited by Peregrine Horden, 109–19. Aldershot, U.K.: Ashgate, 2000.

Paresys, Cécile, Dominique Castex, Cédric Roms, Isabelle Richard, and Stéphanie Degobertière. "Un nouvel cas de sépultures multiples à Troyes, Place de la Libération (Aube, Moyen Âge)." *Bulletins et mémoires de la Société d'anthropologie de Paris,* n.s. 20, no. 1–2 (2008): 125–36.

Parisse, Michel, ed. *Les chanoines réguliers: Émergence et expansion (XIe–XIIIe siècles). Actes du sixième colloque international du CERCOR, Le Puy en Velay, 29 juin–1ᵉʳ juil-let 2006.* Saint-Étienne, France: Publications de l'Université de Saint-Étienne, 2009.

Pasztor, Edith. *Donne e sante: Studi sulla religiosità femminile nel medio evo.* Rome: Edizioni Studium, 2000.

Patault, Anne-Marie. *Hommes et femmes de corps en Champagne méridionale à la fin du moyen âge*. Nancy, France: Université de Nancy-II, 1978.

Peixoto, Michael Joseph. "Growing the Portfolio: Templar Investments in the Forests of Champagne." In *L'économie templière en occident: Patrimoines, commerce, finances: Actes du colloque international (Troyes—Abbaye de Clairvaux, 24–26 octobre 2012)*, edited by Arnaud Baudin, Ghislain Brunel, and Nicolas Dohrmann, 207–24. Langres, 2013.

Peyroux, Catherine. "The Leper's Kiss." In *Monks and Nuns, Saints and Outcasts: Religion in Medieval Society: Essays in Honor of Lester K. Little*, edited by Sharon Farmer and Barbara H. Rosenwein, 172–88. Ithaca: Cornell University Press, 2000.

Pieper, Lori. "Saint Elizabeth of Hungary: The Voice of a Medieval Woman and Franciscan Penitent in the Sources for Her Life." PhD dissertation, Fordham University, 2002.

Pinker, Steven. "The False Allure of Group Selection," *Edge: Conversations on the Edge of Human Knowledge*, June 18, 2012.

Piron, Sylvain. "Le devoir de gratitude: Émergence et vogue de la notion d'*antidora* au XIIIe siècle." In *Credito e usura fra teologia, diritto e amministrazione: Linguaggi a confronto (sec. XII–XVI)*, edited by Diego Quaglioni, Giacomo Todeschini, and Gian Maria Varanini, 73–101. Rome: École Française de Rome, 2005.

Putnam, Robert D. *Making Democracy Work: Civic Traditions in Modern Italy*. Princeton: Princeton University Press, 1993.

——. "The Prosperous Community: Social Capital and Public Life." *American Prospect* 13 (Spring 1993): 35–42.

Racinet, Philippe. "Les infirmeries monastiques: Perspectives de recherche." In *Hôpitaux et maladreries au moyen âge: Espace et environnement. Actes du colloque international d'Amiens-Beauvais, 22, 23 et 24 novembre 2002*, edited by Pascal Montaubin, 21–34. Amiens, France: Centre d'Archéologie et d'Histoire Médiévales des Établissements Religieux, 2004.

Ragab, Ahmed. *The Medieval Islamic Hospital: Medicine, Religion, and Charity*. Cambridge: Cambridge University Press, 2015.

Rawcliffe, Carole. "Hospital Nurses and Their Work." In *Daily Life in the Late Middle Ages*, edited by Richard Britnell, 43–64. Stroud, U.K.: Sutton Publishing, 1998.

——. *The Hospitals of Medieval Norwich*. Norwich, U.K.: Centre of East Anglian Studies, University of East Anglia, 1999.

——. *Leprosy in Medieval England*. Woodbridge, U.K.: Boydell Press, 2006.

——. *Medicine for the Soul: The Life, Death, and Resurrection of an English Medieval Hospital, St Giles's, Norwich, c. 1249–1550*. Stroud, U.K.: Sutton, 1999.

Reitzel, J. M. "The Medieval Houses of Bons-Enfants." *Viator* 11 (1980): 179–207.

Resl-Pohl, Brigitte. *Rechnen mit der Ewigkeit: Das Wiener Bürgerspital im Mittelalter*. Munich: Oldenbourg Verlag, 1996.

Réveillas, H., and D. Castex. "La gestion des cimetières d'hôpitaux en période de crise épidémique: Apports des données bio-archéologiques." In *Espaces, objets, populations dans les établissements hospitaliers du moyen âge au XXème siècle*, edited by S. Le Clech, 343–64. Dijon: Presses Universitaires de Dijon, 2009.

Richard, Jean. "Hospitals and Hospital Congregations in the Latin Kingdom during the First Period of the Frankish Conquest." In *Outremer: Studies in the History of the Crusading Kingdom of Jerusalem*, edited by B. Z. Kedar, H. E. Mayer, and R. C. Smail, 89–100. Jerusalem: Yad Izhak Ben-Zvi Institute, 1982.

——. "Les Templiers et les Hospitaliers en Bourgogne et en Champagne méridionale (XIIe–XIIIe siècles)." In *Die geistlichen Ritterorden Europas*, edited by Manfred Hellmann and Josef Fleckenstein, 231–42. Sigmaringen, Germany: Thorbecke, 1980.

Richemond, E. *Recherche généalogiques sur la famille des seigneurs de Nemours du XIIe au XVe siècles*. Fontainebleau, France: Maurice Bourges, 1907.

Riley-Smith, Jonathan. "Crusading as an Act of Love." *History* 65, no. 214 (1980): 177–92.

Risse, Guenter B. *Mending Bodies, Saving Souls: A History of Hospitals*. New York: Oxford University Press, 1999.

Robert, Gaston. "Les beguines de Reims et la maison de Saint-Agnès." *Travaux de l'Académie nationale de Reims* 137 (1922–1923): 235–85.

——. "Les chartreries paroissiales et l'assistance publique à Reims jusqu'en 1633." *Travaux de l'Académie nationale de Reims* 141 (1926–27): 127–264.

Rollo-Koster, Joëlle. "Item Lego . . . Item Volo . . . Is There Really an 'I' in Medieval Provençales' Wills?" In *"For the Salvation of My Soul": Women and Wills in Medieval and Early Modern France*, edited by Joëlle Rollo-Koster and Kathryn L. Reyerson, 3–24. St. Andrews, Scotland: St. Andrews Studies in French History and Culture, 2012.

Rosenthal, Joel. *The Purchase of Paradise: Gift Giving and the Aristocracy, 1307–1485*. London: Routledge, 1972.

Rosenwein, Barbara H. *To Be the Neighbor of Saint Peter: The Social Meaning of Cluny's Property, 909–1049*. Ithaca: Cornell University Press, 1989.

Rosenwein, Barbara H., and Lester K. Little. "Social Meaning in the Monastic and Mendicant Spiritualities." *Past and Present*, 63, no. 1 (1974): 4–32.

Roserot, Alphonse. *Dictionnaire historique de la Champagne méridionale, Aube: Des origines à 1790*. Angers, France: Edition de l'Ouest, 1948.

Rothrauf, Elizabeth. "Charity in Medieval Community: Politics, Piety, and Poor Relief in Pisa, 1257–1312." PhD dissertation, University of California, Berkeley, 2012.

Rouse, Richard H., and Mary A. Rouse. *Preachers, Florilegia, and Sermons: Studies on the "Manipulus florum" of Thomas of Ireland*. Toronto: Pontifical Institute of Mediaeval Studies, 1979.

Rousseau, Louis. "Les ressources casuelles de l'hôtel-Dieu de la Madeleine de Rouen (XIIe–XVIe siècles)." In *Assistance et Assistés jusqu'à 1610. Actes du 97ᵉ congrès des Sociétés savantes, Nantes 1972*, 157–73. Paris: Bibliothèque Nationale, 1979.

Rubin, Miri. *Charity and Community in Medieval Cambridge*. Cambridge: Cambridge University Press, 1987.

——. "Imagining Medieval Hospitals: Considerations on the Cultural Meaning of Institutional Change." In *Medicine and Charity before the Welfare State*, edited by Colin Jones and Jonathan Barry, 14–25. London: Routledge, 1991.

Ruiz, Teofilo F. *From Heaven to Earth: The Reordering of Castilian Society, 1150–1350*. Princeton: Princeton University Press, 2014.

——. "The Business of Salvation: Castilian Wills in the Late Middle Ages." In *On the Social Origins of Medieval Institutions: Essays in Honor of Joseph F. O'Callaghan*, edited by Donald J. Kagay and Theresa M. Vann, 63–90. Leiden: Brill, 1998.

Saint-Denis, Alain. *L'hôtel-dieu de Laon, 1150–1300*. Nancy, France: Presses Universitaires de Nancy, 1983.

——. "Médecins et médecine dans l'hôtel-Dieu de Laon aux XIIème et XIIIème siècles." *Colloque international d'histoire de la médecine médiévale: Orléans, 4 et 5 mai, 1985*, 125–40. Orléans, France: Société Orléanaise d'Histoire de la Médecine Centre Jeanne d'Arc, 1985.

Saint-Denis, Alain. "Soins du corps et médecine contre la souffrance à l'hôtel-Dieu de Laon au XIIIe siècle." *Médiévales* 8 (1985): 33–42.

Saunier, Annie. *"Le pauvre malade" dans le cadre hospitalier médiéval: France du Nord, vers 1300–1500*. Paris: Éditions Arguments, 1993.

Schenk, Jochen. *Templar Families: Landowning Families and the Order of the Temple in France, c.1170–1307*. Cambridge: Cambridge University Press, 2012.

Scheutz, Martin, Andrea Sommerlechner, Herwig Weigl, and Alfred Stefan Weis, eds. *Europäisches Spitalwesen: Institutionelle Fürsorge in Mittelalter und Früher Neuzeit*. Vienna: R. Oldenbourg, 2008.

Schofield, Philipp. "Approaching Poverty in the Medieval Countryside." In *Poverty and Prosperity in the Middle Ages and the Renaissance*, edited by Cynthia Kosso and Anne Scott, 95–112. Turnhout, Belgium: Brepols, 2012.

Seif, Jonathan A. "Charity and Poor Law in Northern Europe in the High Middle Ages: Jewish and Christian Approaches." PhD dissertation, University of Pennsylvania, 2013.

Shaffern, Robert W. *The Penitents' Treasury: Indulgences in Latin Christendom, 1175–1375*. Scranton, PA: University of Scranton Press, 2007.

Shoham-Steiner, Ephraim. *On the Margins of a Minority: Leprosy, Madness, and Disability among the Jews of Medieval Europe*. Translated by Haym Watzman. Detroit: Wayne State University Press, 2014.

Simons, Walter. *Cities of Ladies: Beguine Communities in the Medieval Low Countries, 1200–1565*. Philadelphia: University of Pennsylvania Press, 2001.

Sneider, Matthew Thomas. "The Bonds of Charity: Charitable and Liturgical Obligations in Bolognese Testaments." In *Poverty and Prosperity in the Middle Ages and Renaissance*, edited by Cynthia Kosso and Anne Scott, 129–42. Turnhout, Belgium: Brepols, 2012.

Soskis, Benjamin. "Both More and No More: The Historical Split Between Charity and Philanthropy." Hudson Institute, October 15, 2014. Available at www.hudson.org/research/10723-both-more-and-no-more-the-historical-split-between-charity-and-philanthropy.

——. "The Problem of Charity in Industrial America, 1873–1915." PhD dissertation, Columbia University, 2010.

Stern, Ken. "Why the Rich Don't Give to Charity." *The Atlantic*, April 2013.

Swanson, R. N. *Indulgences in Late Medieval England: Passports to Paradise?* Cambridge: Cambridge University Press, 2007.

——, ed. *Promissory Notes in the Treasury of Merits: Indulgences in Late Medieval Europe*. Leiden: Brill, 2006.

Sweetinburgh, Sheila. *The Role of the Hospital in Medieval England: Gift-Giving and the Spiritual Economy*. Dublin: Four Courts Press, 2004.

Tabuteau, Emily. *Transfers of Property in Eleventh-Century Norman Law*. Chapel Hill: University of North Carolina Press, 1988.

Tarbé, Prosper. *Reims: Essais historique sur les rues et ses monuments.* Reims, France: Librairie de Quentin-Dailly, 1844.

Terpstra, Nicholas. *Lay Confraternities and Civic Religion in Renaissance Bologna.* Cambridge: Cambridge University Press, 1995.

Terrasse, Véronique. *Provins: Une commune du comté de Champagne et de Brie (1152–1355).* Paris: L'Harmattan, 2005.

Thomas, Christopher, Barney Sloane, and Christopher Phillpotts. *Excavations at the Priory and Hospital of St. Mary Spital, London.* London: Lavenham Press, 1997.

Thompson, Augustine. *Cities of God: The Religion of the Italian Communes, 1125–1325.* University Park: Pennsylvania State University Press, 2005.

Tierney, Brian, "The Decretists and the 'Deserving Poor.'" *Comparative Studies in Society and History* 1, no. 4 (June 1959): 360–73.

Todeschini, Giacomo. *Franciscan Wealth: From Voluntary Poverty to Market Society.* New York: Franciscan Institute, St. Bonaventure University, 2009.

——. *Les marchands et le temple: La société chrétienne et le cercle vertueux de la richesse du moyen âge à l'époque moderne.* Translated by Ida Giordano and Mathieu Arnoux. Paris: Albin Michel, 2017.

——. *Il prezzo della salvezza: Lessici medievali del pensiero economico.* Rome: La Nuova Italia Scientifica, 1994.

——. "I vocabolari dell'analisi economica fra alto e basso medioevo: Dai lessici della disciplina monastica ai lessici antiusurari." *Rivista storica Italiana* 110, no. 3 (1998): 781–833.

Touati, François-Olivier. "Aime et fais ce que tu veux: Les chanoines réguliers et la révolution de charité au moyen âge." In *Les chanoines réguliers: Émergence et expansion (XIe–XIIIe siècles),* edited by Michel Parisse, 159–210. Saint-Étienne: Publications de l'Université de Saint-Étienne, 2009.

——, ed. *Archéologie et architecture hospitalières de l'antiquité tardive à l'aube des temps modernes.* Paris: La Boutique de l'Histoire, 2004.

——. *Archives de la lèpre: Atlas des léproseries entre Loire et Marne au moyen âge.* Paris: Edition du C.T.H.S., 1996.

——. "Domus judaeorum leprosorum: Une léproserie pour les Juifs à Provins au XIIIe siècle." In *Fondations et oeuvres charitables au moyen âge,* 97–106. Edited by Jean Dufour and Henri Platelle. Paris: Éditions du CTHS, 1999,

——. "Un dossier à rouvrir: L'assistance au moyen âge." In *Fondations et oeuvres charitables au moyen âge.* Edited by Jean DuFour and Henri Platelle, 23–38. Paris: Éditions du CTHS, 1999.

——. "La géographie hospitalière médiévale (Orient-Occident, IVe–XVe siècles): Des modèles aux réalités." In *Hôpitaux et maladreries au moyen âge: Espace et environnement. Actes du colloque international d'Amiens-Beauvais, 22, 23, et 24 novembre 2002,* edited by Pascal Montaubin, 7–20. Amiens, France: Publications du Centre d'Archéologie et d'Histoire Médiévales des Établissements Religieux, 2004.

——. "Les groupes des laïcs dans les hôpitaux et les léproseries au moyen âge." In *Les mouvances laïques des ordres religieux,* edited by Nicole Bouter, 137–62. Saint Étienne: Publications de l'Université de Saint-Étienne, 1996.

——. *Maladie et société au moyen âge: La lèpre, lépreux et les léproseries dans la province ecclésiastique de Sens jusqu'au milieu du XIVe siècle.* Paris: De Boeck Université, 1998.

——. "La terre sainte: Un laboratoire hospitalier au moyen âge?" *Sozialgeschichte mittelalterlicher Hospitäler*, edited by Neithard Bulst and Karl-Heinz Spieß, 169–212. Vorträge und Forschungen, vol. 65. Ostfildern, Germany: Jan Thorbecke Verlag, 2007.

——. *Yves de Chartres (1040–1115): Aux origines de la révolution hospitalière médiévale.* Paris: Les Indes Savantes, 2017.

Van Leeuwen, Marco H. D. "Logic of Charity: Poor Relief in Preindustrial Europe." *Journal of Interdisciplinary History* 24, no. 4 (April 1994): 589–613.

Vauchez, André. "Assistance et charité en occident, XIII–XVe siècles." In *Domanda e consumi: Livelli e strutture nei secoli (XIII–XVIIIe)*, edited by V. Barbagli Bagnoli, 151–62. Florence: Olschki, 1978.

——. "Charité et pauvreté chez sainte Elisabeth de Thuringe d'après les actes du procès de canonisation." In *Études sur l'histoire de la pauvreté*, edited by Michel Mollat, 163–73. Vol. 1. Paris: Publications de la Sorbonne, 1974.

——. *Sainthood in the Later Middle Ages.* Translated by Jean Birrell. Cambridge: Cambridge University Press, 1997.

——. *La spiritualité du moyen âge occidental (VIIIe–XIIIe siècle).* 2nd ed. Paris: Seuil, 1994.

Veissière, Michel. "L'hôpital provinois du Saint-Esprit." *Bulletin philologique et historique* (1963, année 1961): 581–606.

——. "Provins et ses environs à la fin du XIIIe siècle: À propos d'une publication récente (Censier de l'hôtel-Dieu de Provins)." *Provins et sa région: Bulletin de la Société d'histoire et d'archéologie de Provins* 131 (1977): 31–34.

Venarde, Bruce. *Women's Monasticism and Medieval Society: Nunneries in France and England, 890–1215.* Ithaca: Cornell University Press, 1997.

Verdier, François. *L'aristocratie de Provins à la fin du XIIe siècle.* Provins, France: Société d'Histoire et d'Archéologie de l'Arrondissement de Provins, 2016.

Vervaet, Lies. "Goederenbeheer in een veranderende samenleving: Het Sint-Janshospital van Brugge ca. 1275–ca. 1575." PhD dissertation, University of Ghent, 2015.

——. "Lease Holding in Late Medieval Flanders: Towards Concentration and Engrossment? The Estates of the St John's Hospital of Bruges." In *Beyond Lords and Peasants: Rural Elites and Economic Differentiation in Premodern Europe*, edited by Frederic Aparisi and Vicent Royo, 111–38. Valencia: Publicacions de la Universitat de València, 2014.

Vincent, Catherine. *Des charités bien ordonnées: Les confréries en Normandie de la fin du XIIIe siècle au début du XVIe siècle.* Paris: Éditions Rue d'Ulm, 1988.

——. *Les confréries médiévales dans le royaume de France XIIIe–XVe siècle.* Paris: Albin Michel, 1994.

——. "Y-a-t-il une mathématique du salut dans les diocèses du nord de la France à la veille de la réforme?" *Revue d'histoire de l'Église de France* 77, no. 198 (1991): 137–49.

Vincent, Nicholas. "Some Pardoners' Tales: The Earliest English Indulgences." *Transactions of the Royal Historical Society*, series 6, vol. 12 (2002): 23–58.

Watson, Sethina. "City as Charter: Charity and the Lordship of English Towns, 1170–1250." In *Cities, Texts, and Social Networks, 400–1500: Experiences and Perceptions of Medieval Urban Space*, 235–62. Edited by Caroline Goodson, Anne E. Lester, and Carol Symes. Farnham, U.K.: Ashgate, 2010.

——. "Fundatio, Ordinatio, and Statuta: The Statutes and Constitutional Documents of English Hospitals to 1300." Doctoral thesis, St. Hilda's College, Oxford University, 2003.

——. "A Mother's Past and Her Children's Futures: Female Inheritance, Family, and Dynastic Hospitals in the Thirteenth Century." In *Motherhood, Religion, and Society in Medieval Europe, 400–1400: Essays Presented to Henrietta Leyser*, edited by Conrad Leyser and Lesley Smith, 213–50. Farnham, U.K.: Ashgate, 2011.

——. *On Hospitals: Welfare, Law, and Christianity in Western Europe, 400–1320*. Oxford: Oxford University Press, 2020.

Webster, Margaret, and Nicolas Orme. *The English Hospital, 1070–1570*. New Haven: Yale University Press, 1995.

Wei, Ian P. *Intellectual Culture in Medieval Paris: Theologians and the University of Paris, c. 1100–1330*. Cambridge: Cambridge University Press, 2012.

White, Stephen. *Custom, Kinship, and Gifts to Saints: The Laudatio Parentum in Western France, 1050–1150*. Chapel Hill: University of North Carolina Press, 1988.

White, William. "Excavations at St. Mary Spital: Burial of the 'Sick Poore' of Medieval London, the Evidence of Illness and Hospital Treatment." In *The Medieval Hospital and Medical Practice*, edited by Barbara S. Bowers, 59–64. Aldershot, U.K.: Ashgate, 2007.

Wolf, Kenneth Baxter, ed. and trans. *The Life and Afterlife of St. Elizabeth of Hungary: Testimony from Her Canonization Hearings*. Oxford: Oxford University Press, 2010.

Young, Spencer E. "More Blessed to Give and Receive: Charitable Giving in Thirteenth and Early Fourteenth-Century *Exempla*." In *Experiences of Charity, 1250–1650*, edited by Anne M. Scott, 63–78. Farnham, U.K.: Ashgate, 2015.

——. *Scholarly Community at the Early University of Paris: Theologians, Education, and Society, 1215–1248*. Cambridge: Cambridge University Press, 2014.

INDEX

Page numbers followed by n indicate notes. *Italicized* page numbers indicate illustrations